# Introduction to Veterinary Genetics

# Introduction to Veterinary Genetics

F. W. Nicholas

*Department of Animal Science,*
*University of Sydney*

OXFORD   NEW YORK   TOKYO
OXFORD UNIVERSITY PRESS
1996

Oxford University Press, Walton Street, Oxford OX2 6DP

Oxford   New York
Athens   Auckland   Bangkok   Bombay
Calcutta   Cape Town   Dar es Salaam   Delhi
Florence   Hong Kong   Istanbul   Karachi
Kuala Lumpur   Madras   Madrid   Melbourne
Mexico City   Nairobi   Paris   Singapore
Taipei   Tokyo   Toronto
and associated companies in
Berlin   Ibadan

Oxford is a trade mark of Oxford University Press

Published in the United States
by Oxford University Press Inc., New York

A catalogue record for this book is available from the British Library

Library of Congress Cataloging in Publication Data
Nicholas, F. W.
Introduction to veterinary genetics/Frank W. Nicholas.
Includes bibliographical references and index.
1. Veterinary genetics.   I. Title.
SF756.5.N52     1996       636.08'21—dc20       95–14972
ISBN 0 19 854293 3 (Hbk)
ISBN 0 19 854292 5 (Pbk)

Typeset by Footnote Graphics, Warminster, Wilts
Printed in Great Britain on acid-free paper by
Biddles Ltd, Guildford and King's Lynn

To my family

# Preface

The aim of this book is to provide an introductory overview of those aspects of genetics that are relevant to animal diseases and to animal production; it provides an introduction to many topics that are covered in greater detail in *Veterinary genetics* (Clarendon Press, Oxford, 1987). As with most areas of biology, molecular techniques are creating a revolution in our understanding of animal genetics, and this revolution is reflected in the substance of this book—molecular biology makes its presence felt in many chapters. The wish to keep the book to a reasonable size has meant omitting references from the text, and mathematical/statistical derivations from the appendices. I hope that the many researchers whose work is described anonymously will gain some satisfaction from seeing the fruits of their labours contributing to the telling of such a marvellous story. A list of general references at the end of each chapter provides a starting point for further reading. The derivations can still be found in *Veterinary genetics*.

Despite the restrictions on space, an attempt has been made to satisfy the strong demand for an extended (but still very incomplete) list of single-locus disorders (Appendix 3.1), concentrating on those disorders for which the deficient protein has been identified, or which have been characterized at the molecular level. This list has been extracted from a database of inherited disorders maintained by the author. An updated list of references and (in some cases) further details for each entry, is available on the Internet.

I wish to record my gratitude to friends and colleagues who have read drafts of various chapters. These include Ken Beh, Andrew Blattman, Martin Combs, Ian Hughes, Muladno, Mick Murphy, Mohammad Shariflou, Pradeepa Silva, and Rasoul Torshizi. Ian Hughes deserves particular thanks for his detailed, constructive comments on the early chapters. To Paul Le Tissier I am deeply indebted for numerous, helpful suggestions following his reading of the entire manuscript. Thanks also to Peter Harwin for providing an idyllic retreat. Chris Moran continues to be a stimulating colleague with whom it is a great pleasure to share the adventure of keeping up to date in such a rapidly developing field. I am very grateful to him for holding the fort while I completed the task.

Finally, I thank my family for patiently accepting the fact that taking leave does not necessarily mean taking a holiday.

*Sydney*                                                                                                  F.W.N.
January 1995

# Acknowledgements

Various figures and tables throughout this book are reproduced with permission from the sources listed below.

FIGURES: **1.1:** courtesy of P. Muir. **1.2** and **1.3:** ISCNDA (1989), *Cytogenetics and Cell Genetics*, **53**, 65–79, courtesy of S. Karger AG, Basel. **1.6:**(a) Suzuki, Griffiths, and Lewontin (1981), *An introduction to genetic analysis* (2nd edn). © W. H. Freeman and Co., all rights reserved; (b) after Symons (1981), in *The biological manipulation of life* (ed. H. Messel) pp. 13–30, Pergamon, Sydney. **1.7:** (a) and (b) after Symons (1981), as for 1.6 (b). **1.13:** *Nature* (1949), **163**, 676–7, © 1949 Macmillan Magazines Ltd. The cat, pig, goat, and sheep karyotypes in Appendix 1.1 from Ford *et al.* (1980), *Hereditas*, **92**, 145–62; the dog karyotype is from Stone *et al.* (1991), *Genome*, **34**, 407–12; the horse karyotype is from Richer *et al.* (1990) *Hereditas*, **112**, 289–93; the chicken karyotype is reproduced courtesy of M. Thorne. **2.1:** (a) Grobstein (1977), *Scientific American*, **237**(1), 22–33 (courtesy of J.D. Griffith); (b) and (c) Old and Primrose (1985), *Principles of gene manipulation* (3rd edn), Blackwell, Oxford. **2.10:** Barendse *et al.* (1994), *Nature Genetics*, **6**, 227–35. **2.11:** courtesy of J. Murray. **3.3:** Evans *et al.* (1989), *Proceedings of the National Academy of Sciences, USA*, **86**, 10095–9. **3.4:** drawn from data in Sharp *et al.* (1992), *Genomics*, **13**, 115–21. **4.2:** Hageltorn *et al.* (1973), *Hereditas*, **75**, 147–51. **4.4:** *Nature* (1964), **203**, 990, © 1964 Macmillan Magazines Ltd. **4.5:** Chapman and Bruere (1977), *Canadian Journal of Genetics and Cytology*, **19**, 93–102. **5.1:** courtesy of K. Bell. **6.2:** courtesy of R. Zammit and G. Allan. **6.5:** after Patterson *et al.* (1972), in *The cardiovascular system* (ed. D. Bergsma), part XV, Williams & Wilkins, Baltimore, for the National Foundation – March of Dimes, BD:OAS, **8**(5), 160–74. **6.6** and **6.7:** Patterson *et al.* (1974), *American Journal of Cardiology*, **34**, 187–205. **7.1:** redrawn from Gardner *et al.* (1975), *Journal of Heredity*, **66**, 318–22, © 1975 American Genetic Association. **8.3:** drawn from data in Bijnen *et al.* (1980), *Transplantation*, **30**, 191–5. **9.1:** after Gonzalez and Nerbet (1990), *Trends in Genetics*, **6**, 182–6, using data from Idle and Smith (1979), *Drug Metabolism Review*, **9**, 301–17. **9.2:** Vogel and Motulsky (1979), *Human genetics: problems and approaches*, © Springer-Verlag, Berlin. **11.1:** photograph courtesy of I. P. Hughes. **12.2:** Hermans *et al.* (1991), *New Zealand Veterinary Journal*, **39**, 61–4, by kind permission of the editor of the journal. **15.1:** data from Barlow *et al.* (1978), *Wool Technology and Sheep Breeding*, **26**(11), 5–12. **17.2:** after Bichard (1978) in *New developments in scientific pig breeding* (supplement to *Pig Farming*, **27**(11)), 2–6. **18.1:** after Cundiff (1982), in *Beef research program progress report No. 1*

(ARM-NC-21), pp. 3–5, Roman L. Hruska US Meat Animal Research Center, Nebraska.  **20.1:** Smith (1989), *Animal Production*, **49**, 49–62.

TABLES: **5.1:** data adapted from Adalsteinsson *et al.* (1979), *Carnivore Genetics Newsletter*, **3**, 359–72.  **18.3:** cattle figures from data presented by Gregory and Cundiff (1980), *Journal of Animal Science*, **51**, 1224–42; sheep figures from data presented by Ch'ang and Evans (1982), in *Proceedings of the 2nd World Congress on Genetics Applied to Livestock Production*, Vol. 8, pp. 796–801; pig data adapted from Bichard (1977), *Livestock Production Science*, **4**, 245–54.

Every effort has been made to identify copyright holders and to acknowledge the source of copyright material. Any inadvertent omissions from the above listing will be rectified in any future reprinting or edition of this work.

# Contents

# Basic genetics

This chapter provides a review of basic genetics. It concentrates on the general principles that apply to normal, healthy animals. The exceptions to these principles are often the basis of genetic diseases, which are discussed in subsequent chapters.

## Chromosomes

When a culture of rapidly dividing white blood cells is treated with the alkaloid colchicine (which halts cell division), and the cells are then stained and viewed under a light microscope, structures called **chromosomes** become clearly visible. They are scattered randomly within clusters, and each cluster contains all the chromosomes from just one cell. The area of genetics concerned with chromosomes is called **cytogenetics**.

In order to study chromosomes more closely, a suitable cluster is chosen and photographed, as shown in Fig. 1.1a. Each unit in the figure consists of two rod-like structures joined together at a constricted point. Each rod-like structure is a **chromatid**, and the constriction is a **centromere**. The two chromatids that are joined at the centromere have just been formed from one original chromosome. If the cell division had been allowed to proceed, the centromere would have split and each separate chromatid would then be called a new chromosome. For convenience, we talk of each pair of chromatids joined at the centromere as being just one chromosome, referring in fact to the chromosome that has just given rise to them.

From the photographic print, all chromosomes are cut out individually with scissors, and arranged in order of size on a sheet of paper. An arrangement such as this provides a picture of the complete set of chromosomes or **karyotype** of a cell (Fig. 1.1b). If many such arrangements are examined from normal, healthy individuals of both sexes of any species of mammal or bird, two facts become evident: each species has a characteristic karyotype, and within any species, each sex has a characteristic karyotype.

Karyotypes of different species differ in the shape, size and number of their chromosomes. Within any species, all the chromosomes occur in pairs. In individuals of one sex, both members of each chromosome pair have the same size and shape. In the other sex, all but two chromosomes occur in such pairs, with the remaining pair consisting of two chromosomes of different size and shape. In this unequal pair, one chromosome has the same shape and size as members of one of the pairs in the opposite sex.

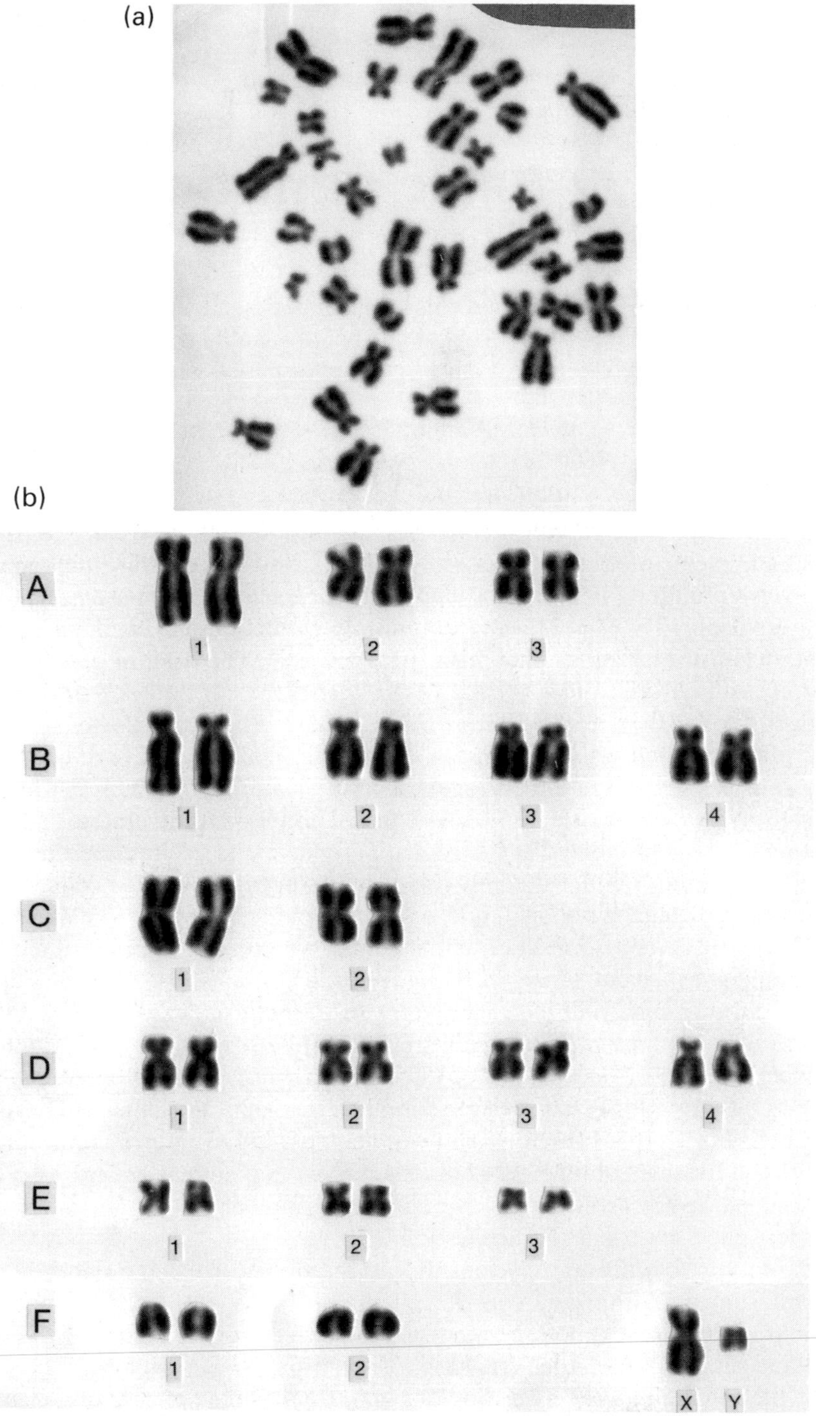

**Fig. 1.1** (a) The chromosomes of a male cat, as seen through a light microscope. (b) The karyotype of a male cat, as obtained by rearranging individual chromosomes cut out from a photographic print of (a).

The difference in karyotype between the two sexes is the key to sex determination. In mammals, the two chromosomes that form the unequal pair occur in males, and are called the X and Y chromosomes. In female mammals, one of the pairs of chromosomes consists of two X chromosomes. Thus in mammals, males are XY and females are XX. The X and the Y chromosomes are known as **sex chromosomes**. In birds, the sex chromosomes are given different names, and their relationship to sex is the opposite to that in mammals: male birds are ZZ and female birds are ZW. For convenience, we shall refer only to mammals in the following discussion, although all statements apply equally to birds if the names of the sexes are reversed.

Chromosomes other than the sex chromosomes are called **autosomes**. Within any species, males and females have the same set of autosomes, occurring in pairs. The sex chromosomes plus the autosomes constitute a **genome**, which is the total set of chromosomes in a cell. Genomes in which chromosomes occur in pairs are said to be **diploid**, and the two members of a pair are called **homologues**. In order to emphasize that chromosomes occur in pairs, the total number of chromosomes is called the $2n$ number, where $n$ is the number of pairs. For example, the number of chromosomes in the karyotype illustrated in Fig. 1.1 is $2n = 38$. To enable identification of each pair of chromosomes in a karyotype, the autosome pairs are labelled according to an internationally-agreed convention, as shown in Fig. 1.1b. The two sex chromosomes are placed at the end.

In order to describe karyotypes more fully, chromosomes are often classified according to whether the centromere is at one end (**acrocentric**), closer to one end than the other (**sub-metacentric**) or in the middle (**metacentric**). In this book, we shall follow common practice in using metacentric to cover both metacentric and sub-metacentric. The short arm of each chromosome is designated p (think of petite = small), and the long arm is designated q. (If the centromere is in the centre of the chromosome, the designation of which arm is called p is arbitrary, but is agreed by international convention; for acrocentric chromosomes, e.g. cattle autosomes, there is no need to distinguish between arms, and so neither p nor q is used.) A summary description of the karyotypes of common domestic species is given in Table 1.1. Avian karyotypes are different from mammalian karyotypes, because in addition to several large autosomes, they possess a number of very small autosomes called **microchromosomes**.

## Banding

When karyotypes were first investigated, individual pairs of chromosomes could be identified only according to their shape and size. Since then, various methods of staining chromosomes have been developed, giving rise to alternating light and dark regions called bands. The main types of bands are broadly classified as G, Q, R, C, T, and N.

As an example of banding, the G bands of cattle are illustrated in Fig. 1.2.

**Table 1.1** A summary description of the karyotypes of some domestic species

| Species | Total diploid number ($2n =$) | Autosomal pairs | |
|---|---|---|---|
| | | Metacentrics | Acrocentrics |
| Cat, *Felis catus* | 38 | 16 | 2 |
| Dog, *Canis familiaris* | 78 | 0 | 38 |
| Pig, *Sus scrofa domesticus* | 38 | 12 | 6 |
| Goat, *Capra hircus* | 60 | 0 | 29 |
| Sheep, *Ovis aries* | 54 | 3 | 23 |
| Cattle, *Bos taurus* | 60 | 0 | 29 |
| Horse, *Equus caballus* | 64 | 13 | 18 |
| Donkey, *Equus asinus* | 62 | 24 | 6 |
| Alpaca, *Lama pacos* / Llama, *Lama glama* | 74 | 16 | 20 |
| Rabbit, *Oryctolagus cuniculus* | 44 | 19 | 2 |

Since the position, width and number of bands are different for each pair of chromosomes, each chromosome pair can be identified by its banding pattern. By studying many cells treated in the same way, it is possible to draw up an **idiogram**, which is a representation of the characteristic banding pattern for each pair of chromosomes. The bands are uniquely identified according to a convention known as the International System for Cytogenetic Nomenclature of Domestic Animals (ISCNDA). Each arm is divided into a small number of regions which are numbered sequentially starting from the centromere. Then, in each region, the bands are numbered sequentially starting nearest the centromere. For example, the second band in the third region of chromosome 1 in cattle is designated 132, while the second band in the fourth region of the long arm of the X chromosome is Xq42. The ISCNDA idiogram for cattle is illustrated in Fig. 1.3. Banded karyotypes of other domestic species are illustrated in Appendix 1.1.

## Meiosis and mitosis

For many thousands of years, humans have observed two phenomena in relation to sex determination in animals: first, that there is considerable variation in the numbers of each sex among the offspring of pairs of parents; and second, that despite this variation, the overall numbers of males and females across families are approximately equal.

As noted above, the difference in sex chromosomes between the two sexes is the key to sex determination. The reason why XX individuals are females

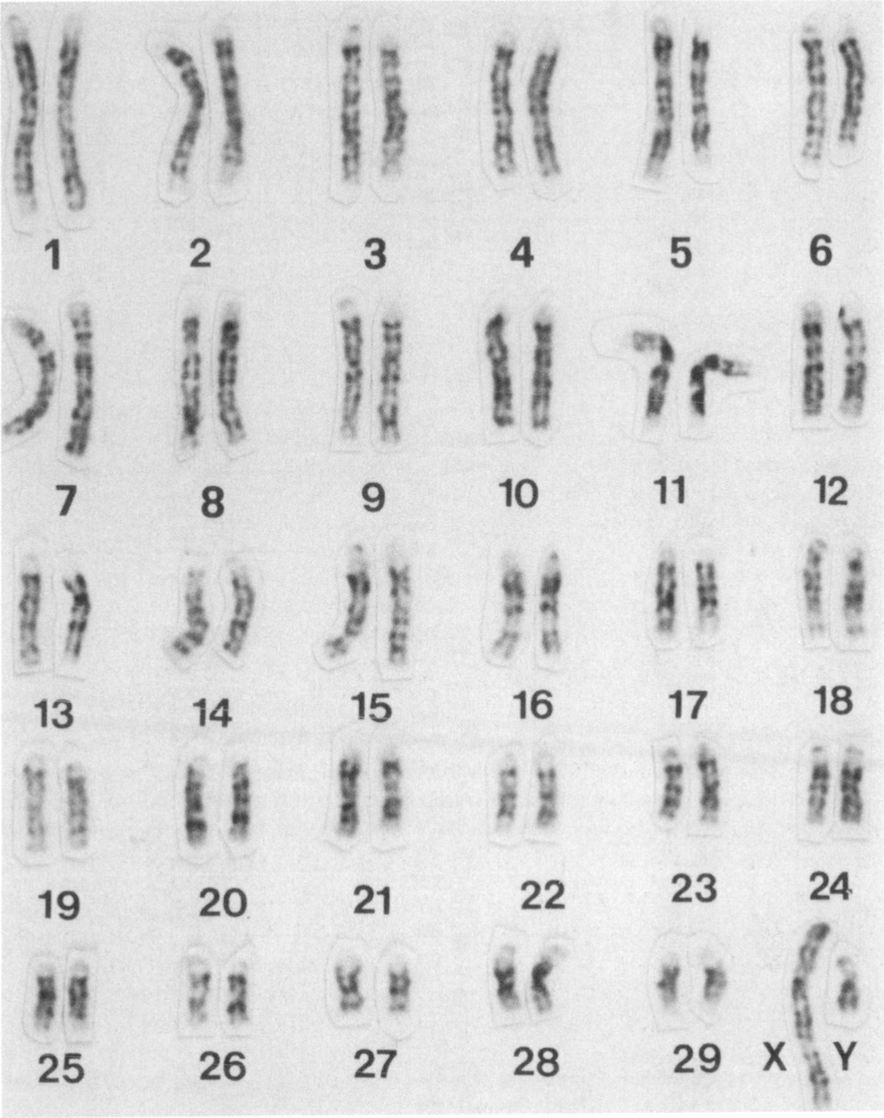

**Fig. 1.2** The standard G-banded cattle karyotype.

and XY individuals are males is explained in Chapter 4. For the present, we shall ask simply: why is there so much variation in the numbers of XX and XY individuals in the offspring of pairs of parents, and yet at the same time approximately equal numbers of each sex overall? The answer lies in an understanding of gamete formation.

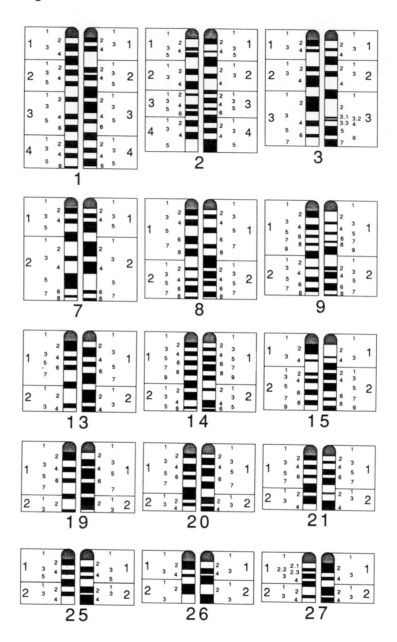

**Fig. 1.3** The standard cattle idiogram, showing both G-bands (*left*) and R-bands (*right*).

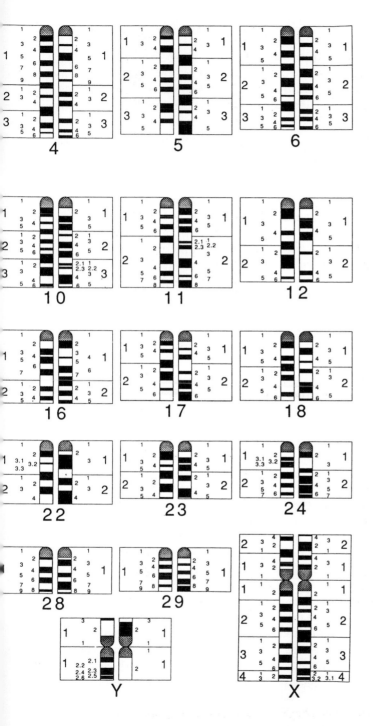

## Meiosis

Meiosis is the process of gamete formation in which sperms are formed in testes of males, and ova are formed in ovaries of females. The main result of meiosis is that each sperm and each ovum contains one member of each pair of chromosomes. Containing exactly one half of the usual diploid number of chromosomes, gametes are said to be **haploid**. The union of a sperm with an ovum at fertilization produces a **zygote** with the usual diploid number of chromosomes.

The process of meiosis commences with a normal cell containing the usual diploid set of chromosomes. To make the explanation easier, we shall consider what happens to just one pair of chromosomes (the sex chromosomes) in one sex (females), as illustrated in Fig. 1.4a. In order to distinguish the two X chromosomes in females, we shall refer to them as $X_p$ (paternal: originating from the father) and $X_m$ (maternal: originating from the mother).

Meiosis occurs in two stages. Meiosis I begins with each chromosome duplicating itself, giving rise to two identical chromatids joined at the centromere. Then homologous chromosomes, in our case $X_p$ and $X_m$, line up next to each other in the centre of the cell, in a process known as **pairing** or **synapsis**. This is facilitated by a protein structure called the **synaptonemal complex**, which 'zips' the two homologues together. Because each chromosome has already duplicated itself into two chromatids, there are now four chromatids side by side in the cell; two $X_p$ chromatids and two $X_m$ chromatids. The two $X_p$ chromatids are still joined at their centromere, as are the two $X_m$ chromatids. At this stage, a process called **recombination** or **crossing-over** occurs, in which homologous chromatids each break at the same site and, in the process of re-uniting, exchange segments. This produces cross-like structures called **chiasmata**. In order to simplify the present discussion, we shall continue to refer to the chromatids as $X_p$ or $X_m$, realizing that, as a result of crossing-over, any one chromatid may in fact consist of parts of both $X_p$ and $X_m$. (A full discussion of the genetic implications of crossing-over is presented later in this chapter.) In the next stage of meiosis I, the two centromeres are pulled to opposite ends or **poles** of the cell, with the result that the two $X_p$ chromatids move to one pole of the cell and the two $X_m$ chromatids move to the other pole. Since this process involves the two pairs of chromatids disjoining from their previous paired arrangement, it is known as **disjunction**. In the final stage of meiosis I, the original cell divides into two cells; one contains the two $X_p$ chromatids still joined at their centromere, and the other contains the two $X_m$ chromatids, still joined at their centromere.

Following disjunction in females, only one cell continues to function normally; the other degenerates into a dark-staining structure known as the **first polar body**. It is entirely a matter of chance as to which of the cells remains functional. Consequently, there is an equal chance of either the two $X_p$ chromatids or the two $X_m$ chromatids ending up in the functional cell. (In Fig. 1.4a, it happens to be the $X_p$ chromatids that have survived.)

In meiosis II, the two chromatids in the functional cell move apart (disjoin) and the cell divides into two cells, each containing one chromatid which is now called a chromosome. Once again, only one of the two cells remains functional; the other degenerates into the **second polar body**. And once again, it is entirely a matter of chance as to which of these two cells becomes the second polar body.

It is evident that in females, only one functional gamete results from each cell that originally underwent meiosis. It is also obvious that, irrespective of which cell ultimately remains functional, all gametes produced by females are the same in the sense that each contains one X chromosome. For this reason, females are known as the **homogametic** sex.

In males, meiosis is basically the same as described above: a disjunction followed by a cell division in meiosis I, and the same in meiosis II (Fig. 1.4b). There are, however, two important differences. The first is that the X and Y chromosomes have only a small homologous region at the end of one arm (called the **pseudo-autosomal region**) where synapsis occurs; for the re-mainder of their length, the arms are not joined together. Despite this unusual arrangement, their subsequent disjunction is normal, and gives rise to two functional cells at the end of meiosis I: one contains two X chromatids still joined at their centromere, and the other contains two Y chromatids still joined at their centromere. The second difference between meiosis in females and in males is that polar bodies are not formed in males. Instead, both of the cells formed at the end of meiosis I undergo a cell division in meiosis II, giving rise to four functional gametes (sperms), two of which contain an X chromo-some and two of which contain a Y chromosome. Since males produce two different types of gametes, they are known as the **heterogametic** sex.

Having now produced the gametes, the next stage is fertilization which, genetically speaking, is largely a matter of chance.

## Chance and variation

Since all female gametes contain an X chromosome, the chance of a female gamete containing an X chromosome is one. In contrast, males produce equal numbers of X-bearing gametes and Y-bearing gametes. There is, therefore, a chance of ½ that a particular sperm contains an X and the same chance that it contains a Y. It follows that the chance of obtaining an XY zygote is $1 \times \frac{1}{2}$ which equals ½. Similarly, the chance of obtaining an XX zygote is $1 \times \frac{1}{2}$, or ½. We can represent this situation by using a common genetic device called a checkerboard or **Punnett square**, in which the proportion at the head of each column is multiplied by the proportion at the head of each row, to give the expected proportions of offspring in the body of the checkerboard:

|  | Male gametes | |
|---|---|---|
|  | ½ X | ½ Y |
| Female gametes all X | ½ XX | ½ XY |

(a)

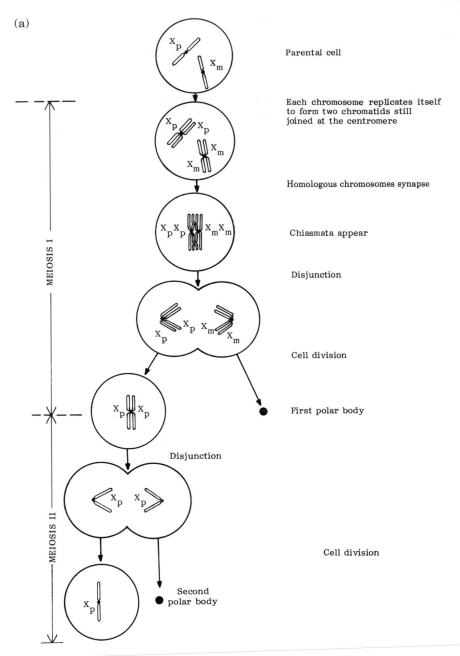

Parental cell

Each chromosome replicates itself to form two chromatids still joined at the centromere

Homologous chromosomes synapse

Chiasmata appear

Disjunction

Cell division

First polar body

Disjunction

Cell division

Second polar body

MEIOSIS I

MEIOSIS II

**Fig. 1.4** Meiosis in a female (a) and in a male (b), illustrated in terms of the sex chromosomes. With the exception of the unusual pairing in males, exactly the same processes occur for all pairs of autosomes.

(b)

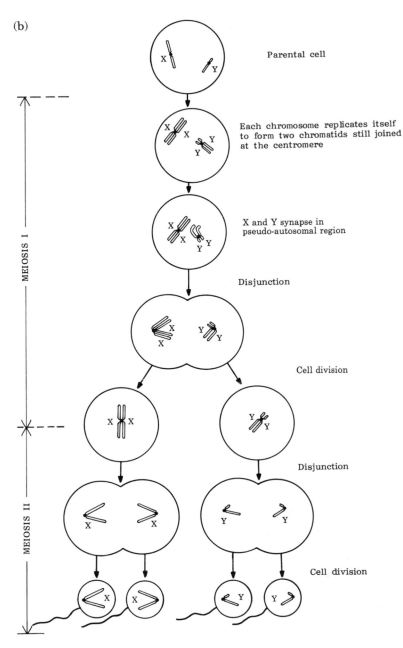

Parental cell

Each chromosome replicates itself
to form two chromatids still joined
at the centromere

X and Y synapse in
pseudo-autosomal region

Disjunction

Cell division

Disjunction

Cell division

MEIOSIS I

MEIOSIS II

We have now seen how meiosis enables the production of an expected
equal proportion of each sex, which accounts for one of our original observations. How can we account for the second observation, concerning the considerable variation in numbers of each sex among the offspring of different
pairs of parents? There is just one fact that enables us to explain this variation:

each fertilization is an independent event. By this we mean that irrespective of whether an X-bearing or Y-bearing sperm is successful with a particular ovum, the result of that fertilization has no bearing on subsequent fertilizations, even if they occur at the same time. For example, in a female that ovulates four ova, the chance that the last ovum is fertilized by a Y-bearing sperm is exactly ½ irrespective of which type of sperm fertilized the other ova. In fact, any particular sequence of sexes, e.g. MMFM, is just as likely as any other sequence, e.g. FFFF.

We have now provided adequate explanations for each of the observations described earlier. In so doing, we have discussed chromosomes, simple inheritance and chance, each of which is basic to an understanding of genetics. In order to complete the cycle of reproduction on which we embarked when discussing meiosis, we need to pass, by a process known as mitosis, from the zygote to an adult capable of producing its own gametes.

## Mitosis

The growth of a single-celled zygote into a multicellular adult involves a mechanism whereby the number of cells can be expanded rapidly, while at the same time ensuring that each cell has exactly the same set of chromosomes as the original single-celled zygote. Mitosis is such a mechanism. For convenience we shall consider just two chromosomes (the sex chromosomes) in a male; but the process is exactly the same for all chromosomes in both sexes. As shown in Fig. 1.5, mitosis begins when each chromosome duplicates itself to form two chromatids still joined at their centromere. Each duplicated chromosome moves to the centre of the cell but does not, as in meiosis, synapse with its homologue. This stage, which is known as **metaphase**, is the one at which chromosomes are most readily visible. Karyotypes, therefore, consist of metaphase chromosomes. After metaphase, the centromere splits and the chromatids separate (disjoin), one going to each pole of the cell. A constriction forms in the centre of the cell and two cells are formed, each containing both an X and a Y. In this way, the two cells have exactly the same set of chromosomes as did the original cell.

In both meiosis and mitosis, chromosomes are duplicated. How does this happen? Fortunately, we now have sufficient knowledge of the biochemical nature of chromosomes to be able to answer this question and to explain a few other processes as well.

## The biochemistry of inheritance

Chemically, chromosomes consist of mostly deoxyribonucleic acid (DNA) with a small amount of a protein called histone. The latter has a binding and structural function, while the former constitutes the genetic information that

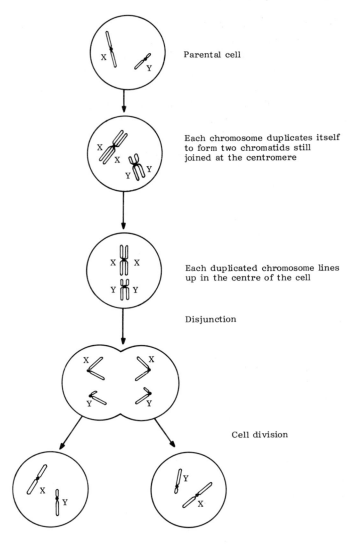

Parental cell

Each chromosome duplicates itself to form two chromatids still joined at the centromere

Each duplicated chromosome lines up in the centre of the cell

Disjunction

Cell division

Two daughter cells, each identical to the parental cell

**Fig. 1.5** Mitosis in a male, illustrated in terms of the sex chromosomes. The process is exactly the same for all chromosomes, and in all cells of each sex.

is passed from 'parent' cell to 'offspring' cell during mitosis, and from one generation to the next, via meiosis.

## DNA

DNA consists of two strands, each of which is a linear arrangement of **nucleotides**. All nucleotides of DNA contain an identical pentose sugar molecule

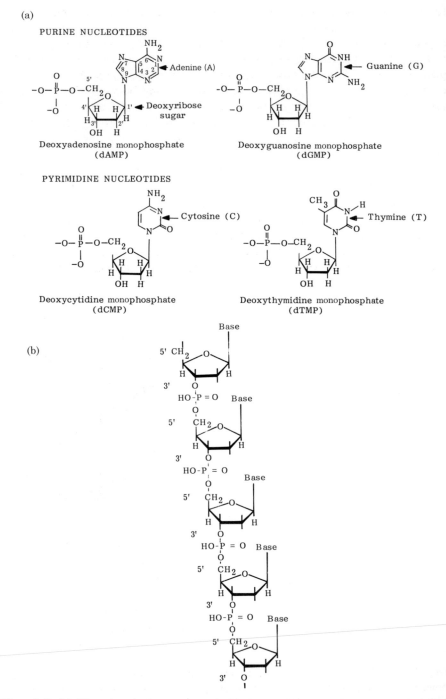

**Fig. 1.6** (a) The chemical structure of the four nucleotides that are the building blocks of DNA. (b) The basic structure of a strand of DNA.

(deoxyribose) and an identical phosphate group. Their third component, a nitrogenous base, exists in four different forms (adenine: A; guanine: G; thymine: T; cytosine: C), giving rise to four different nucleotides, as illustrated in Fig. 1.6a. The bases A and G have a similar structure and are called **purines**; T and C have a similar structure and are called **pyrimidines**. A strand of nucleotides is held together by covalent bonding between the phosphate attached to the 5′ carbon of one nucleotide and the OH attached to the 3′ carbon of the adjacent nucleotide, as shown in Fig. 1.6b. It follows that a strand of DNA has a 5′ phosphate at one end (called the **5′ end**) and a 3′ OH at the other end (called the **3′ end**).

The two strands that constitute DNA are held together by very specific hydrogen bonding between purines and pyrimidines (A with T, and G with C; Fig. 1.7a), giving rise to the **base pairs** A : T and G : C. Since A binds only with T, and G binds only with C, one strand of DNA is complementary to the other; the sequence of bases in one strand can be predicted from the sequence in the other strand. A further consequence of the pairing arrangements is that the two strands occur together in a helix. Because two strands are involved, it

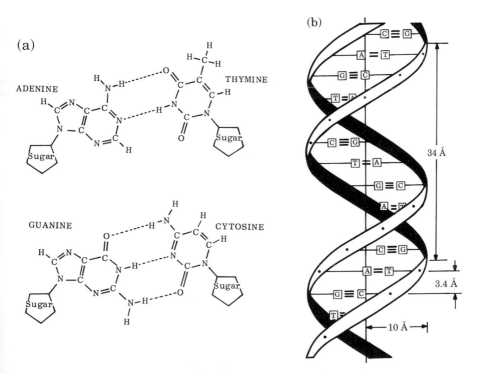

**Fig. 1.7** (a) The two types of pyrimidine : purine base pairs formed by hydrogen bonding between the two strands of DNA. (b) A double helix of DNA. The two ribbons represent the sugar–phosphate 'backbones'. The structure repeats every 10 base pairs.

is known as a **double helix** (Fig. 1.7b). The length of a short segment of DNA is usually measured in terms of the number of base pairs (bp). Longer segments are measured in terms of kilobases (1 kb = 1000 bases) or even megabases (1 Mb = 1000 kb).

The most important aspect of DNA structure is that it immediately suggests a mechanism for replication. If the double helix begins to unwind and the two strands separate, free nucleotides present in the cell are able to pair with the bases of each strand, forming a new and complementary strand for each of the original strands. As the unwinding proceeds (Fig. 1.8), two double helixes are produced from one original double helix; DNA has been replicated. The formation of each new strand by the addition of nucleotides is accomplished with the aid of the enzyme **DNA polymerase**. However, this enzyme can add nucleotides only at the 3′ end of a growing strand, which means that replication can occur only in the 5′ to 3′ direction. Consequently, one new strand (top of Fig. 1.8) is synthesized continually, while the other strand (bottom of Fig. 1.8) is assembled in small segments (called **Okazaki fragments**) which are each synthesized in the 5′ to 3′ direction. The Okazaki fragments are subsequently joined together by another enzyme called **DNA ligase**. The ability of these two enzymes to perform these functions has been put to good use in molecular biology, as described in Chapter 2.

It remains now to relate our knowledge of the structure of DNA to the structure of a chromosome as seen through a microscope. The total length of DNA in a mammalian cell is 1.74 metres, which is more than 7000 times the total length of metaphase chromosomes viewed through a microscope! Obviously, therefore, a chromosome is composed of DNA that is very tightly folded or coiled. This raises the question as to how such a tight coil is unwound each time a chromosome replicates itself. The histone proteins are

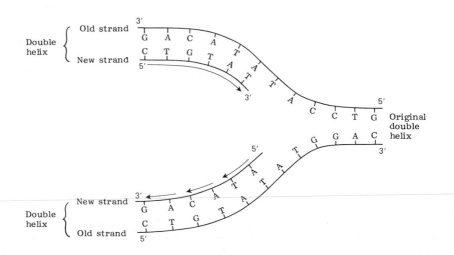

**Fig. 1.8** Replication of DNA.

certainly involved in chromosome replication, but the actual mechanism has not yet been fully revealed.

The structure of DNA is the key to understanding the way in which genetic information is stored in the chromosomes, and is transmitted to the cell in such a way as to produce a particular effect. In fact, the sequence of bases in DNA has a very specific meaning recorded in the form of a code.

## *The genetic code*

Proteins are chemical compounds with a wide range of specific roles in living organisms. Some are involved in transport (e.g. haemoglobin), support (e.g. collagen), or immunity (e.g. antibodies); some are enzymes that catalyse the innumerable biochemical reactions that occur in living cells (e.g. alcohol dehydrogenase). Some are hormones (e.g. growth hormone); some are receptors for hormones (e.g. oestrogen receptor). Some control the flow of molecules or ions in and out of cells (e.g. calcium release channel). In addition, the commercial products commonly obtained from animals either consist almost solely of protein, e.g. meat and wool, or have protein as an important component, e.g. milk and eggs.

Proteins consist of one or more polypeptides, each of which is a chain of amino acids. There are 20 different amino acids. Each polypeptide has a specific sequence of amino acids that confers upon it a specific set of physical and chemical properties.

The information necessary for producing a specific sequence of amino acids is contained in code-form within the sequence of bases in a segment of DNA. This code, which is called the **genetic code**, exists as triplets of bases (Table 1.2). With $4 \times 4 \times 4 = 64$ different possible triplets and only 20 amino acids, there is obviously some **redundancy**; in fact, the first two bases of a triplet are often sufficient to specify a particular amino acid, e.g. the triplets GTT, GTC, GTA, and GTG all specify valine. Three triplets (TAA, TAG, and TGA) do not code for any amino acid, and are known as **stop** triplets; they bring about the termination of a polypeptide chain. Another triplet (ATG) acts as a **start** signal for polypeptide synthesis. (It also codes for methionine.) The DNA between and including the start and stop triplets is called an **open reading frame** or ORF, within which the base sequence is 'read' in triplets, each of which encodes an amino acid.

Equipped with the genetic code, we can now follow the processes involved in the synthesis of proteins.

## *Protein synthesis*

As shown in Fig. 1.9, the synthesis of polypeptides begins with the relevant segment of DNA unwinding, and the two strands separating. The sequence of DNA bases in one of the strands (called the **template** strand) acts as a template for the synthesis of a different nucleic acid (ribonucleic acid, RNA,

**Table 1.2** The genetic code

| Triplet in DNA coding strand[1] | mRNA codon | Amino acid[2] | Triplet in DNA coding strand[1] | mRNA codon | Amino acid[2] |
|---|---|---|---|---|---|
| TTT<br>TTC | UUU<br>UUC | Phenylalanine<br>(Phe; F) | TAT<br>TAC | UAU<br>UAC | Tyrosine<br>(Tyr; Y) |
| TTA<br>TTG | UUA<br>UUG | | TAA<br>TAG | UAA<br>UAG | STOP |
| CTT<br>CTC | CUU<br>CUC | Leucine<br>(Leu; L) | CAT<br>CAC | CAU<br>CAC | Histidine<br>(His; H) |
| CTA<br>CTG | CUA<br>CUG | | CAA<br>CAG | CAA<br>CAG | Glutamine<br>(Gln; Q) |
| ATT<br>ATC<br>ATA | AUU<br>AUC<br>AUA | Isoleucine<br>(Ile; I) | AAT<br>AAC | AAU<br>AAC | Asparagine<br>(Asn; N) |
| | | | AAA<br>AAG | AAA<br>AAG | Lysine<br>(Lys; K) |
| ATG | AUG | START/Methionine (Met; M) | | | |
| GTT<br>GTC<br>GTA<br>GTG | GUU<br>GUC<br>GUA<br>GUG | Valine<br>(Val; V) | GAT<br>GAC | GAU<br>GAC | Aspartic acid<br>(Asp; D) |
| | | | GAA<br>GAG | GAA<br>GAG | Glutamic acid<br>(Glu; E) |
| TCT<br>TCC<br>TCA<br>TCG | UCU<br>UCC<br>UCA<br>UCG | Serine<br>(Ser; S) | TGT<br>TGC | UGU<br>UGC | Cysteine<br>(Cys; C) |
| | | | TGA | UGA | STOP |
| | | | TGG | UGG | Tryptophan<br>(Trp; W) |
| CCT<br>CCC<br>CCA<br>CCG | CCU<br>CCC<br>CCA<br>CCG | Proline<br>(Pro; P) | CGT<br>CGC<br>CGA<br>CGG | CGU<br>CGC<br>CGA<br>CGG | Arginine<br>(Arg; R) |
| ACT<br>ACC<br>ACA<br>ACG | ACU<br>ACC<br>ACA<br>ACG | Threonine<br>(Thr; T) | AGT<br>AGC | AGU<br>AGC | Serine<br>(Ser; S) |
| | | | AGA<br>AGG | AGA<br>AGG | Arginine<br>(Arg; R) |
| GCT<br>GCC<br>GCA<br>GCG | GCU<br>GCC<br>GCA<br>GCG | Alanine<br>(Ala; A) | GGT<br>GGC<br>GGA<br>GGG | GGU<br>GGC<br>GGA<br>GGG | Glycine<br>(Gly; G) |

[1] Following the usual convention, DNA sequences are written in the DNA-equivalent of RNA, which is the sequence in the non-template (coding) strand.
[2] The symbols in brackets after each amino acid name are the standard three-letter and single-letter abbreviations.

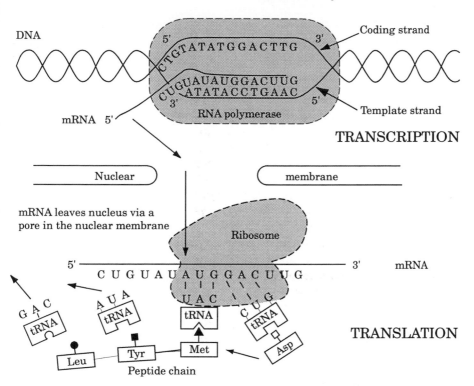

**Fig. 1.9** Synthesis of polypeptide in eukaryotes, by means of transcription and translation.

so-called because its nucleotides contain ribose rather than deoxyribose). The synthesis is catalysed by the enzyme **RNA polymerase**, which, like DNA polymerase, adds nucleotides at the 3′ end of the growing strand, i.e. RNA is also synthesized in the 5′ to 3′ direction. Three of the bases in RNA are the same as in DNA, and the fourth, uracil (U), occurs instead of thymine. The formation of a complementary strand of RNA on the DNA template is called **transcription** (because the base sequence in DNA has been transcribed to RNA).

Before the next stage can commence, the RNA has to move from the nucleus, where the chromosomes are, to structures called **ribosomes** in the cytoplasm, where polypeptides are synthesized. (Obviously, this step is necessary only in organisms whose cells have a nucleus, i.e. eukaryotes. In pro-karyotes, which have no nucleus, ribosomes become attached directly to RNA even before transcription has finished.) Because the RNA carries the code between DNA and protein, it is called **messenger RNA** or **mRNA**. Its triplets are called **codons** (shown in Table 1.2).

As also shown in Fig. 1.9, the second stage of protein synthesis involves a second type of RNA known as **transfer RNA** or **tRNA**. For each of the 20 amino acids, there is one or more specific tRNA molecules which bind to the relevant amino acid and which have a nucleotide triplet (called an **anticodon**) that is complementary to an mRNA codon. Being complementary, a tRNA anticodon pairs with the relevant mRNA codon, bringing the correct amino acid into position in the polypeptide chain. This second and final stage of protein synthesis is called **translation**, because the base sequence has been translated (via the genetic code) to a sequence of amino acids.

## What is a gene?

From the above account, it is evident that particular segments of DNA code for particular polypeptides, which are produced via mRNA. A segment of DNA including all the nucleotides that are transcribed into mRNA is called a **structural gene** (Fig. 1.10).

Since it is the mRNA sequence that is actually translated into polypeptide, and since translation starts at the 5′ end of mRNA, there is a convention that the base sequence of a gene is written as the DNA equivalent of the mRNA sequence, in the 5′ to 3′ direction. Recalling that the base sequence of mRNA is complementary to the sequence in the DNA strand from which it was transcribed, it follows that the DNA strand whose sequence is equivalent to the mRNA sequence is not the template strand, but the other strand. For this reason, the non-template strand is called the **sense** or **coding** strand, while the template strand is called the **antisense** or **anticoding** strand.

Obviously a structural gene includes all of the nucleotides that are eventually translated into polypeptide, i.e. everything from the first nucleotide of the start triplet to the third nucleotide of the stop triplet. But it includes more than this. In fact, transcription starts before the start triplet and finishes after the stop triplet. This means that mRNA has **untranslated regions** at each end. The region that occurs before the start triplet (the **leader sequence**) is where ribosomes become attached. The untranslated region at the other end (the **trailer sequence**) is required for processing of mRNA. The definition of a structural gene includes the sections of DNA that correspond to these regions. Thus, the first nucleotide of a structural gene is the nucleotide at the point where transcription actually commences, i.e. at the **transcription initiation site**. The end of a structural gene is called the **transcription termination site**. By convention, nucleotides of a structural gene are numbered from the start of the transcription initiation site, and bases preceding the site are numbered negatively, i.e. $-1$, $-2$, etc.

The region immediately preceding, i.e. **upstream** from, the transcription initiation site is particularly important, because it is the site to which RNA polymerase becomes attached prior to the initiation of transcription. This region is called the **promoter**. It contains specific sequences that are highly conserved, by which we mean that the same or very similar base sequence occurs in most genes. By studying the sequence at these conserved regions in

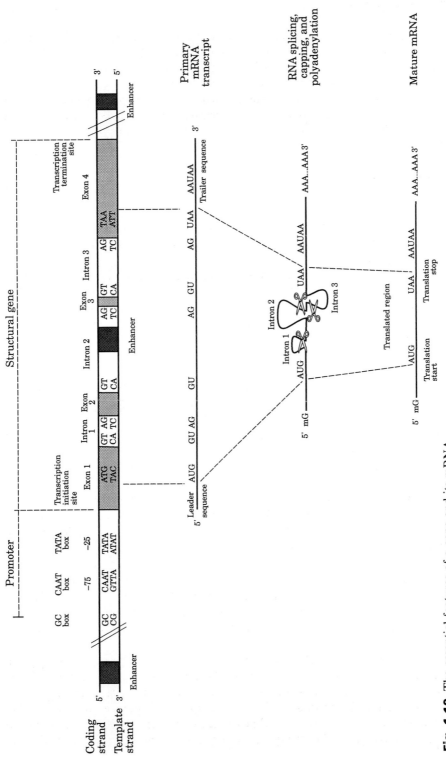

**Fig. 1.10** The essential features of a gene and its mRNA.

many genes in many species, a **consensus sequence** can be deduced, consisting of the most common base at each position. The first such sequence in the promoter of eukaryotic genes is TATAAAA (called the **TATA box**), which is located approximately 25 bases upstream, i.e. at around position $-25$. Further upstream is the sequence GGCCAATCT (the **CAAT box**) at around position $-75$, and GGGCGG (the **GC box**) at around $-90$. These boxes are the site for recognition and binding of regulatory proteins called **transcription factors**, which enable RNA polymerase to be positioned correctly for the initiation of transcription. In this way, they exert control over transcription. Prokaryotes have similarly conserved sequences in their promoters, namely TATAAT and TTGACA.

Termination of transcription is less well understood than initiation. It is known, however, that transcription actually extends beyond what we have called the termination site. Then an unidentified enzyme cleaves the transcript at the termination site. There is no conserved sequence corresponding to this site, but there is a highly conserved region with consensus sequence AATAAA (AAUAAA in the mRNA) located 10–30 bases before the termination site, which appears to be a recognition site in mRNA for a factor that controls the cleavage.

## Split genes

Until 1977, it was thought that structural genes were just long enough to encode the mRNA that is involved in translation. But it is now known that in eukaryotes, most structural genes are longer than this—they contain sections that are not represented in the mRNA by the time it undergoes translation. These sections are called **introns** (because they were originally called *intragenic regions*). Sections that are represented in the final (**mature**) version of mRNA are called **exons** (**ex**pressed regi**ons**). Genes that contain introns are said to be **split**. The original (**primary**) mRNA is a copy of the whole of a structural gene, i.e. exons and introns. Before the mRNA moves from the nucleus to the cytoplasm, the introns are removed and the exons are spliced together (in a process called **RNA splicing**), so that the mature mRNA consists solely of exons. The recognition and removal of introns is aided by the fact that in each intron, the first two bases at the 5′ end and the last two bases at the 3′ end are highly conserved—the same bases (GU and AG respectively in the mRNA) occur at these sites in most, if not all, introns. Recalling that sequences are usually expressed in terms of the coding strand of DNA, this is called the **GT–AG rule**. The base sequence immediately on either side of the highly conserved sequences, i.e. across the boundaries between introns and exons, is also conserved, but to a lesser degree. These boundaries are called **splice sites**, with the 5′ site being called the **donor site** and the 3′ site the **acceptor site**.

Structural genes range in size from around 1000 bases (1 kb) to greater than two million bases (2000 kb), with an average of around 100 000 bases (100 kb).

In contrast, the number of amino acids in polypeptides ranges from around 200 to around 5000, with an average of around 330, which means that mature mRNA ranges in size from around 600 bases (0.6 kb) to around 15 000 bases (15 kb), with an average of around 1000 bases (1 kb). It is obvious from these figures that exons constitute only a small proportion of structural genes; most of the DNA in structural genes is in introns. The existence of so much 'non-functional' DNA remains one of the great unsolved mysteries of biology. We should not be surprised, however, if the solution to the mystery is that introns really do have important functions, which are just waiting to be discovered. (We already have some hints, in that introns tend to act as spacers between functional units, i.e. many exons correspond to functional units which can be assembled in different combinations to produce different polypeptides. But this is not a satisfactory explanation for the quantity of DNA that exists in introns.)

Apart from the excision of introns, the primary mRNA transcript is also modified in two other ways. Its 5′ (front) end is protected by the addition of a **5′ cap**, which consists of a methylated guanine nucleotide. At the other end, a **poly-A tail** is added, consisting of a variable number (typically 100–200) of adenine nucleotides. Since the cap and the tail are such important features of mature mRNA, the translation initiation and termination sites of a gene are sometimes called the **cap site** and the **poly-A site**. The AAUAAA sequence that occurs 10–30 bases upstream from the poly-A site is called the **polyadenylation signal**.

The type of gene described above is by far the most common. However, it is important to realise that there are segments of DNA whose sole function is the production, via transcription, of either tRNA or **ribosomal RNA (rRNA**, which is the major constituent of ribosomes). These are also called genes. Since a large quantity of rRNA is required for the construction of sufficient ribosomes to satisfy each cell's requirements for translation, there are hundreds of genes for rRNA in the genome. They occur in several clusters of tandemly repeated rRNA genes. Each cluster produces a **nucleolus**, which is a discrete structure found within the nucleus (see Fig. 1.13), and which consists mainly of ribosomal RNA plus the enzymes necessary for the assembly of ribosomes. A cluster of rRNA genes is called a **nucleolar organizer region** (NOR).

We can incorporate all the different types of genes into a single definition by saying that a gene is a stretch of DNA that produces a functional RNA molecule.

# Gene regulation

It is obvious that there would be complete chaos if all genes were transcribed in all cells all of the time. In fact, only a small proportion of genes are transcribed at any one time in any one cell. From the moment of fertilization until death, the development of each living organism is determined by genes being switched on and off at the appropriate time(s) in the appropriate cell(s). This switching is achieved by various proteins (sometimes in association with steroid hormones) becoming attached to, or being released from, specific sequences of DNA that are often highly conserved. We have already encountered three such sequences in promoters. Sequences having a similar function but which are not located within promoters are called **enhancers**. These are located upstream, downstream and sometimes even within structural genes (i.e. within introns). Some are located in the near vicinity of the structural gene, but others are quite some distance (20 kb or even further) away.

The regulatory proteins that exert control over transcription by binding to promoters or enhancers have in common one or more amino-acid sequences (called amino-acid **motifs**) that have been given some rather exotic names. For example, **zinc fingers** are structures that result from the repeated occurrence of a pair of cysteine molecules separated by two or three other amino acids, followed 10 or so amino acids later by a pair of histidine molecules, also separated by two or three other amino acids. In combination with a zinc atom, the two cysteines link with the two histidines, and the intervening amino acids form a finger-like loop which binds with DNA. Another example is the **leucine zipper**, which contains a periodic repeat of leucine every seventh amino acid, giving rise to a helix with the leucines aligned along one face. Two such molecules readily join together (in the manner of a zipper), creating a dimer. One end of this dimer binds to DNA.

In general, it is the binding of regulatory proteins (sometimes in conjunction with steroid hormones) to promoters or enhancers that enables RNA polymerase to attach to the promoter of a gene, and which therefore exerts control over the first step in transcription. This is the way in which genes are switched on and off.

For example, early embryonic development is controlled firstly by a set of **segmental** genes (which divide the undifferentiated embryo into segments) and then by a set of **homeotic** genes (each of which determines the developmental fate of one segment, e.g. hindbrain or spinal cord). Proteins encoded by segmental and homeotic genes have DNA-binding motifs such as zinc fingers or leucine zippers. Many of these genes also have a highly conserved 180-bp region called the **homeobox**, which encodes a DNA-binding motif called the **homeo domain** that is highly conserved throughout eukaryotes. Thus the genes that control early embryonic development encode regulatory proteins that switch genes on and off in a controlled manner.

A specific example of gene regulation later in life is provided by the way in which oestrogen controls the transcription of the ovalbumin gene in chickens. Molecules of the hormone enter a cell and bind with a protein called the oestrogen receptor. The complex of oestrogen plus receptor then binds to a region approximately 250 bases upstream from the TATA box of the gene for ovalbumin, switching it on.

Not surprisingly, groups of genes that all need to be controlled in a similar manner have a region of their promoters in common. These regions are called **response elements**. For example, all genes that need to be activated by glucocorticoids have a glucocorticoid response element, to which the gluco-corticoid receptor binds, following activation by glucocorticoid. Its consensus sequence is TGGTACAAATGTTCT.

From the above discussion, it is clear that the sequences on either side of a gene are just as important as the gene itself. In fact, when the word 'gene' is used on its own, it is often taken to include the promoter and enhancer regions as well as the region in between.

## Mutation

We have seen how DNA replicates, and how it gives rise to protein. Although the processes involved are remarkably elegant and usually operate faultlessly, mistakes do occur from time to time. Many mistakes have no effect at all, as they are corrected by the cell's own repair mechanisms. Uncorrected mistakes in DNA replication, however, result in an alteration in the DNA in at least one of the new cells. And because DNA replication is usually so faultless, the altered DNA is passed on unchanged to all descendent cells; until the next mistake occurs. Uncorrected mistakes in DNA replication are called **mutations**.

We shall start by considering **point mutations** (also called **gene mutations**), which involve the substitution of one nucleotide for another, or the addition or deletion of one or a few nucleotides. Other types of mutation will be considered in subsequent chapters.

There are several different possible consequences of point mutations. At one extreme, a base substitution can change a functional triplet into a stop triplet (called a **nonsense** mutation). For example, TAT codes for tyrosine; but if T in the third position is replaced with A, the resulting triplet (TAA) means stop (check this in Table 1.2). If the new stop triplet occurs before the usual stop triplet, the resultant polypeptide is shorter than usual, and is therefore probably not functional. If a base substitution changes a triplet so as to cause an amino acid substitution, it is called a **mis-sense** mutation. For example, substituting A for T at the third position of CAT (histidine) results in CAA (glutamine).

At the other extreme, many base substitutions have no effect on the amino acid sequence of the gene product, because the mutant triplet happens to specify the same amino acid as the original triplet. These so-called **silent** mutations are a direct consequence of the redundancy in the genetic code. For example, substituting C for T at the third position of CAT (histidine) results in CAC, which still codes for histidine (check this in Table 1.2).

Another type of point mutation involves the deletion or insertion of one or two bases. These are called **frameshift** mutations, because each of the triplets which occurs downstream from the site of such a mutation is shifted out of phase from the original open reading frame. At the very least, a frameshift mutation results in a completely different sequence of amino acids down-stream from the site of mutation. For example, consider the following case (check it against Table 1.2):

Original coding strand TCCGAGTATCAGTCCCAG . . .
Amino acid sequence   Ser  Glu  Tyr  Gln  Ser  Gln  . . .

If the second base is deleted, we have:

Mutant coding strand TCGAGTATCAGTCCCAG . . .
Amino acid sequence  Ser  Ser  Ile  Ser  Pro . . .

The mutant amino acid sequence is obviously very different from the original sequence. In some cases, one of the 'new' triplets is a stop triplet, causing premature termination of translation. Whether or not a new stop triplet is created, it is most unlikely that the mutant polypeptide will be functional.

If a mutation occurs in cells other than those that give rise to sex cells, it is called a **somatic mutation**. The stage of development of the animal when a somatic mutation occurs determines the total number of cells that contain the altered or mutant DNA; in general, the earlier the mutation occurs, the larger the number of cells affected.

In contrast, a mutation that occurs in cells that give rise to sex cells is known as a **germ-line mutation**, which may lead to the formation of a gamete that contains the altered DNA. If this gamete is successful in fertilization, the mutation is passed on to the resultant offspring, in every cell of whom it is faithfully reproduced.

## Genes, alleles, and loci

The different forms of a segment of DNA that can exist at a particular site in a chromosome are called **alleles**. The particular site of a gene in a chromosome is called the **locus** (plural **loci**). The word 'gene' is commonly used in the sense of either allele or locus. When used in this way, the appropriate meaning of the word is usually quite evident from its context.

If an offspring results from the union of a sperm with normal DNA and an ovum with an altered or mutant DNA segment in one of its chromosomes, that offspring has one normal chromosome and one mutant chromosome making up the pair of homologues. More specifically, there is one normal allele and one mutant allele at the relevant locus. In the examples below, we shall give these two alleles the symbols *B* and *b* respectively. Animals with two different alleles at a particular locus are said to be **heterozygous** at that locus. In contrast, if an animal has two copies of the same allele, the animal is **homozygous** at that locus.

Although any one animal can have a maximum of only two different alleles at a locus, the number of different alleles in a population of animals can be much greater than two. If more than two alleles exist in a population at a particular locus, that locus is said to have **multiple alleles**.

## Simple or Mendelian inheritance

The passage of genes from one generation to the next is called **inheritance**. One of the major breakthroughs in science was the realization that the results of inheritance can be predicted. The first person to formulate these predictions was the Augustinian monk Gregor Mendel, who conducted his research in a monastery in Brün (now Brno in the Czech Republic) in the middle of last century.

### Single locus

Consider, for example, the mating of a heterozygote (*Bb*) with a homozygote (*bb*). This is exactly analogous to the situation with sex chromosomes. Consequently, the results of the mating *Bb* × *bb* can be represented in exactly the same way as that used for the inheritance of sex discussed earlier, with the aid of a checkerboard:

$$
\begin{array}{cc}
 & \text{Gametes from} \\
 & \text{heterozygous parent} \\
 & \tfrac{1}{2}\,B \qquad\qquad \tfrac{1}{2}\,b \\
\end{array}
$$

|  | | Gametes from heterozygous parent | |
|---|---|---|---|
|  |  | ½ *B* | ½ *b* |
| Gametes from homozygous parent | all *b* | ½ *Bb* | ½ *bb* |

The result of the mating *Bb* × *bb* is expected to be an equal proportion of *Bb* and *bb* offspring. The separation of alleles at a locus during meiosis is called **segregation**, and the ratio of different types of offspring is known as the **segregation ratio**. For the mating *Bb* × *bb*, the segregation ratio is ½ *Bb*: ½ *bb*, which is often written as 1 *Bb*: 1 *bb*.

A checkerboard can be used to predict the outcome of any particular mating involving a single locus. The segregation ratios expected from all possible types of mating with respect to a single locus are listed in Table 1.3.

### More than one locus

In the absence of any evidence to the contrary, it is assumed that segregation at one locus is independent of segregation at other loci. This was the assumption made by Mendel, and it is true for many situations observed in animals today. If segregation at each locus is independent of segregation at other loci,

**Table 1.3** Segregation ratios expected in the offspring arising from all possible types of mating in relation to a single autosomal locus, as obtained from a checkerboard

| Type of mating | Segregation ratio | | | | |
| --- | --- | --- | --- | --- | --- |
| | *BB* | | *Bb* | | *bb* |
| *BB* × *BB* | 1 | : | 0 | : | 0 |
| *BB* × *Bb* | 1 | : | 1 | : | 0 |
| *BB* × *bb* | 0 | : | 1 | : | 0 |
| *Bb* × *Bb* | 1 | : | 2 | : | 1 |
| *Bb* × *bb* | 0 | : | 1 | : | 1 |
| *bb* × *bb* | 0 | : | 0 | : | 1 |

the chance of obtaining a gamete with a particular allele (say *B*) at the first locus and a particular allele (say *d*) at the second locus is simply the product of the probabilities associated with each allele independently. For example, if an individual is heterozygous at two loci (*BbDd*), there are four possible types of gametes, *BD*, *Bd*, *bD*, and *bd*, which are produced with equal frequency.

The results of independent segregation at two loci can also be shown in a checkerboard:

|  |  | Gametes from one parent | | | |
| --- | --- | --- | --- | --- | --- |
|  |  | ¼ *BD* | ¼ *Bd* | ¼ *bD* | ¼ *bd* |
| Gametes | ¼ *BD* | *BBDD* | *BBDd* | *BbDD* | *BbDd* |
| from | ¼ *Bd* | *BBDd* | *BBdd* | *BbDd* | *Bbdd* |
| other | ¼ *bD* | *BbDD* | *BbDd* | *bbDD* | *bbDd* |
| parent | ¼ *bd* | *BbDd* | *Bbdd* | *bbDd* | *bbdd* |

Combining all cells of the checkerboard having identical offspring, and realizing that the offspring in each cell occur with a frequency of ¼ × ¼ = 1/16, the segregation ratio is:

1 *BBDD* : 2 *BBDd* : 1 *BBdd* : 2 *BbDD* : 4 *BbDd* : 2 *Bbdd* : 1 *bbDD* : 2 *bbDd* : 1 *bbdd*

Although checkerboards quickly become rather large, in principle they can be used to derive expected segregation ratios for any type of mating involving any number of independently segregating loci.

## Sex-linkage

The above patterns of inheritance illustrate simple autosomal inheritance because they describe what happens in relation to loci on autosomes. Some loci, however, are on the sex chromosomes and consequently have different patterns of inheritance. Such loci are said to be **sex-linked**. The inheritance patterns of **X-linked** loci can be illustrated in a checkerboard:

|  |  | Male gametes | |
|  |  | $\frac{1}{2}\,X^H$ | $\frac{1}{2}\,Y$ |
| Female | $\frac{1}{2}\,X^H$ | $\frac{1}{4}\,X^H X^H$ | $\frac{1}{4}\,X^H Y$ |
| gametes | $\frac{1}{2}\,X^h$ | $\frac{1}{4}\,X^H X^h$ | $\frac{1}{4}\,X^h Y$ |
|  |  | (female offspring) | (male offspring) |

and are summarized in Table 1.4. Very few loci have been identified on Y chromosomes (**Y-linked**).

**Table 1.4** Segregation ratios expected from all possible types of matings in relation to an X-linked locus, as obtained from a checkerboard

| Type of mating | Segregation ratio | | | | | | | | |
|  | Among females | | | | | | Among males | | |
|  | $X^H X^H$ | | $X^H X^h$ | | $X^h X^h$ | | $X^H Y$ | | $X^h Y$ |
| $X^H X^H \times X^H Y$ | 1 | : | 0 | : | 0 | | 1 | : | 0 |
| $X^H X^h \times X^H Y$ | 1 | : | 1 | : | 0 | | 1 | : | 1 |
| $X^h X^h \times X^H Y$ | 0 | : | 1 | : | 0 | | 0 | : | 1 |
| $X^H X^H \times X^h Y$ | 0 | : | 1 | : | 0 | | 1 | : | 0 |
| $X^H X^h \times X^h Y$ | 0 | : | 1 | : | 1 | | 1 | : | 1 |
| $X^h X^h \times X^h Y$ | 0 | : | 0 | : | 1 | | 0 | : | 1 |

At the beginning of this section it was implied that sometimes segregation at two or more loci is not completely independent. We shall now examine why this is so.

## Linkage

There are at least many thousands of different genes, but there are only a relatively few chromosomes. Inevitably, therefore, each chromosome consists of many different genes, each of which has a specific position (locus) on that chromosome. If chromosomes were inherited as integral units, then for all the loci on a particular chromosome, the alleles present in that chromosome would always segregate together. Consider, for example, one chromosome containing allele $B$ at one locus and allele $D$ at another locus, and its homologue containing alleles $b$ and $d$ respectively. If chromosomes segregated as integral units, only two types of gametes would result, namely *BD* and *bd*, with equal frequency.

In practice, chromosomes are not inherited as integral units. Instead, as described earlier, recombination or crossing-over occurs when homologous chromosomes are synapsed during the first stage of meiosis. During synapsis, breakage and rejoining of chromatids occur. If the two segments of a broken chromatid rejoin, that chromatid is still inherited as an integral unit. If, however, a break occurs in the same position in two adjacent chromatids, sometimes the segments change partners, forming **recombinant** chromatids. If the two chromatids originated from just one homologue, i.e. are joined at the centromere (called **sister chromatids**), the cross-over has no effect, since sister chromatids are exact copies of each other. If, however, the two chromatids are **non-sister chromatids** (one from one homologue and one from the other), the cross-over results in the reciprocal exchange of genes between homologous chromosomes, as shown in Fig. 1.11. To the extent that break-

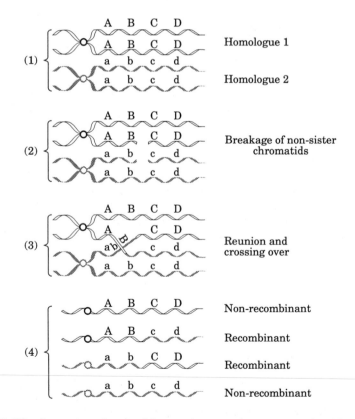

**Fig. 1.11** The four stages involved in crossing-over between a pair of homologous chromosomes.

ages occur more or less randomly along the length of each chromosome, there is a direct relationship between the physical distance separating two loci on a chromosome, and the average number of cross-overs between them. Unfortunately, this number cannot be directly measured. However, by observing the progeny of certain matings, we can calculate the **recombination fraction**, which is the proportion of gametes from one parent that can only have resulted from crossing-over during meiosis in that parent. Fig. 1.12 illustrates the concept of recombination fraction, for the two extreme cases of complete linkage and independence, and for one example of actual data.

If two loci are very close together on a chromosome, the recombination fraction is quite low and the loci are said to be tightly linked. The further apart two loci are on the same chromosome, the greater is the chance of a cross-over occurring between them, and hence the greater is the recombination fraction. For loci that are far apart on the same chromosome, recombinant gametes are just as frequent as non-recombinant ones, which results in the maximum value of recombination fraction, namely 50 per cent. (The reason why the maximum recombination frequency is 50 per cent is evident from Fig. 1.11, which shows that a cross-over results in two recombinant gametes and two non-recombinant gametes.) Loci that are sufficiently far apart on the same chromosome to have a recombination fraction of 50 per cent are said to be effectively unlinked, even though they are actually located on the same chromosome. They are said to be effectively unlinked because they segregate independently, as if they were on different chromosomes.

The relationship between the recombination fraction and the distance between two loci enables the construction of **linkage maps**, in which loci are positioned according to the recombination fraction between them. In such maps, the distance between loci is expressed as **map distance** (in units called **centimorgans**, cM), which equals 100 times the recombination fraction. By estimating the recombination fractions among many pairs of loci within a species, groups of linked loci (**linkage groups**) can be deduced. Since the loci within each group are linked, they must be located on the same chromosome. It follows, therefore, that if sufficient loci have been subjected to linkage analysis in a species, the number of linkage groups equals the number of chromosome pairs. The construction of linkage maps, which have very important practical applications, is discussed in Chapter 2.

## Inactivation

### X-inactivation and dosage compensation

Among the many coat colours seen in cats, the mosaic of orange and non-orange, which is known as tortoiseshell (Fig. 1.13a) is one of the most attractive. The orange hairs result from the action of an X-linked allele $O$, which prevents the production of dark pigment (black and brown), but enables the production of yellow pigment. The non-orange hairs are due to

One parent
(double heterozygote)

*B* *D*
*b* *d*

Four different types of gametes

| | Non-recombinant | Recombinant | Recombinant | Non-recombinant | % recombinants (= map distance) |
|---|---|---|---|---|---|
| | *B* *D* / *b* *d* | *B* *d* / *b* | *b* *D* / *b* | *b* *d* / *b* | |
| Complete linkage | 0.50 | 0 | 0 | 0.50 | 0% = 0 cM |
| Independence | 0.25 | 0.25 | 0.25 | 0.25 | 50% = 50 cM |
| Real data | 82 | 16 | 20 | 79 | $\dfrac{(16 + 20)}{(82 + 16 + 20 + 79)}$ = 18 cM |

Other parent
(double homozygote)

*b* *d*
*b* *d*

All gametes the same

*b* *d*

(a)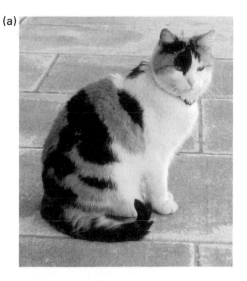

(b)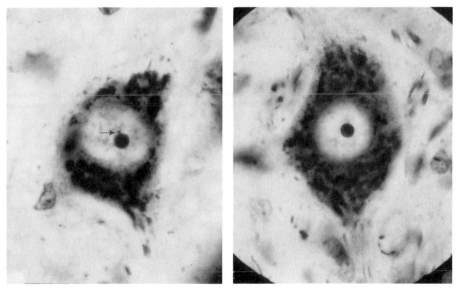

**Fig. 1.13** (a) A tortoiseshell cat with white spotting. The white spotting is due to an allele at an autosomal locus (see Chapter 12). (b) Motor neurones from the hypoglossal nucleus of a mature female cat (left) and a mature male cat (right). The large dark-staining body in each cell is a nucleolus. The small dark-staining body (arrowed) in the female cell is a Barr body.

**Fig. 1.12** The concept of recombination fraction, illustrated with a checkerboard. The first and second lines at the bottom show theoretical expectations for the extremes of zero and 50 per cent recombination. The last line shows some actual data, giving an estimated map distance of 18 cM.

the normal (**wild-type**) allele at the same locus, $o$, which enables the production of dark pigment, in whatever manner is determined by alleles at other coat-colour loci. (See Chapter 12 for more information on the genetics of coat colour.) Since both alleles must obviously be present in order to produce the mosaic of orange and non-orange, tortoiseshell cats must be heterozygous, $X^O X^o$, at this X-linked locus. But why do some parts of the body express the effect of the orange allele, while other parts express that of the non-orange allele? And why are the patches of non-orange and orange approximately equal in total area, and why are they scattered more or less randomly throughout the coat?

The answers to these questions lie partly in another observation, first made in cats, by Barr and Bertram, who in 1949 reported that the nucleus of non-dividing nerve cells in females usually contains a small dark-staining body, whereas that in males does not (Fig. 1.13b). This dark-staining body is now called a **Barr body** or **sex chromatin**. Although it had been observed by many previous researchers, Barr and Bertram were the first to note that the dark-staining body occurs in only female cells. In an attempt to explain their observations, they speculated that it might be an X chromosome which had become very highly condensed. Other researchers showed that they were correct; a Barr body is, in fact, an X chromosome that is late in replicating during mitosis.

Drawing on similar observations in mice, Mary Lyon suggested in 1961 that the highly condensed X chromosome seen in female cells is the result of one of the X chromosomes (chosen at random) becoming inactive in each cell of all female embryos at an early stage of development. This is the **Lyon hypothesis**. (In fact, it is now known that not all genes on the inactivated X chromosome are inactivated; those in and near the pseudo-autosomal region remain functional in both X chromosomes.)

Since the Lyon hypothesis postulates that the choice of X for inactivation is entirely random, it follows that each of the X chromosomes in normal females is active in approximately one-half of that female's cells.

The process of **random X-inactivation** provides an adequate explanation for tortoiseshell coat colour in cats; each patch of orange represents the cells that descended from a cell in which the non-orange allele was inactivated, and vice versa. In addition, the apparently random distribution of patches, and the approximately equal total area of orange and non-orange, are to be expected if the inactivated X is chosen at random.

In passing, it should be noted that since tortoiseshell cats are heterozygous at an X-linked locus, they must have two X chromosomes, in which case they should be female. Normal male cats, having only one X chromosome, can be either orange ($X^O Y$) or non-orange ($X^o Y$), but not tortoiseshell. It is therefore a fairly safe bet that any tortoiseshell cat is a female. Occasionally male tortoiseshells are reported, but they often turn out to be abnormal males having an extra X chromosome, as described in Chapter 4.

The result of random X-inactivation is that each female is a **mosaic**, consisting of two distinct populations of cells derived from a common source; in one population of cells the maternal X chromosome is inactive, and in the other cell population, the paternal X is inactive.

The only well-documented exception to random X-inactivation occurs in marsupials, where it is the paternal X chromosome that is inactivated, and often only incompletely so. The reason for this is not known.

Obviously the result of X-inactivation in females is that each female cell has the same quantity of gene product from X-linked genes as do males. Thus, X-inactivation is a mechanism that compensates for the difference in gene 'dosage' between males and females in relation to X-linked genes. This effect of X-inactivation is called **dosage compensation**.

Finally, an important difference between mammals and birds must be noted: while X-inactivation appears to occur in all mammals, Z-inactivation does not occur in birds. The reasons for this are not known.

## Imprinting

Inactivation is not confined to the X chromosome. At certain loci on other chromosomes, the extent to which an allele is expressed (or even whether it is expressed at all) depends on the parent from which it came. This differential expression of alleles is called **genomic imprinting**. As might be imagined, this can be a source of frustration in attempts to determine the mode of inheritance of disorders, because imprinting can result in atypical inheritance patterns.

## Inactivation results from methylation

At the molecular level, inactivation is associated with the addition of a methyl group ($CH_3$) to cytosine molecules that occur immediately on the 5' side of guanine molecules, i.e. inactivation is associated with methylation of cytosines in so-called **CpG islands**, where p stands for the phosphate link between the two adjacent bases. Within an individual animal, all descendants of each cell in which inactivation first occurred have the same inactive gene or chromosome, because after each replication of a methylated strand of DNA, the new strand is automatically methylated at the same CpG sites as in the original strand. In meiosis, however, or in early embryonic development, the methylation patterns are reset.

Not all methylation patterns are set for the lifespan of the animal. In fact, in regions that are not subjected to X-inactivation or imprinting, methylation of CpG islands in promoters is a common attribute of inactive genes, and de-methylation is a prerequisite for transcription of many genes. Thus methylation is another means by which genes are regulated.

## Types of DNA

Despite the obvious importance of genes, not all DNA consists of genes. In fact, only a small proportion of the genome of animals consists of genes;

probably less than 10 per cent and maybe as little as 1 per cent. How can we categorize total DNA, and where do genes fit into the picture?

The most common category of DNA consists of **unique** or **single-copy** sequences, which account for 60–70 per cent of the genome of mammals. These single-copy sequences are dispersed throughout the genome. A small proportion of this DNA accounts for most genes.

Some genes occur in **multigene families**, which consist of sets of identical or very similar genes, whose individual members are usually scattered around the genome, or, in some cases, occur as sets of adjacent genes. Not surprisingly, the genes which occur in multigene families are those whose products are required in relatively large quantities, e.g. histone, keratin, collagen, ribosomal RNA, and transfer RNA.

The third major category of DNA is **repetitive** DNA, which consists of multiple copies of particular sequences called **repeat units**, which range in size from a single base to several thousand bases. Repetitive DNA has assumed increasing importance in recent years, with the realization that it holds the key to some important inherited diseases, and provides a major tool for the practical application of molecular biology to animal health and improvement. We shall discuss these aspects of repetitive DNA in following chapters.

There is one other category of chromosomal DNA that should be mentioned. Scattered throughout the genome are small DNA fragments called **transposable genetic elements (TGEs)** or **jumping genes**. A notable property of a TGE is that the nucleotide sequence at one end is an **inverted repeat** (or occasionally a **direct repeat**) of the sequence at the other end. In cattle, for example, there is a TGE which is 611 bases long. Its terminal sequences are:

5′ GCCGGGGA . . . TCCCCGGC 3′
3′ CGGCCCCT . . . AGGGGCCG 5′

Notice that the sequence TCCCCGGC at the 3′ end of the top strand is really a repeat of the GCCGGGGA sequence at the other end of the same strand, only in an inverted (i.e. reverse) and complementary form. Another way to look at this is to note that reading the sequence in the top strand from 5′ to 3′ is exactly the same as reading the bottom sequence from 5′ to 3′. Because they contain exactly the same message when read in either direction, inverted repeats are said to be **palindromes** (by analogy with palindromic sentences such as ABLE WAS I ERE I SAW ELBA).

The repeats are homologous, and are therefore able to pair with each other, just as homologous chromatids pair during meiosis I. In the case of TGEs, the pairing of the repeats results in the TGE itself being formed into a loop. Often when this occurs, the whole of the TGE excises itself from wherever it happens to be, and moves to another section of the same or a different chromosome, into which it then inserts itself by the reverse process. Sometimes, the TGE is replicated, and the resultant copy moves elsewhere, leaving the original one in its original position. As we shall see in Chapter 10,

TGEs are extremely important in relation to the rapid spread of multiple antibiotic resistance in bacteria. In eukaryotes, TGEs are surprisingly ubiquitous: there are hundreds of thousands of them in the mammalian genome, making up from 1 to 5 per cent of total DNA. In cattle, for example, the TGE described above occurs 35 000 times. Many of the copies of this and other TGEs have lost the ability to move from one site to another (to transpose). However, those that are able to transpose themselves are extremely important, because if a TGE inserts itself into a structural gene, it will most likely inactivate that gene. Alternatively, if a TGE inserts itself in the control region of a gene, it may interfere with normal control, resulting in the gene being expressed at inappropriate times and places, or not being expressed when it should be. Because of these effects, TGEs are important sources of mutation. The mutations they create are called **insertion mutations**. TGEs are also important causes of cancer, as we shall see in Chapter 12.

## Further reading

### General

Alberts, B., Bray, D., Lewis, J., Raff, M., Roberts, K., and Watson, J. D. (1994). *Molecular biology of the cell*, (3rd edn). Garland Publishing, New York.

King, R. C. and Stansfield, W. D. (1990). *A dictionary of genetics*, (4th edn). Oxford University Press, New York.

Lewin, B. (1994). *Genes V*. Oxford University Press, New York.

### Chromosomes

Barch, M. J. (ed.) (1991). *The ACT cytogenetics laboratory manual*, (2nd edn). Raven Press, New York.

McFeely, R. A. (ed.) (1990). *Domestic animal cytogenetics*, Advances in Veterinary Science and Comparative Medicine, Vol. 34. Academic Press, San Diego.

### Meiosis and mitosis

Handel, M. A. and Hunt, P. A. (1992). Sex-chromosome pairing and activity during mammalian meiosis. *Bioessays*, **14**, 817–22.

Moens, P. B. (1994). Molecular perspectives of chromosome pairing at meiosis. *Bioessays*, **16**, 101–6.

### Biochemistry of inheritance

Jukes, T. H. (1993). The genetic code—function and evolution. *Cellular and Molecular Biology Research*, **39**, 685–8.

Kornberg, A. and Baker, T. A. (1992). *DNA replication*, (2nd edn). Freeman, New York.

## What is a gene?

Dibb, N. J. (1993). Why do genes have introns? *FEBS Letters*, **325**, 135–9.
Portin, P. (1993). The concept of the gene—short history and present status. *Quarterly Review of Biology*, **68**, 173–223.

## Gene regulation

Cowell, I. G. (1994). Repression versus activation in the control of gene transcription. *Trends in Biochemical Sciences*, **19**, 38–42.
Das, A. (1993). Control of transcription termination by RNA-binding proteins. *Annual Review of Biochemistry*, **62**, 893–930.
Duboule, D. (ed.) (1993). *Guidebook to the homeobox genes*. Oxford University Press, Oxford.
Harrison, S. C. and Sauer, R. T. (ed.) (1994). Protein-nucleic acid interactions. *Current Opinion in Structural Biology*, **4**, 1–66.
O'Halloran, T. V. (1993). Transition metals in control of gene expression. *Science*, **261**, 715–25.

## Inactivation

Lyon, M. F. (1992). Some milestones in the history of X-chromosome inactivation. *Annual Review of Genetics,* **26**, 17-28.
Lyon, M. F. (1993). Epigenetic inheritance in mammals. *Trends in Genetics*, **9**, 123–8.
Peterson, K. and Sapienza, C. (1993). Imprinting the genome—imprinted genes, imprinting genes, and a hypothesis for their interaction. *Annual Review of Genetics*, **27**, 7–31.
Tycko, B. (1994). Genomic imprinting—mechanism and role in human pathology. *American Journal of Pathology*, **144**, 431–43.

## Appendix 1.1.

*Banded karyotypes of domestic species*

Cat

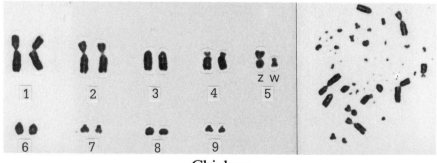

Dog

Chicken

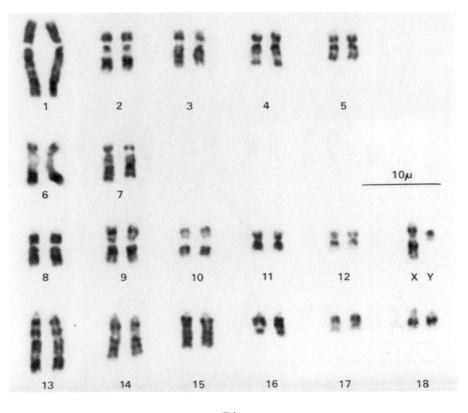

Pig

Goat

Sheep

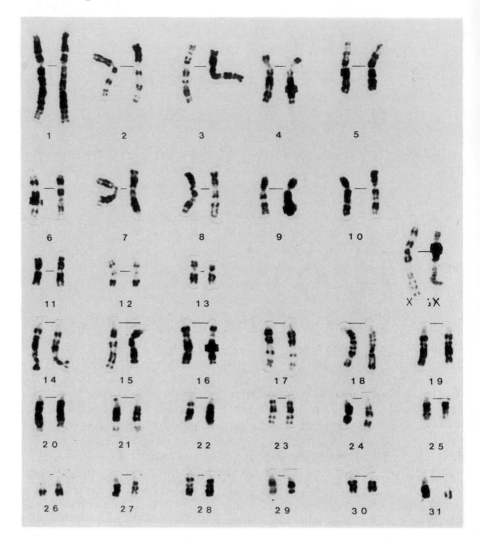

Horse

# Molecular biology 2

Molecular biology is a general term encompassing the manipulation of DNA and RNA in the laboratory. As well as providing powerful research tools, molecular biology is already being applied in vaccine production, veterinary diagnosis, manufacture of therapeutic proteins, detection of carriers of harmful genes, and in gene therapy. In the future, it will be increasingly difficult to find areas of animal health and production that are not substantially affected by this technology. In the following account, we shall review the most important features of this rapidly expanding field.

## Restriction enzymes

In 1970, it was discovered that bacteria produce enzymes that are able to degrade foreign DNA that enters the bacterial cell. Because these enzymes play a key role in a phenomenon known as host restriction (whereby a bacteria protects itself from viruses by cutting the viral DNA into segments), they are called **restriction enzymes**. Hundreds of restriction enzymes are now known, and a standard method of naming them has been developed: the first letter of the genus name, followed by the first two letters of the species name, followed by letters indicating strain, order of discovery, etc. For example, the enzyme *Bam*HI is obtained from *Bacillus amyloliquefaciens*, with H indicating a particular strain, and I indicating that it is the first enzyme obtained from this strain. Restriction enzymes bind to specific sequences of bases called **recognition sequences**, and each enzyme cuts the DNA at a specific **cleavage site** that is usually located within the recognition sequence. In most cases, recognition sequences are palindromes, which, as we saw in Chapter 1, contain exactly the same sequence when read in either direction. A list of commonly used restriction enzymes, together with their recognition sequences and cleavage sites, is given in Table 2.1. Check the table for palindromes: the sequence in the top strand when read from 5′ to 3′ is exactly the same as the sequence in the bottom strand when read from 5′ to 3′.

Some restriction enzymes, such as *Sma*I, cut both strands of the double helix at the same place, leaving two **blunt ends**. Others, such as *Eco*RI, cut each strand at a different position, leaving some nucleotides unpaired. Because complementary nucleotides readily bind to these unpaired nucleotides, enzymes such as *Eco*RI are said to create **sticky ends**.

When a restriction enzyme is added to DNA, the DNA is cleaved in as

**Table 2.1** Some common restriction enzymes

| Source | Enzyme | Recognition sequence, and cleavage site ( ↑  ↓ ) |
|---|---|---|
| *Arthrobacter luteus* | *Alu*I | ↓<br>5'. . .-A-G-C-T-. . .3'<br>3'. . .-T-C-G-A-. . .5'<br>↑ |
| *Bacillus amyloliquefaciens* H | *Bam*HI | ↓<br>5'. . .-G-G-A-T-C-C-. . .3'<br>3'. . .-C-C-T-A-G-G-. . .5'<br>↑ |
| *Escherichia coli* R | *Eco*RI | ↓<br>5'. . .-G-A-A-T-T-C-. . .3'<br>3'. . .-C-T-T-A-A-G-. . .5'<br>↑ |
| *Haemophilus influenzae* $R_d$ | *Hind*III | ↓<br>5'. . .-A-A-G-C-T-T-. . .3'<br>3'. . .-T-T-C-G-A-A-. . .5'<br>↑ |
| *Haemophilus aegyptius* | *Hae*III | ↓<br>5'. . .-G-G-C-C-. . .3'<br>3'. . .-C-C-G-G-. . .5'<br>↑ |
| *Providencia stuartii* | *Pst*I | ↓<br>5'. . .-C-T-G-C-A-G-. . .3'<br>3'. . .-G-A-C-G-T-C-. . .5'<br>↑ |
| *Serratia marcescens* | *Sma*I | ↓<br>5'. . .-C-C-C-G-G-G-. . .3'<br>3'. . .-G-G-G-C-C-C-. . .5'<br>↑ |

many positions as there are cleavage sites for that enzyme; the DNA is **digested** into fragments. Since cleavage sites are not positioned at regular intervals along a DNA molecule, the fragments are of different lengths and hence different weights. If the mixture of fragments is placed at one end of a gel and subjected to electrophoresis, the fragments migrate along the gel at a rate inversely proportional to the logarithm of their weights. At any given time after the electric field was first applied, there are as many different bands of DNA fragments in the gel as there were different-sized fragments in the original mixture. And the position of each band indicates the size of each fragment.

Consider, for example, a relatively small DNA molecule such as that of the bacterial virus called bacteriophage lambda (abbreviated to phage λ), whose total DNA consists of a single molecule 49 kilobases (kb) long (Fig. 2.1a). If the

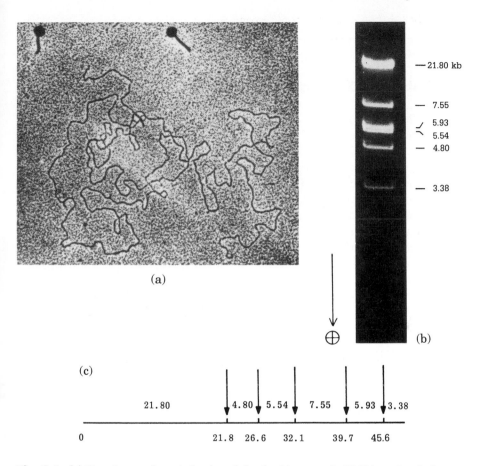

**Fig. 2.1** (a) Two intact phage λ (top) and the double-stranded DNA molecule from a third phage. The two ends of the DNA molecule are clearly visible. (b) The result of electrophoresis of DNA from phage λ, after digestion with *Eco*RI. (c) An *Eco*RI restriction map of DNA from phage λ. Cleavage sites are indicated by arrows. The numbers under each arrow indicate the location of each site in terms of the number of kb from the left-hand end of the molecule. Numbers above the line indicate the size of each fragment in kb, and correspond to the numbers in (b).

total DNA from this virus is digested with the enzyme *Eco*RI, and if the resultant fragments are subjected to electrophoresis and stained with ethidium bromide (which binds to DNA and fluoresces under ultraviolet light), a picture like that in Fig. 2.1b emerges. Each band corresponds to a different fragment, whose size in kb is given beside the gel. The existence of six fragments indicates that there are five *Eco*RI cleavage sites in the DNA of phage λ. To determine the order of the *Eco*RI fragments, the DNA has to be separately digested with that enzyme and with one other enzyme, and with a mixture of the two enzymes. By comparing fragments resulting from each of the three digestions, the order of the fragments for each enzyme can be determined. This enables a **restriction map** to be drawn (Fig. 2.1c).

## Recombinant DNA and DNA cloning

One of the main processes in molecular biology is the production of an un-limited number of copies of a particular segment of DNA. This mass produc-tion of a DNA segment is a necessary prerequisite for determining the segment's base sequence (which provides the key to its function) and for many other molecular techniques. It can be achieved in two ways. The first is called gene cloning or DNA cloning, and the second is called the polymerase chain reaction (PCR). We shall start with DNA cloning; PCR will be con-sidered in a later section.

**DNA cloning** is achieved by joining the DNA that is to be cloned (called **foreign** or **insert** DNA) to a **vector** which is capable of replication within a **host**. The initial requirement for this process is that the insert and vector DNA must have compatible ends (generated by an appropriate restriction enzyme). When insert and vector DNA are mixed together with the enzyme DNA ligase (described in Chapter 1), the end of the insert DNA binds with the end of the vector DNA, in a process called **splicing** or **ligation**. The resultant DNA molecule is one example of **recombinant DNA**. (The term applies to the result of ligating any two segments of DNA from different sources.)

One type of commonly used vector is a **plasmid**, which is a circle of double-stranded DNA, typically 1–3 kb in length, that exists in certain bacterial cells (hosts) independently of the main bacterial chromosome. Plasmids are very useful for cloning relatively small fragments of DNA—up to around 10 kb. A general outline of DNA cloning using plasmids is given in Fig. 2.2.

Another popular vector is the phage λ, which we have already encountered. Up to around 20 kb of the central region of its 49 kb DNA molecule can be removed without interfering with the phage's ability to infect a bacterial cell. If this central region is replaced with an insert of approximately the same size, the resultant recombinant DNA molecule is sufficiently close in total size to a normal phage λ DNA molecule that it can be 'packaged' *in vitro* into phage particles which then obligingly follow their usual practice of attaching to bacterial cell walls and injecting their DNA (in this case, recombinant DNA) into the bacterial (host) cell. Once inside the host, the two ends of the phage DNA join together to form a circle, which replicates in the host. In practice, phage vectors can accommodate inserts in the range of around 10–20 kb.

Larger fragments can be cloned if just the two ends of phage λ DNA (called **cos** ends because they are cohesive, i.e. they join together in the host) are added to a plasmid, forming a **cosmid** vector. Since the phage normally packages a DNA molecule of 49 kb with cos ends, and since the total length of

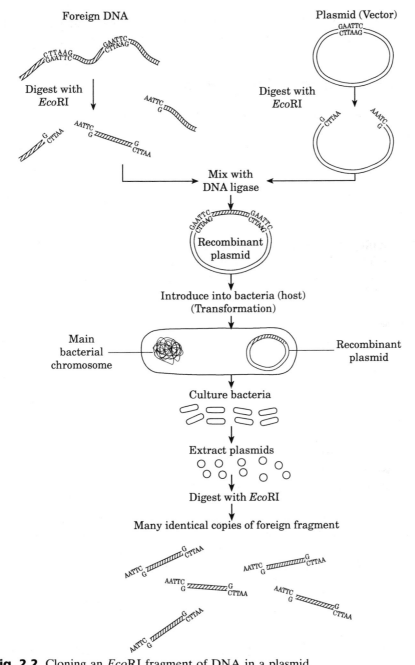

**Fig. 2.2** Cloning an *Eco*RI fragment of DNA in a plasmid.

the cos ends plus the plasmid is only relatively small, cosmids can be used for cloning fragments in the range 40–50 kb.

Even larger fragments of foreign DNA (from several hundred kb up to 1 Mb) can be cloned in yeast, in a **yeast artificial chromosome (YAC)**, which consists of the insert flanked by the essential parts of a yeast chromosome, namely the two ends (called **telomeres**), a centromere, and a site where replication begins (called the **origin of replication**).

In many cases, the aim of cloning may simply be to generate an unlimited number of copies of a particular segment of DNA, in preparation for sequencing or some other molecular procedure.

But there are other uses for DNA cloning. For example, if all of the DNA from some white blood cells of a cow is digested with one or more restriction enzymes, all of the resultant fragments can be cloned, resulting in a **genomic library** (Fig. 2.3). In principle, such a library contains all of the DNA for that particular species. (In practice, some small segments may be missing.)

One particularly important use of genomic libraries is to create an ordered set of overlapping clones (called **contigs**, from contiguous) which together cover a particular region of a chromosome or even whole chromosomes or whole genomes. As explained in Chapters 11 and 14, such a set of contigs is especially useful in tracking down particular genes, once their general location has been determined through linkage to one or more DNA markers.

## Complementary DNA

There is a class of viruses whose entire genome consists only of RNA. Because RNA is not capable of replication, the only way for these viruses to propagate is for their RNA to be transcribed 'backwards' into DNA. Because of this, they are called **retroviruses**. The DNA then replicates and acts as a template for the synthesis of more RNA. The enzyme that catalyses the reverse transcription of RNA into DNA is called **reverse transcriptase**. It is extremely important in molecular biology because, among other things, it enables rapid isolation of the coding regions of a gene.

A tissue that is producing polypeptides contains relatively high concentrations of mature mRNA for those polypeptides. If mRNA is extracted from that tissue, and if nucleotides and the enzyme reverse transcriptase are added to the mRNA, a complementary strand of DNA (called **complementary DNA** or **copy DNA** or **cDNA**) can be synthesized. Then, by adding more nucleotides and the enzyme DNA polymerase, the single-stranded cDNA can be replicated into double-stranded cDNA.

This cDNA corresponds to the genes that were active in the tissue at the time the mRNA was extracted. Recalling that mature mRNA consists solely of exons, it is evident that cDNA is equivalent to genes from which the introns have been removed.

cDNA fragments can be cloned, creating a **cDNA library** (Fig. 2.3). Such

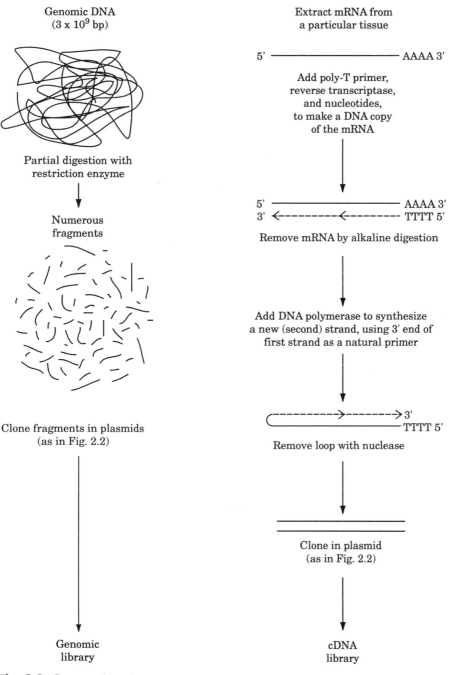

**Fig. 2.3** Construction of genomic and cDNA plasmid libraries.

libraries contain cDNA copies of all the genes that were functional in the tissue at the time the mRNA was extracted. Note, however, that whereas a genomic library contains all the DNA of a species (including exons and introns of all structural genes, plus all of the other DNA), a cDNA library contains only the exons of those structural genes that happened to be functioning (i.e. producing protein) at the time when the tissue was sampled.

## DNA sequencing

One of the major breakthroughs in molecular biology has been the development of methods for rapidly sequencing fragments of DNA. In fact, DNA sequencing has become so commonplace that it is often one of the first steps taken in studying a segment of DNA. Increasingly, it is also being used for diagnostic purposes.

There are two methods: the **Sanger** or **dideoxy** or **chain-terminating** method, and the **Maxam–Gilbert** or **chemical** method, with the former being more commonly used. Each method involves the creation of a series of labelled single strands of varying length, starting from one end of the fragment being sequenced. Electrophoresis of the strands in a polyacrylamide gel separates them according to size, creating a 'ladder' of labelled bands, with each band corresponding to an occurrence of a base. If the labelling is radioactive, the gel is then dried and placed next to an X-ray film, which records the presence of each band on the resultant autoradiograph. Increasingly, fluorescent labelling (which is activated by a laser beam) is replacing radioactivity. Once the bands have been visualized with either system of labelling, the sequence of bases in the fragment can be read directly from the ladder of bands. Both methods are illustrated in Fig. 2.4. The size of fragment that can be sequenced is between 250 and 350 with the Sanger method and up to around 250 bases with the Maxam–Gilbert method. Longer sequences are assembled by combining the sequences obtained from overlapping fragments.

The whole process of sequencing is becoming increasingly automated, and sequence data are being accumulated at an ever-increasing rate. Databases such as Genbank (USA) and the EMBL Data Library (Europe) have been established specifically to record such data, and on-line access to them is available throughout the world. Many research journals now insist that sequence information be submitted to at least one of these databases, as a prerequisite for publication. With each mammalian genome containing approximately $3 \times 10^9$ base pairs (i.e. three million kb or 3000 Mb), the rapid expansion of sequencing is posing substantial challenges to information scientists. However, much progress has been made, especially in terms of the development of powerful software for searching and analysing sequences. Already the entire sequence has been determined for some microorganisms, and for the whole of one chromosome of baker's yeast (*Saccharomyces*

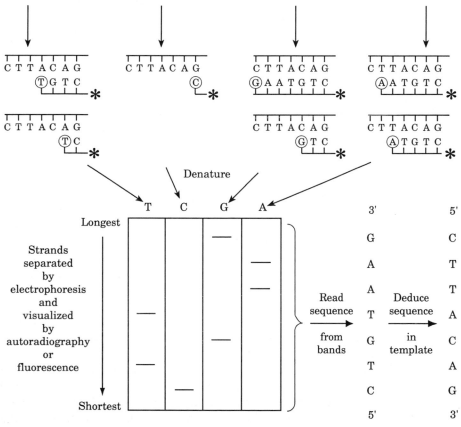

**Fig. 2.4** Sequencing DNA by the dideoxy method (*this page*) and the chemical method (*next page*).

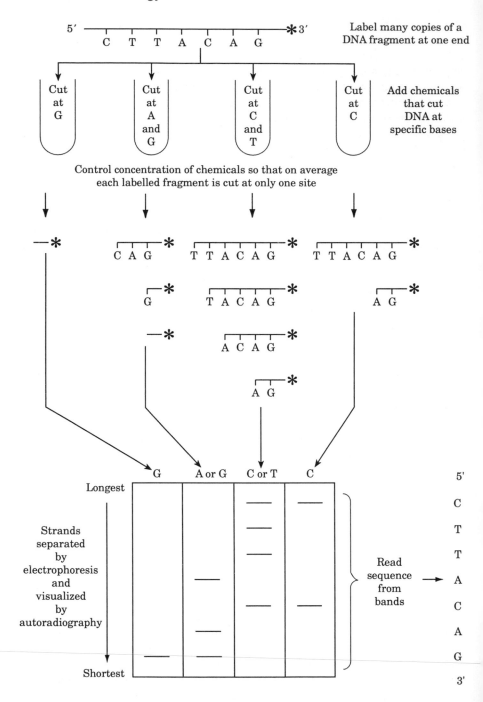

*cerevisiae*). Work is also underway on the **human genome project**, a vast collaborative project with the aim, among other things, of sequencing the entire human genome. It is important to note that there are *no* plans to sequence the entire genome of any domestic species, mainly because it is agreed that the limited funds available for molecular research in these species can be better spent in concentrating on genes of interest or apparent importance. Also, in view of the high degree of homology between mammalian genomes (discussed later in this chapter), the fact that one mammalian species (human) is being sequenced, substantially reduces the value of obtaining the entire sequence of another mammal. In the fullness of time, many of the discoveries that emerge from the human genome project will be directly applicable to domestic animals.

There are many uses to which sequence information can be put. For example, it is possible to search sequence data, looking for long open reading frames (explained in Chapter 1), which indicate structural genes. This is one way of discovering hitherto unknown genes. In such situations, researchers then have the sequence of a gene without knowing anything about its polypeptide. By comparing the sequence in their newly discovered gene with sequences from genes of known function, it is often possible to determine the type and function of the polypeptide, long before it has ever been isolated. For example, if a newly discovered gene contains sequences that give rise to zinc fingers (described in Chapter 1), it is likely to encode a regulatory protein. Another important use of sequence data is in comparing sequences from the same gene in different species, which enables evolutionary trees to be constructed (see Chapter 5).

Of equal importance is the sequencing of the genomes of parasites and pathogens. The knowledge gained from this work is providing valuable new insights into potential means of controlling these organisms.

## Polymerase chain reaction (PCR)

One of the most powerful tools in molecular biology is the **polymerase chain reaction (PCR)**. Developed in 1985 by Kary Mullis and colleagues, it is now used extensively in research. Increasingly, it is also being applied in diagnosis and in the detection of particular genes (both favourable and harmful) in domestic animals. In the future, it will have widespread use in many areas of veterinary practice and in animal improvement programmes.

The DNA on which PCR is performed (the **template** DNA) can be genomic DNA (extracted from white blood cells or a sample of spleen or other tissue) or a fragment of DNA from any source. PCR creates approximately a million copies of a small segment of the template DNA; sufficient to enable that segment to be cloned or sequenced or analysed in other ways described below. The basic requirement is to know the sequence of the segment, or, at the very least, the sequence at each end of the segment, that

we wish to amplify. Using this sequence information, two strings of nucleotides (called **oligonucleotides**, or **oligos** for short), each around 20 bases in
length, are synthesized: one is complementary to the 3' end of one of the
strands of the segment to be amplified; and the other is complementary to the
3' end of the other strand of the segment. Because the role of these oligonucleotides is to prime the synthesis of new strands of DNA, they are called
**primers**.

The essential features of PCR are illustrated in Fig. 2.5. The template
DNA is placed in a tube, together with the primers, a quantity of deoxynucleotides, and some DNA polymerase. The mixture is heated to around
95 °C in order to separate (**denature**) the two strands of template DNA. (The
DNA polymerase has to be heat-stable so that it can withstand the high
temperature of the denaturation phase. A commonly used form is *Taq* **polymerase**, so called because it comes from the thermophilic bacterium *Thermus
aquaticus*.) The temperature is then decreased to around 50 °C–60 °C, to allow
the primers to bind (**anneal**) to their complementary sequences in the template DNA (i.e. to either end of the segment that we wish to amplify). Once

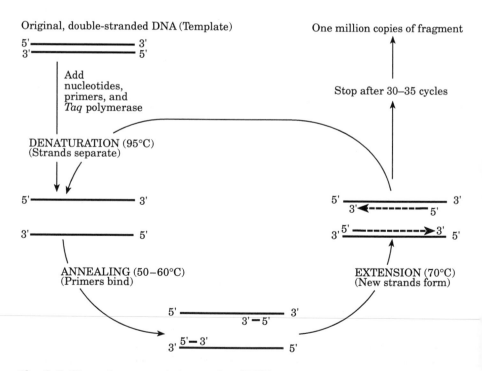

**Fig. 2.5** The polymerase chain reaction (PCR).

the primers have bound, the temperature is increased to around 70°C, this being optimum for the DNA polymerase, which adds the appropriate nucleotides at the 3' end of each primer, thereby **extending** the new DNA strands. After allowing sufficient time for the new strands to be synthesized, the temperature is increased to 95°C again, thereby commencing a new cycle of denaturation, annealing and extension. The length of one cycle (called an **amplification cycle**) is typically about 5 minutes, consisting of 15 seconds for denaturation, 30 seconds for annealing, 90 seconds for extension, plus the minimum time required to change temperatures between phases (30–60 seconds for each change).

The amplification cycle is usually performed between 30 and 35 times in custom-built PCR machines (thermal cyclers), which provide exact, programmable control over the length and temperature of each step in each cycle. In theory, the result is between $2^{30}$ and $2^{35}$ times the original number of copies of the segment—equivalent to between one billion and 35 billion identical segments (called the **PCR product**). In practice, the exponential amplification is not perfect. It is still quite possible, however, to acheive at least a million-fold amplification, and to obtain 1 μg of PCR product.

The range and power of PCR is remarkable. For example, PCR products can be obtained from DNA in living organisms, in animal products such as meat and eggs, or in museum or archaeological specimens; and the sample can be as small as a single sperm or a single hair follicle. PCR products can even be obtained from milk, because milk contains somatic cells.

Many variations on the basic PCR theme are now in use. For example, several pairs of primers can be included in the one **multiplex** PCR reaction. The main requirement is that the primers be designed so that the amplified fragments differ sufficiently in size to be distinguishable in a single lane of the gel. In another variation, primers with a random sequence are constructed, giving rise to **random amplified polymorphic DNA** or **RAPD**. (The word 'polymorphic' refers to the existence of more than one type or form.) In some species, RAPDs are a useful source of random DNA markers for genetic maps or (in the case of parasites) for species identification. Another variation involves reverse transcription of a sample of RNA to produce cDNA, which is then amplified by PCR. Known as **reverse transcription PCR (RT-PCR)**, this is a powerful means of identifying and studying genes without having to go through the cloning process.

An important application of PCR has been to combine it with dideoxy DNA sequencing, giving rise to a procedure called **cycle sequencing**. Just one primer is used, so that only one strand is amplified. In addition to the usual deoxynucleotides, the PCR mixture also contains some dideoxynucleotides, which, as already explained in Fig. 2.4, terminate the extension of any new strand into which they are incorporated. The result is a graded series of PCR products (exactly the same as those produced in dideoxy sequencing), which can be electrophoresed and visualized as bands from which the sequence can be read, in the usual manner. The advantages of cycle sequencing (and other combinations of PCR and sequencing) are that it can be performed on very small quantities of DNA, and there is no need to clone the DNA before it is sequenced.

## Southern analysis and related technologies

Another important molecular technique is Southern analysis, which is named after Ed Southern who developed its central component in 1975. As with PCR, we start with genomic DNA or DNA from some other source. The first step involves digesting this DNA with a restriction enzyme, producing thousands of fragments of various lengths. The fragments are then separated according to their size, by means of gel electrophoresis (as described earlier in this chapter), denatured into single strands, and transferred (blotted) onto a membrane of nitrocellulose or nylon, either by capillary action or under vacuum. (This last step is **Southern blotting**.) The membrane is then baked in an oven at 80°C (to firmly attach the DNA fragments), and bathed in a solution containing labelled denatured DNA. The bathing is called **probing**, and the labelled DNA is called a **probe**, which is typically derived from a cloned DNA fragment, either genomic or cDNA. Being single-stranded, the probe binds strongly to any complementary DNA fragment on the membrane. Unattached probe is then washed off, and the fragments to which the probe has bound are visualized by autoradiography or fluorescence (see Fig. 2.6).

The same basic steps have since been adapted to a wide range of circumstances: electrophoresis of RNA followed by probing with DNA is called **northern blotting**; electrophoresis of protein followed by probing with labelled antibody is called **western blotting**; and a more complex procedure in which protein is probed with DNA is called **south-western blotting**.

## The detection of variation in base sequence

Molecular technology can distinguish between alleles that differ by as little as a single base substitution. In order to illustrate how this is done, we shall consider a practical example.

In a herd of cattle, one animal is homozygous for the sequence AGCT at a particular site in its genome, another animal is homozygous for the sequence AGTT at the same site, and a third animal is heterozygous at this site (Fig. 2.7). By referring to Table 2.1, you will see that AGCT is the recognition sequence for the restriction enzyme *Alu*I. In this herd of cattle, all animals have other *Alu*I recognition sequences 4 kb on one side of this site, and 2 kb on the other side.

Both PCR and Southern analysis are extremely powerful means of differentiating between these three animals.

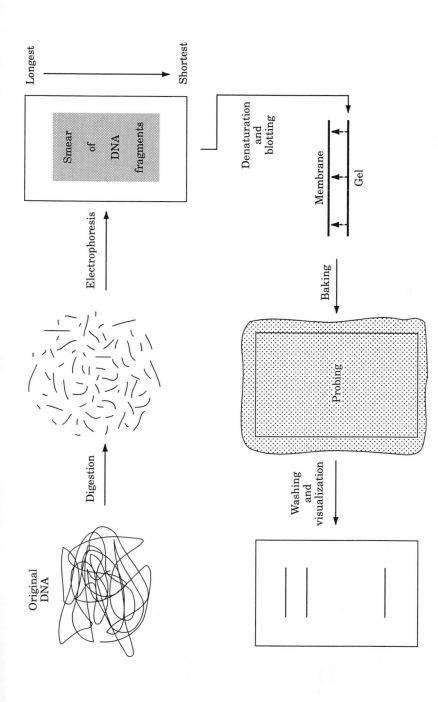

**Fig. 2.6** Southern analysis.

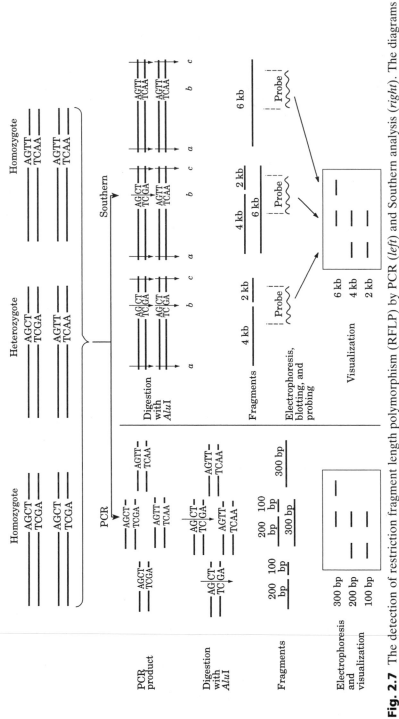

**Fig. 2.7** The detection of restriction fragment length polymorphism (RFLP) by PCR (*left*) and Southern analysis (*right*). The diagrams are not drawn to scale. Short vertical arrows are cleavage sites for the enzyme *Alu*I. Since sites *a* and *c* are the same in all animals, their nucleotide sequence (AGCT) is not shown. For the Southern analysis, readers are left to verify that if the probe had corresponded only to the region between *a* and *b*, or to the region between *b* and *c*, in both cases excluding *b* itself, the three animals would still be distinguishable.

## PCR

As mentioned earlier, to use PCR it is necessary to know the base sequence in the immediate vicinity of the region of interest. Using this information, a pair of primers is synthesized so as to amplify a fragment that includes the site containing the four bases at which the animals differ. In this example, the primers are chosen so that the fragment is 300 bp long and the site is located 100 bases from one end of the fragment.

After amplification, the PCR product from each animal is digested with AluI. All of the PCR products from the first animal contain the sequence AGCT, and are therefore cut by the enzyme at this site, yielding fragments of 100 bp and 200 bp. The second animal produces two types of PCR product: the first is amplified from the chromosome in which the sequence is AGCT, and the other is amplified from the chromosome in which the sequence is AGTT. The former is cut by AluI, but the latter is not, since AGTT is not a recognition sequence for this enzyme. Digestion of the PCR product from the second animal therefore produces fragments of 100 bp, 200 bp, and 300 bp. By similar reasoning, none of the PCR products from the third animal is cut, which means that it has only 300 bp fragments.

After digestion, the fragments are electrophoresed and then stained in the gel with either ethidium bromide or silver nitrate. As shown in Fig. 2.7a, the three animals can be differentiated readily.

## Southern analysis

For Southern analysis, the simplest situation is to have a probe that includes the site of the four nucleotides. (The analysis will also work, however, if the probe does not overlap the site, provided one end of the probe is very near to the site. See the caption to Fig. 2.7.) The probe in this example is 3 kb long, with the site occurring right in the middle, i.e. 1.5 kb from each end.

Genomic DNA is extracted from each animal, digested with AluI, transferred to a membrane, probed, and autoradiographed. In the first animal, of all the different-sized fragments produced by digestion with AluI, only those immediately on either side of the site contain a section that is complementary to the probe. Since the two nearest AluI sites are 4 kb on one side and 2 kb on the other, the two fragments containing sequence that is complementary to the probe are 4 kb and 2 kb long. All other fragments have no sequence in common with the probe. Thus, only a 4 kb fragment and a 2 kb fragment are detected (Fig. 2.7b). In the second animal, the chromosome containing the AGCT sequence yields the same detectable fragments as obtained from the first animal. Its other chromosome (the one with the sequence AGTT) yields only one 6 kb fragment to which the probe hybridizes, because AGTT is not cut by the AluI. This animal therefore shows three bands. By similar reasoning, the third animal shows only the 6 kb band. Once again, the three animals are readily distinguishable.

## Restriction fragment length polymorphism (RFLP)

With both PCR and Southern analysis, the readily visible difference in band patterns between animals arises from the smallest of all possible genetic differences: the two alleles differ by just a single base substitution. This illustrates the power of these techniques.

The difference in band pattern between the three animals is called a **restriction fragment length polymorphism** or **RFLP**. Recalling that the word 'polymorphism' refers to the existence of more than one form or type, the origin of the term is obvious: the gel or autoradiograph reveals polymorphism in the length of DNA fragments resulting from digestion with a restriction enzyme.

Although the above example concerns a single base substitution, other types of genetic differences can be detected as RFLPs. In principle, any mutation that destroys or creates a recognition sequence for a restriction enzyme can be detected as an RFLP. For example, insertions, deletions or base substitutions within a recognition sequence alter that sequence so that it is no longer recognisable by the enzyme. New recognition sequences can be created by base substitutions, by insertions, or (in rare cases) by deletions. Also, deletions or insertions between recognition sequences alter the length of the fragment between the two sequences, and therefore give rise to an RFLP. In practice, the size of fragment that can be detected by Southern analysis typically ranges from 300 bp to 15 kb, with differences in size as small as 50 bp being detectable, depending on the type of gel and the electrophoresis conditions used. The range for PCR products is typically 60 bp–2 kb, with differences as low as a few bases being detectable, again depending on the conditions used.

What about base substitutions that neither destroy nor create a recognition sequence? Fortunately, there are methods for their detection as well. In fact, there are methods which, in principle, enable the detection of any difference in DNA sequence. These all involve PCR as the initial step in amplifying the DNA fragment of interest.

## Other methods and cycle sequencing

In one method, the PCR product is denatured into single strands, which are then electrophoresed in a gel. Strands which differ by as little as a single base substitution adopt different shapes (and hence travel at different speeds) when moving through the gel. When the electrophoresis is stopped, each different strand has travelled a different distance, and can be visualized as a different band after adding a DNA stain to the gel. The polymorphism revealed by this technique is called **single-stranded conformational polymorphism** or **SSCP**.

In another method, the double-stranded PCR product is electrophoresed in a gel, through a gradient of some factor which is capable of denaturing double-stranded DNA. (The method is therefore called **denaturation gradient gel electrophoresis** or **DGGE**). One of the most practical forms of denaturing gradient is temperature, giving rise to **temperature gradient gel electrophoresis** or **TGGE**. As soon as the strands start to separate, they become clogged in the gel. Two fragments of double-stranded DNA that differ by as little as a single base substitution start to separate at different temperatures, and therefore give rise to different bands that are readily visible after staining.

A variation on Southern blotting is the **dot blot**. There are various types of dot blot, but one of its most powerful forms is where PCR is used to amplify a segment of DNA from each of a group of animals or pathogens. The segment is chosen so as to include one or more sites at which allelic variation is known to occur. The amplified segment from each animal is placed as a small dot on a membrane, which is probed with a labelled synthetic oligonucleotide whose sequence corresponds to a particular allele at the locus. It is possible to control the conditions such that the labelled probe will hybridize only if its sequence is exactly the same as in the amplified segment. By preparing several replicate membranes, each with the same set of dots (from the same group of animals or pathogens), and probing each membrane with a different labelled oligonucleotide corresponding to a different allele, it is possible to determine which alleles exist at that locus in each animal or pathogen. An oligonucleotide used in this type of analysis is called an **allele-specific oligo** or **ASO**. If there are many ASOs, often the procedure is reversed: all ASOs are dotted onto a single membrane, which is then screened with the labelled amplified DNA from a single animal or pathogen. This is called a **reverse dot blot**. Yet another variation is to design primers that are unique to each known allele at a locus, and then to run the PCR under conditions such that amplification of a particular allele occurs only if a perfectly matched primer is present. This is called **allele-specific amplification** (**ASA**).

Increasingly, many of these variations are being replaced by automated cycle sequencing, which can detect *all* base variation in an amplified fragment, i.e. alleles are identified according to their base sequence. If a different fluorescent label is used for each of the four sequencing reactions (A, C, T, G), the products of the four reactions can be placed in a single lane.

## Veterinary diagnosis

The techniques described in the previous section are creating a revolution in veterinary diagnosis: time-consuming and inexact diagnostic tests are being replaced by DNA-based tests which are far quicker and much more sensitive. Most of these tests rely on PCR. The original sample can be from living animals (solid tissue, blood, swabs, semen, faeces), from animal products (eggs, milk, meat), from post-mortem tissue (either fresh or archival), or from water suspected of being contaminated. By appropriate choice of primers and/or probes, the tests can identify the presence of particular species/strains/

serogroups of viruses, retroviruses, bacteria, fungi, protozoa, roundworms, or tapeworms. They can also be used to distinguish between meat from different species of animals. The simplest tests involve amplification of a particular segment of DNA, followed by electrophoresis and staining of the gel, which results in a diagnostic band. For RNA viruses, an initial round of reverse transcription is performed before the PCR.

The specificity of these tests depends on the region that is amplified (i.e. depends on the choice of primers): the less conserved the region, the more specific is the test. The whole range of possibilities has been exploited, from primers that amplify a fragment that is found in only one strain or serogroup, to primers that amplify a fragment that is common to several genera. In the latter case, digestion of the PCR product with a restriction enzyme often produces a banding pattern that is diagnostic of one species or strain or serogroup. Alternatively, the undigested PCR product can be dot-blotted with oligonucleotides that are diagnostic of species, strain or serogroup. The possibilities are limitless, and the power of the overall approach ensures that PCR will be an extremely important diagnostic tool for many years to come.

## Variable number of tandem repeats (VNTR), DNA fingerprints, and microsatellites

While substitutions, deletions and insertions are very important sources of genetic differences between alleles and between animals, they are not the only type of genetic difference. Another important category involves variation in the number of tandem repeats in repetitive DNA. Before discussing how repetitive DNA can be detected using molecular techniques, we must first expand upon the information provided in Chapter 1.

### Repetitive DNA

There are two types of repetitive DNA: **dispersed** and **tandemly repeated**.

Dispersed repetitive DNA is classified according to the size of the repeat unit: the longer repeat units are called **long interspersed elements (LINEs)**, being typically more than 1000 bases long. The shorter forms are called **short interspersed elements (SINEs)**, which are usually shorter than 500 bases. Typically, LINEs occur about 10 000 times in the genome, while SINEs occur about 100 000 times. Considered together, LINEs and SINEs account for about 20 per cent of mammalian DNA. In essence, LINEs are cDNA copies of functional genes present in the same genome. Known as **processed pseudogenes**, these nonfunctional segments of DNA most probably arose from the unintended action of reverse transcriptase during a retroviral infection. Interestingly, some LINEs appear also to have a degenerate open reading frame for the enzyme reverse transcriptase, suggesting that at some time in the past, they had the capacity for their own transposition, i.e. they were transposable genetic elements (TGEs—explained in Chapter 1). This would help to explain the occurrence of so many copies. Most SINEs also appear to have arisen from the unintended action of reverse transcriptase, but in this case, the DNA is a copy of certain tRNA molecules. For example, a typical SINE is a 73-bp sequence, which occurs in cattle and goats, and which is a DNA copy of the tRNA for glycine.

In tandemly repeated DNA, the repeat unit occurs end-on-end. If there are many copies (typically thousands) of the repeat unit in tandem at one site, the DNA is called **satellite** DNA. The size of the repeat unit in satellite DNA typically falls in the range from 5 to 500 bp, with the total number of repeat units at any one site ranging between 1000 and 50 000. In some cases, the longer repeat units include many imperfect repeats of a smaller repeat unit. An example of satellite DNA is a 23-bp repeat unit which occurs at several locations in the genome of cattle, with a total of approximately 7 000 000 copies. Another example is a 483-bp repeat unit in cats, which includes about 25 imperfect (i.e. slightly variable) copies of a 6-bp repeat unit (TAACCC), and which comprises 1–2 per cent of the cat genome. A similar, slightly longer repeat unit exists in dogs.

As the size and number of tandem repeats at any one site decreases, the terms **minisatellite** and **microsatellite** are used to describe them.

Minisatellite repeat units typically range in size from 10 to 100 bases. They are more widespread in the genome than satellite DNA, but their distribution still tends to be concentrated in certain regions such as telomeres and sites with an unusually high frequency of recombination (**recombination hotspots**). Indeed, it is thought that minisatellite DNA may actually be involved in the initiation of recombination.

The term microsatellite refers to the smallest repeat units (around five bases or less, e.g. ACCGG, ATTT, GGC, AC, T, etc.), with the number of repeat units at any one site typically varying from just a few up to around 30. Microsatellites occur throughout the genome. In fact, it seems that almost every gene has at least one microsatellite, located in an intron or in the 5′ or 3′ regions which flank the coding sequence. A typical example of a microsatellite is the repeat unit AC, which occurs at approximately 100 000 different sites in a typical mammalian genome.

## VNTR and DNA fingerprints

A major characteristic of repetitive DNA is that there is considerable variation in the number of repeat units at any one site: a site on one chromosome might have, say, 24 tandem copies of a certain repeat, while at the same site on the homologous chromosome in the same animal, there may be 21 tandem copies. In another animal, there might be 23 copies at the same site on one chromosome, and 15 copies on the homologous chromosome. With some important and notable exceptions, which are discussed in Chapter 3, this variation in the number of repeat units does not seem to have any adverse effect.

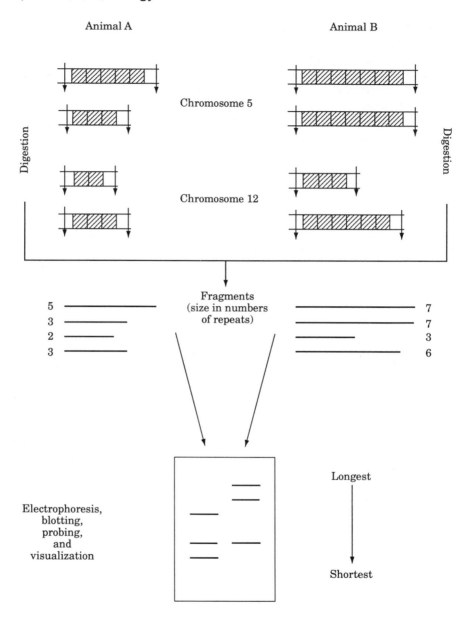

**Fig. 2.8** Detection of variable number of tandem repeats (VNTR) in two animals, using Southern analysis. Short vertical arrows indicate cleavage sites for a restriction enzyme that does not cut the repeat sequence. In this example, the repeat sequence occurs at two different sites (loci) in the genome. With the exception of the locus on chromosome 5 in animal B, each animal is heterozygous for the number of repeat units (shown alongside the fragment) at each locus. The ladder of bands is called a DNA fingerprint. In practice, there are usually more than two loci, and hence more bands than shown in this example.

**Variable *number* of *tandem* *repeats*** (abbreviated to **VNTR**) can be detected by Southern analysis, using a restriction enzyme that does *not* cut within the repeat unit, and probing with a tandem set of the repeat unit (Fig. 2.8). The size of repeat units most suitable for this type of analysis is in the minisatellite range of 10–20 bases. Since these repeat units tend to be located at several sites in different chromosomes, and since there is a different number of repeats at almost every site, the repeat-unit probe detects many bands (in theory, two bands at each site, assuming a detectably different number of repeats on each homologous chromosome at each site). The result is a relatively large number of bands. Since there is so much variation in the number of repeat units at any one site, each animal has an almost unique set of bands—a **DNA fingerprint**. Although each band is inherited from a parent, it is not easy to follow the inheritance of DNA fingerprint patterns, because they are jointly determined by so many loci. They are still, however, of substantial practical benefit in providing a means of checking pedigrees, as discussed in Chapter 12. An alternative way to detect minisatellite VNTR is to use a probe corresponding to unique-sequence DNA adjacent to a particular minisatellite site. The result is a far simpler band pattern which shows single-locus inheritance.

Notice that even though we are not dealing here with functional genes, we can still use the terms locus and allele: a locus is a site where the repeat units occur, and each different number of repeat units can be regarded as a different allele at that locus.

## Microsatellites

As we saw above, microsatellites involve tandem repeat units at the smallest end of the size range, typically from one base to five bases. They are detected using PCR, with primers corresponding to the unique-sequence DNA that flanks the tandem repeats (Fig. 2.9). Also, electrophoresis has to be conducted in circumstances that allow bands to be distinguished which differ by as little as just one base. Since the electrophoresis conditions used for sequencing DNA fulfil this requirement, microsatellite PCR products are electrophoresed in sequencing gels. In fact, the whole procedure is very similar to that used for sequencing: labelled primers are used, and bands are visualized either by autoradiography or fluorescence. As with sequencing, the detection of microsatellites is becoming increasingly automated.

As its name suggests, the unique-sequence DNA to which the primers correspond occurs only once in the entire genome. This means that even if a particular microsatellite repeat unit occurs at many different sites in the genome, the PCR will amplify only just one site, namely the site whose flanking sequence corresponds to the sequence in the pair of primers. Such sites are called **sequence-tagged sites** or **STS**. The length of the PCR product varies according to the number of repeat units at that site.

As with any PCR product amplified from unique-sequence primers, only

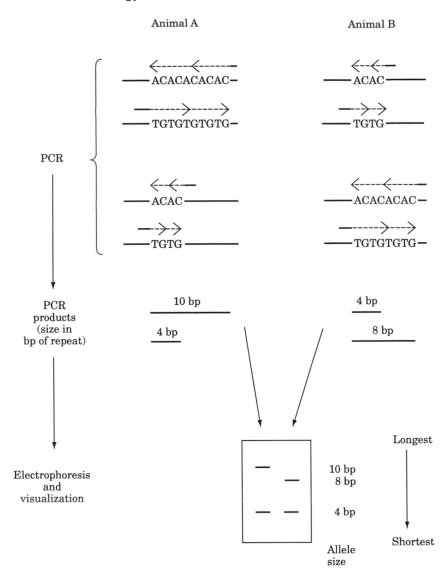

**Fig. 2.9** Detection of a microsatellite in two animals, using a single pair of primers, i.e. at a sequence-tagged site. The repeat unit is AC. PCR products are identified according to the size of the fragment.

one or two bands are produced from an animal; one band if the animal is homozygous, and two bands if it is heterozygous. This means that microsatellite PCR products do not give rise to the large number of bands per animal which are characteristic of DNA fingerprints. As we shall see below, microsatellite PCR products are extremely useful in gene mapping, because each pair of primers corresponds to a specific site on a chromosome, and because there are many different alleles at each site, i.e. they are extremely polymorphic.

## Gene mapping

There are probably between 50 000 and 100 000 genes in each species of mammal and bird. Ultimately, we would like to be able to identify each of these genes, to ascertain their function, and to document the extent of their allelic variation. A major first step along this path of discovery is the creation of a genetic map for each species.

There are two complementary forms of a genetic map. The first is a **linkage map**, which consists of lists of linked genes (linkage groups) arranged in linear order according to the recombination fraction between them. The second is a **physical map**, which indicates the location of each gene on its chromosome.

Both forms of genetic map have existed for many years in a very incomplete form for several domestic species, and in a quite substantial form for chickens. Until recently, the expansion of these maps was limited by the relatively low levels of polymorphism detectable at most loci by conventional means such as visual assessment of traits or biochemical assays. All this has changed with the development and widespread use of molecular technology, and in particular, with microsatellites, which, among other things, enable the detection of extensive DNA polymorphism at thousands of locations (loci) throughout the genome.

The creation of a linkage map involves estimating the recombination fraction between all pair-wise combinations of as many loci as can possibly be identified. A popular way to do this is to cross two populations that are as genetically different as possible (to create a first-cross or **F1** generation). The F1s are then mated either with other F1s, to produce an **F2** generation, or with members of one of the parental populations, producing a **backcross (BC)** generation. The reason for choosing parental populations as different as possible is to maximize the chance of them having different alleles at each locus. This in turn maximizes the chance of the F1s being heterozygous at each locus, which consequently maximizes the chance of being able to estimate the recombination fraction for each pair of loci. As an indication of how such an estimate is obtained, the mating between an F1 animal and a member of one of the parental populations is equivalent to the mating shown in Fig. 1.12.

When recombination fraction is estimated from genotype frequencies in the offspring of a known mating, we are really inferring the frequencies of the gametes produced by one or both parents. Basically, we are trying to estimate the proportion of gametes that resulted from recombination, but we have to do this indirectly, by looking at progeny genotypes. Recently, a method of linkage mapping has been developed in which we can look at the gametes directly, and thereby obtain direct estimates of recombination frequency.

Known as **single-sperm typing**, the method involves flow-sorting sperm cells by **fluorescence activated cell sorting (FACS)**, which results in a single sperm cell being placed in each well of a microtitre plate. Each sperm cell is then lysed to expose its DNA, and is subjected to PCR for each of the loci of interest. The identity of the allele at each locus in each sperm is then determined by appropriate analysis of the PCR product. In contrast to traditional linkage analysis which requires the genotyping of parents and offspring from particular matings, single-sperm typing requires no matings; all that is required is a sample of sperm cells from a single male that is heterozygous at the loci of interest.

While all of the methods of detecting DNA polymorphisms have been tried in gene mapping, the detection of microsatellites by PCR is proving to be the most effective and hence the most popular method, both within structural genes and at anonymous sites throughout the genome. Hundreds of microsatellite markers have already been mapped in each of the major domestic species. In most cases, the base sequence of the primers for each microsatellite marker is publicly available, which means that anyone can generate their own set of mapped markers, simply by preparing the appropriate PCR primers.

The other type of map—the physical map—is being generated in several ways. One involves the use of a panel of somatic-cell hybrids, where each hybrid is a cell line with a different mixture of chromosomes from two species, e.g. hamster and cattle, derived from an original fusion of cells from the two species. The presence of any particular locus in a particular cell line can be detected by various means, including Southern analysis or PCR. DNA markers that are always **concordant** (all present, or all absent) in each cell line must be located on the same chromosome; the presence or absence of the concordant group of markers corresponds to the presence or absence of their chromosome. Even finer location of markers is possible in cell lines which contain only portions of certain chromosomes. Loci that are shown in this manner to be located on the same chromosome are said to be **syntenic**, and the group to which they belong is called a **syntenic group**. In the end, each syntenic group should correspond exactly to a linkage group.

Another method of physical mapping involves *in situ* hybridization of cloned DNA to its corresponding site on the chromosome. Initially, this involved radioactive labelling of the cloned DNA, but now a non-radioactive method known as **fluorescence *in situ* hybridization (FISH)** is proving to be much more effective.

A development that shows much promise is the preparation of chromosome-specific DNA libraries, i.e. libraries consisting of DNA from just one chromosome. These can be obtained from chromosomes separated by FACS or by **microdissection**, which involves using a micromanipulator or laser to pick up just a single chromosome from a spread of chromosomes like that shown in Fig. 1.1. In either case, all of the DNA from that chromosome can be amplified by PCR and then cloned in the usual manner. This is called **micro-cloning**. With microdissection, it is even possible to pick up only small portions of an individual chromosome, and hence to create a microclone library corresponding just to that portion of the chromosome. To check that each library contains DNA from just a particular chromosome, or a certain part of a chromosome, a sample of the entire DNA from the library can be hybridized to a complete chromosome spread using FISH. If the library contains what it should contain, then the entire relevant chromosome, or the relevant part of the chromosome, will fluoresce. This procedure is called **chromosome painting**.

The result of this technology is a set of DNA libraries covering each region of each chromosome. Each of these libraries can be divided into a series of overlapping YAC clones, with the final result being a contiguous set of YAC clones covering the entire genome. As soon as a gene is shown to be located within a particular YAC clone, its physical location is automatically pinpointed to within several hundred kb (the size of the YAC clone). It is then possible, given time and resources, to eventually isolate the gene.

In most of the major domestic species there is now a substantial effort, often involving global collaboration, to create a genetic map which combines the information from linkage and physical maps. An example of the results of such collaboration is given in Fig. 2.10, which shows a genetic map for chromosome 1 in cattle.

One of the most striking features to emerge from the creation of genetic maps is the remarkable conservation of groups of loci across widely divergent

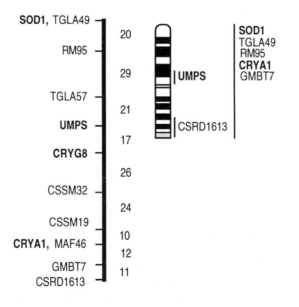

**Fig. 2.10** A genetic map of chromosome 1 in cattle. On the left is the linkage map, showing the map distance (in cM) between loci. On the right is the physical mapping information: only two of the genes have been localized to specific regions.

species. For example, many of the genes located on human chromosome 12 are on cattle chromosome 12 and cat chromosome 5. And the X chromosome shows even higher conservation. In fact, if a gene is X-linked in one species of mammal, it is almost certainly X-linked in every other species of mammal. This high degree of conservation has spurred considerable interest in **comparative gene mapping**—the comparison of genetic maps between species. Apart from its evolutionary interest, comparative gene mapping also has substantial practical importance, because the high degree of conservation of chromosomal segments across species means that a well-mapped region in one species can provide very useful information about the location of the same genes in other species, long before they have actually been mapped in the other species. Comparative mapping holds much promise as a means of tracking down disease loci in domestic animals, based on information from mice and humans.

Keeping track of the rapidly expanding genetic maps, and of comparative mapping information, is proving to be quite a challenge. By far the most useful reference for this information is the publication *Genetic Maps*, edited by Steve O'Brien, which contains details of linkage maps and physical maps of all species, from viruses to humans. Increasingly, *Genetic Maps* is being complemented by databases providing up-to-date information on genetic maps of all of the major domestic species, which are freely accessible on international computing networks.

## Production of polypeptide from cloned DNA

When foreign DNA is cloned in bacteria or some other microorganism, the sole aim is to produce unlimited copies of that foreign DNA. If the foreign DNA is a gene, it is possible to go one step further than this; it is possible to arrange for that foreign DNA to produce its corresponding polypeptide in that host. To achieve this, it is necessary to incorporate an appropriate promoter, and possibly some other control regions.

There is one important difference between prokaryotic and eukaryotic control arising from the absence of split genes in the former. Having no split genes, prokaryotes have no need for the elaborate splicing mechanisms required by eukaryotes for converting a primary mRNA transcript into mature mRNA. Because of this, the only eukaryotic genes that can be transcribed and translated in prokaryotes are those consisting solely of exons.

Also, since there are substantial differences in control mechanisms between species, the control regions used should be those of the host cell.

In practice, this is usually achieved by ensuring that the foreign DNA is the coding sequence only, and by inserting this immediately downstream from a leader sequence and promoter in the vector DNA. This 'tricks' the host into thinking that the foreign DNA is, in fact, part of its own DNA. In some cases, it is easier to insert the foreign DNA into the middle of a vector gene, which results in the production of a hybrid (**fusion**) polypeptide from which the foreign polypeptide can be released by appropriate chemical treatment. Vectors that enable the transcription and translation of a foreign gene are called **expression vectors**, and libraries containing such vectors are called **expression libraries**.

Many different polypeptides from prokaryotes and eukaryotes are being mass-produced in the manner described above, using a wide range of microorganisms (both prokaryotes and eukaryotes) and mammalian cell lines as hosts. Examples include recombinant vaccines (protective polypeptides from pathogens or parasites); therapeutic proteins such as insulin, blood-clotting factors, interferons, immunoglobulins, growth hormone; and the many enzymes used in molecular biology. In addition, the technology is not limited to existing genes: it is possible, for example, to design and produce novel polypeptides for specific purposes, either as variants of existing polypeptides, or as completely original molecules.

From using microorganisms to produce foreign polypeptide in the laboratory, it is only a small extra step (at least in principle) to arrange for the microorganism to produce its foreign polypeptide where it is actually needed, such as inside an animal's body. This has given rise to the concept of **live recombinant vaccines**, typically consisting of a harmless virus or bacterium (the vaccine vector), some of whose genes have been replaced by a functional gene for the protective polypeptide from a pathogen or parasite. Rather than having to provide a means of delivering the protective polypeptide by injection or some other labour-intensive process, the vaccine vector quite naturally infects the animal and automatically manufactures the polypeptide where it is needed—inside the animal. The same approach can be used as a means of combating insect pests. For example, if an insect gene for juvenile hormone esterase is inserted into a virus that is a natural pathogen of insects, and if the recombinant virus infects the insects, the esterase inactivates the insects' juvenile hormone, which causes a substantial reduction in larval feeding, which is the most damaging aspect of many insect pests.

## Transgenesis

We have seen that it is quite possible to insert a gene from one species, e.g. a pig, into the DNA of a microorganism or mammalian cell line. Furthermore, because of the universality of the genetic code, the same polypeptide will be produced by any host. If this can be achieved with microorganisms and mammalian cell lines, in principle it should be possible to achieve the same result by inserting a foreign gene into the DNA of a living animal. The name given to this process is **transgenesis**.

The first step in transgenesis is to combine the cloned gene with an appropriate promoter, producing what is called a **gene construct**. The second step is to introduce the construct into one or more chromosomes of an animal. At

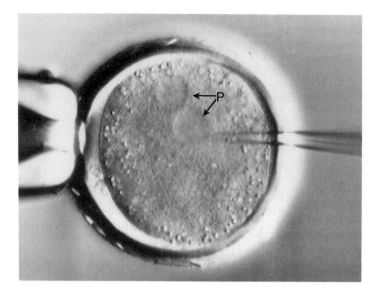

**Fig. 2.11** Producing a transgenic sheep by microinjection of a cloned transgene into one of the two pronuclei (P) of a fertilized ovum.

present, this is most commonly achieved by microinjection of many copies of the construct into either the male or the female **pronucleus** of a newly fertilized ovum (the male pronucleus is the haploid nucleus of the sperm cell, and the female pronucleus is the haploid nucleus of the ovum), as shown in Fig. 2.11. After microinjection, the fertilized ovum is transferred into a suitably prepared recipient female, which carries the resultant embryo through to birth in the usual manner. In a very small proportion of cases (currently less than 1 per cent in domestic animals), the genome of the resultant animal contains one or more copies of the construct. Such animals are said to be **transgenic**, and the inserted construct is called a **transgene**. About one-half of transgenic animals actually express (i.e. produce polypeptide from) the transgene, but almost all of them pass the transgene on to their descendants in a normal manner.

The first transgenic animals were mice produced in 1980. The first application of this technology to farm animals was reported in 1985, when pigs and sheep were made transgenic for the human growth hormone gene. Since then, many different transgenes have been used, from species as diverse as bacteria and humans; and the range of domestic species made transgenic has been expanded to include fish, chickens, goats, and cattle. The microinjection technique has several disadvantages, e.g. there is no control over where the transgene is inserted, nor is there any control over how many copies have been inserted. In the future, we will see more controlled methods used for creating transgenic animals. In mice, for example, undifferentiated and totipotent embryonic cells (called **embryonic stem cells**) can be made transgenic, and are then tested in the laboratory for expression of the transgene. In this way, only those cells that actually express the transgene in the desired manner are transferred to the recipient mouse. This overcomes the problems and expense associated with the very low success rate of microinjection into fertilized ova. Furthermore, by a process called **targeted gene replacement**, it is possible to replace a normal gene in embryonic stem cells with a version of the same gene that has been mutated in a specific manner. By appropriate matings of the resultant transgenic mouse and its descendants, it is possible to establish a strain of transgenic mice that is homozygous for the specific mutation.

What is the purpose of making transgenic animals? By far the most extensive use of transgenesis is in basic research using laboratory animals, especially mice. The technology has proved to be extremely useful in investigating the regulation of gene expression and in testing methods of gene therapy. When used as a means of replacing a functional gene with a nonfunctional one (producing **knockout** mice), it is also a powerful way to investigate gene function and inherited diseases. Also, transgenic mice whose own antibody genes have been inactivated by targeted gene replacement, but which are transgenic for antibody genes from another species, can be used for the production of species-specific monoclonal antibodies. In relation to farm animals, the uses of transgenesis can be considered from two points of view, associated with the two main parts of a transgene, namely the promoter and the coding sequence.

The appropriate choice of a promoter brings transgene expression under human control. For example, one of the promoters commonly used in early transgenesis was from a metallothionein gene. Metallothionein is a protein that occurs naturally in many species; its role is to bind to heavy metals. In normal (non-transgenic) animals, if the concentration of heavy metals becomes too high, the metallothionein gene begins to produce metallothionein which binds to the excess heavy metal, thereby removing the threat of toxicity. If the promoter from a metallothionein gene is attached to the coding sequence of, say, a growth hormone gene, the resultant transgene can be switched on simply by adding heavy metal to the drinking water of the transgenic animal. This means that the production of growth hormone from the transgene can be turned on and off by a simple manipulation of the drinking water. Alternatively, if the aim is to have a transgene expressed in just one tissue, a promoter is chosen from a gene that is naturally expressed only in that tissue. For example, a transgene containing the promoter from a milk-protein gene will be expressed only in the mammary gland of the transgenic animal.

In relation to the coding sequence, transgenesis offers several possibilities. First, it can be used to introduce a novel allele of a gene that already exists in the species. For example, the transgene for an enzyme involved in lactogenesis could be designed and constructed specifically to produce milk that is low in lactose, thereby giving rise to an improved form of animal product. Second, transgenesis offers the possibility of introducing genes that are completely novel to the species. For example, there is a plant enzyme called chitinase which degrades chitin (a major component of the cuticle and digestive tract of insects). If a chitinase gene could be expressed in the skin of sheep or cattle, it could provide them with a nontoxic form of natural resistance to insects. Another example of this approach comes from chickens, in which natural resistance to viral disease has been produced by transgenes that express polypeptide from the virus that causes the disease. Third, transgenesis can be used to produce human proteins required for therapeutic purposes, such as alpha-1-antitrypsin or blood clotting factors. For example, sheep have been made transgenic for the coding sequence of a human gene (e.g. blood clotting factor IX) attached to the promoter from a gene for a protein that occurs naturally in sheep's milk, e.g. β-lactoglobulin. These sheep produce the human polypeptide in their milk, from which it can be extracted readily. (One of the major advantages of transgenesis as a means of producing therapeutic proteins is that eukaryote hosts are much more likely to be able to process the polypeptide into its appropriate tertiary structure than are the alternative hosts, namely prokaryotes such as bacteria.) Fourth, transgenesis can be used to create animals whose organs or tissue are likely to be suitable for transplantation into humans. For example, pigs have been made transgenic for a gene that expresses a human polypeptide on the surface of the cells of the organ or tissue to be transplanted, with the aim of avoiding the problem of rejection. This is seen as an important means of overcoming the critical shortage of human organs for transplantation.

The likely future uses of transgenic animals, and the ethical controversies that surround them, are discussed in Chapter 20.

## Antisense technology

In Chapter 1 we saw how genes are regulated by proteins. In certain prokaryotes (and possibly in eukaryotes), some genes are regulated by RNA: the RNA from a regulator gene is complementary to, and therefore binds with, the RNA from a second gene, thereby inhibiting translation from the second gene.

This raises some intriguing possibilities for artificial control of gene expression. If the promoter of a gene is placed at the other end of that gene, the non-template strand will be transcribed, producing an mRNA whose sequence is the same as that of the template or antisense strand, and which is therefore complementary to the normal or sense mRNA sequence for that gene. This **antisense RNA** will bind to the sense RNA, preventing translation.

There are many potential ways in which antisense RNA could be utilized. For example, bacteria responsible for the fermentation reactions that result in dairy products such as cheese and yoghurt, could be made resistant to the ever-troublesome phages that are a major cause of fermentation failure. This could be achieved by inserting an essential phage-coding sequence into a bacterial plasmid, ensuring that the coding sequence is in reverse orientation, adjacent to a bacterial promoter. When the recombinant plasmid is inserted into the fermentative bacteria, the promoter will produce antisense RNA which could inactivate the phage RNA, and hence combat the phage infection. Another possibility is to make animals transgenic for one of their own genes, but with its promoter at the wrong end (an antisense transgene). If the gene's normal product acts as an inhibitor of other genes, the antisense RNA produced by the transgene could remove the inhibition, and thus possibly increase the animal's performance in say, reproduction. Alternatively, if the coding sequence in the transgene were from a pathogenic virus or bacteria, the antisense RNA produced by the transgene would be directed against the RNA from the pathogen, thereby controlling the infection in the transgenic animal. Another possibility is to design and construct an antisense oligonucleotide directed against, for example, a key region of the genome of a virus, or even against an aberrantly expressed mutant gene in an animal (e.g. a cancer-causing gene), and then to administer the oligonucleotide as a therapeutic drug.

Apart from its substantial use as a research tool, antisense technology is currently showing more promise than practical results. If it can be properly harnessed, however, it may result in some quite important methods of controlling host genes and combating infections.

## Gene shears

**Gene shears** or **ribozymes** are small molecules of RNA that are naturally occurring parasites of certain viruses. They are particularly interesting because they show enzymatic activity: they bind to other molecules of RNA and cut them at particular target sites. In essence, they are small molecules of antisense RNA with built-in scissors. Among other things, their attraction is that a single molecule can cut many copies of the target RNA. In theory, it should be possible to design a gene shears molecule that could bind to, and cut, any known RNA molecule, thereby rendering it inactive, and hence preventing translation of that RNA into its polypeptide. As with antisense RNA, if animals were made transgenic for a fragment of DNA that encodes gene shears RNA, the transgene would give rise to thousands of gene shears, and the transgenic animal could naturally show improved production or resistance to the disease targeted by the gene shears.

There are, of course, many pitfalls along the route from potential to practical reality. But substantial sums of money have been invested in both antisense and gene shears technology, and many people (not the least the investors) are hoping for some useful practical results.

## Further reading

### General

Bernardi, G. (ed.) (1993). Cogene Symposium—From the Double Helix to the Human Genome—40 Years of Molecular Genetics—UNESCO Headquarters, Paris, France, 21–23 April 1993. *Gene*, **135**, (1–2), 1–318.

Berg, P. (1992). *Dealing with genes*. Blackwell Scientific Publications, Oxford.

Martinez, M. L. and Weiss, R. C. (1993). Applications of genetic engineering technology in feline medicine. *Veterinary Clinics of North America—Small Animal Practice*, **23**, 213–26.

Ostrander, E. A., Rine, J., Sack, G. H., and Cork, L. C. (1993). What is the role of molecular genetics in modern veterinary practice? *Journal of the American Veterinary Medical Association*, **203**, 1259–62.

Sambrook, J., Fritsch, E. F., and Maniatis, T. (ed.) (1989). *Molecular cloning: a laboratory manual*, 3 Vols, (2nd edn). Cold Spring Harbor Laboratory Press, Cold Spring Harbor.

### Restriction enzymes

Roberts, R. J. and Macelis, D. (1993). REBASE—restriction enzymes and methylases. *Nucleic Acids Research*, **21**, 3125–37.

### DNA cloning

Nelson, D. L. and Brownstein, B. (ed.) (1993). *YAC libraries: a user's guide*. Freeman, New York.

### DNA sequencing

Brown, T. A. (1994). *DNA sequencing: the basics*. IRL Press, Oxford.

Lagerkvist, A., Stewart, J., Lagerstromfermer, M., and Landegren, U. (1994). Manifold sequencing—efficient processing of large sets of sequencing reactions. *Proceedings of the National Academy of Sciences, USA*, **91**, 2245–9.

Mirzabekov, A. D. (1994). DNA sequencing by hybridization—a megasequencing method and a diagnostic tool. *Trends in Biotechnology*, **12**, 27–32.

Rao, V. B. (1994). Direct sequencing of polymerase chain reaction-amplified DNA. *Analytical Biochemistry*, **216**, 1–14.

### Polymerase chain reaction

Cohen, J. (1994). Molecular biology—long PCR leaps into larger DNA sequences. *Science*, **263**, 1564–5.

Griffin, H. G. and Griffin, A. M. (ed.) (1994). *PCR technology*. CRC Press, Boca Raton.

Mullis, K., Ferre, F., and Gibbs, R. (ed.) (1993). *The polymerase chain reaction*. Birkhauser, Boston.

## Detection of variation in base sequence

Fodde, R. and Losekoot, M. (1994). Mutation detection by denaturing gradient electrophoresis (DGGE). *Human Mutation*, **3**, 83–94.
Prosser, J. (1993). Detecting single-base mutations. *Trends in Biotechnology*, **11**, 238–46.

## Veterinary diagnosis

Barker, R. H. (1994). Use of PCR in the field. *Parasitology Today*, **10**, 117–9.
Batt, C. A., Wagner, P., Wiedmann, M., Luo, J. Y., and Gilbert, R. (1994). Detection of bovine leukocyte adhesion deficiency by nonisotopic ligase chain reaction. *Animal Genetics*, **25**, 95–8.
Belak, S. and Ballagipordany, A. (1993). Application of the polymerase chain reaction (PCR) in veterinary diagnostic virology. *Veterinary Research Communications*, **17**, 55–72.
Binns, M. M. (1993). The application of molecular biology to the study of veterinary infectious diseases. *British Veterinary Journal*, **149**, 21–30.
Chikuni, K., Tabata, T., Kosugiyama, M., Monma, M., and Saito, M. (1994). Polymerase chain reaction assay for detection of sheep and goat meats. *Meat Science*, **37**, 337–45.

## VNTRs, DNA fingerprints, and microsatellites

Bliskovskii, V. V. (1992). Tandem repeats in the vertebrate genome—structure and possible mechanisms of generation and evolution—a review. *Molecular Biology*, **26**, 643–53.

## Gene mapping

Archibald, A. and Haley, C. (1993). Mapping the complex genomes of animals and man. *Outlook on Agriculture*, **22**, 79–84.
Carter, N. P. (1994). Cytogenetic analysis by chromosome painting. *Cytometry*, **18**, 2–10.
Fries, R. (1993). Mapping the bovine genome—methodological aspects and strategy. *Animal Genetics*, **24**, 111–6.
Goodfellow, P. N., Sefton, L., and Farr, C. J. (1993). Genetic maps. *Philosophical Transactions of the Royal Society of London Series B*, **339**, 139–46.
Greulich, K. O. (1992). Chromosome microtechnology—microdissection and microcloning. *Trends in Biotechnology*, **10**, 48–51.
Hoheisel, J. D. (1994). Application of hybridization techniques to genome mapping and sequencing. *Trends in Genetics*, **10**, 79–83.
Libert, F., Lefort, A., Okimoto, R., Womack, J. E., and Georges, M. (1993). Construction of a bovine genomic library of large yeast artificial chromosome clones. *Genomics*, **18**, 270–6.
McKenzie, L. M., Collet, C., and Cooper, D. W. (1993). Use of a subspecies cross for efficient development of a linkage map for a marsupial mammal, the Tammar wallaby (*Macropus eugenii*). *Cytogenetics and Cell Genetics*, **64**, 264–7.

Mark, H. F. L. (1994). Fluorescent in situ hybridization as an adjunct to conventional cytogenetics. *Annals of Clinical and Laboratory Science*, **24**, 153–63.

O'Brien, S. J. (1993). Comparative biology—the genomics generation. *Current Biology*, **3**, 395–7.

O'Brien, S. J., Womack, J. E., Lyons, K. J., Moore, N. A., Jenkins, N. A., and Copeland, N. G. (1993). Anchored reference loci for comparative genome mapping in mammals. *Nature Genetics*, **3**, 103–112.

Scherthan, H., Cremer, T., Arnason, U., Weier, H. U., Limadefaria, A., and Fronicke, L. (1994). Comparative chromosome painting discloses homologous segments in distantly related mammals. *Nature Genetics*, **6**, 342–7.

Womack, J. E. (1993). The goals and status of the bovine gene map. *Journal of Dairy Science*, **76**, 1199–203.

## Human genome project

Hoffman, E. P. (1994). The evolving genome project—current and future impact. *American Journal of Human Genetics*, **54**, 129–36.

## Genetic maps

Barendse, W., Armitage, S. M., Kossarek, L. M., Shalom, A., Kirkpatrick, B. W., Ryan, A. M., *et al.* (1994). A genetic linkage map of the bovine genome. *Nature Genetics*, **6**, 227–35.

Bishop, M. D., Kappes, S. M., Keele, J. W., Stone, R. T., Sunden, S. L. F., Hawkins, G. A., *et al.* (1994). A genetic linkage map for cattle. *Genetics*, **136**, 619–39.

Bumstead, N. and Palyga, J. (1992). A preliminary linkage map of the chicken. *Genomics*, **13**, 690–7.

Fries, R., Eggen, A., and Womack, J. E. (1993). The bovine genome map. *Mammalian Genome*, **4**, 405–28.

Rohrer, G. A., Alexander, L. J., Keele, J. W., Smith, T. P., and Beattie, C. W. (1994). A microsatellite linkage map of the porcine genome. *Genetics*, **136**, 231–45.

Levin, I., Crittenden, L. B., and Dodgson, J. B. (1993). Genetic map of the chicken Z-chromosome using random amplified polymorphic DNA (RAPD) markers. *Genomics*, **16**, 224–30.

Levin, I., Santangelo, L., Cheng, H., Crittenden, L. B., and Dodgson, J. B. (1994). An autosomal genetic linkage map of the chicken. *Journal of Heredity*, **85**, 79–85.

O'Brien, S. J. (ed.) (1993). *Genetic Maps*, (6th edn). Cold Spring Harbor Laboratory Press, Cold Spring Harbor, NY.

Weller, G. L. and Foster, G. G. (1993). Genetic maps of the sheep blowfly *Lucilia cuprina*—linkage-group correlations with other Dipteran genera. *Genome*, **36**, 495–506.

## Production of polypeptide from cloned DNA

Hutchinson, C. R. (1994). Drug synthesis by genetically engineered microorganisms. *Bio/Technology*, **12**, 375–80.

Kimman, T. G. (1992). Risks connected with the use of conventional and genetically engineered vaccines. *Veterinary Quarterly*, **14**, 110–8.

Anon. (ed.) (1993). Recent developments in veterinary vaccines. *Immunology and Cell Biology*, **71**, 355–508.

## Transgenesis

Cameron, E. R., Harvey, M. J. A., and Onions, D. E. (1994). Transgenic science. *British Veterinary Journal*, **150**, 9–24.

Capecchi, M. R. (1994). Targeted gene replacement. *Scientific American*, **270**, (3), 52–9.

Ebert, K. M. and Schindler, J. E. S. (1993). Transgenic farm animals—progress report. *Theriogenology*, **39**, 121–35.

Jiang, Y. (1993). Transgenic fish—gene transfer to increase disease and cold resistance. *Aquaculture*, **111**, 31–40.

Lonberg, N., Taylor, L. D., Harding, F. A., Trounstine, M., Higgins, K. M., Schramm, S. R., *et al.* (1994). Antigen-specific human antibodies from mice comprising four distinct genetic modifications. *Nature*, **368**, 856–9.

Perry, M. M. and Sang, H. M. (1993). Transgenesis in chickens. *Transgenic Research*, **2**, 125–33.

## Antisense technology

Miller, N. and Vile, R. G. (1994). Gene transfer and antisense nucleic acid techniques. *Parasitology Today*, **10**, 92–7.

Stein, C. A. and Cheng, Y. C. (1993). Antisense oligonucleotides as therapeutic agents—is the bullet really magical? *Science*, **261**, 1004–12.

Wahlestedt, C. (1994). Antisense oligonucleotide strategies in neuropharmacology. *Trends in Pharmacological Sciences*, **15**, 42–6.

## Gene shears

Barinaga, M. (1993). Ribozymes—killing the messenger. *Science*, **262**, 1512–14.

Cantor, G. H., McElwain, T. F., Birkebak, T. A., and Palmer, G. H. (1993). Ribozyme cleaves rex/tax messenger RNA and inhibits bovine leukemia virus expression. *Proceedings of the National Academy of Sciences, USA*, **90**, 10932–6.

Pyle, A. M. (1993). Ribozymes—a distinct class of metalloenzymes. *Science*, **261**, 709–14.

# 3 Single-gene disorders

## Inborn errors of metabolism

If a polypeptide acts as an enzyme or is part of an enzyme, a mutation in its gene sometimes results in a deficiency of that enzyme, with a consequent blockage in the biochemical pathway where that enzyme is required. Diseases that result from such blockages are called **inborn errors of metabolism**. A good example of such a disease in animals is citrullinaemia, which occurs in Holstein–Friesian cattle.

Calves with citrullinaemia appear normal at birth, but show signs of depression within just a few hours. By the next day, they exhibit considerable depression, tongue protrusion and an unsteady gait. Deterioration continues during the next few days, with the calves wandering around aimlessly, frothing at the mouth, and pressing their heads against solid objects such as fences. By days 3–5, they collapse and die. The cause of these profound clinical signs is ammonia poisoning, due to a breakdown in the urea cycle, which is the biochemical process by which potentially toxic ammonia (derived from catabolism of proteins) is converted to urea, which is excreted in urine (Fig. 3.1). Calves with citrullinaemia are deficient in one of the enzymes involved in the urea cycle, namely argininosuccinate synthetase (ASS). As can be deduced from Fig. 3.1, the absence of this enzyme leads to a build-up of citrulline and, more seriously, of ammonia, with the latter causing the clinical signs.

What is the cause of the deficiency of ASS? As a result of comparisons between the cDNA sequence of the ASS gene obtained from affected and normal animals, it is now known that the cause of citrullinaemia in Holstein–Friesians is a single base-substitution at the first position in the 86th triplet of the gene for ASS. In the normal allele, this triplet is CGA, which encodes the amino acid arginine. In the mutant allele, the C has been replaced by a T, giving rise to a triplet TGA, which (as can be deduced from the genetic code in Table 1.2), is a stop triplet. Thus, the profound clinical signs and eventual death of calves affected with citrullinaemia are due to the simplest of all possible mutations, namely the substitution of one nucleotide by another.

If tests for ASS activity are conducted among normal cattle within a population known to have produced calves with citrullinaemia, it is found that in some normal animals, including all those that are parents of affected animals, the level of ASS is approximately 50 per cent of that observed in the remainder of normal animals. Not surprisingly, all calves affected by the disease have zero levels of ASS.

The explanation for these observations is that in affected individuals, both

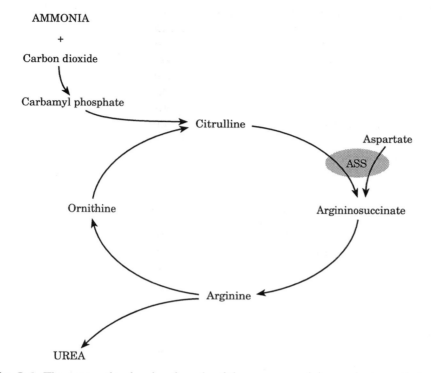

AMMONIA

+

Carbon dioxide

Carbamyl phosphate

Citrulline

Aspartate

ASS

Ornithine

Argininosuccinate

Arginine

UREA

**Fig. 3.1** The urea cycle, showing the role of the enzyme argininosuccinate synthetase (ASS) in converting citrulline plus aspartate to argininosuccinate.

genes responsible for the production of ASS are mutants: affected calves are homozygous for the defective allele. The normal animals with normal ASS activity have two normal ASS alleles: they are homozygous for the normal allele. The normal animals with approximately 50 per cent of normal ASS activity are heterozygotes (often called **carriers**), having one normal allele (producing normal ASS) and one defective allele (producing no ASS). Thus the level of ASS activity is directly proportional to the number of 'doses' of the normal allele.

This is important from a practical point of view, because it provides a means of identifying heterozygotes (carriers). As we shall see in Chapter 11, the detection of carriers on the basis of a biochemical test of enzyme level has been an important means of controlling some inherited disorders. Increasingly, as we shall also see, biochemical testing is being replaced by DNA testing.

As well as illustrating carrier detection by biochemical means, inborn errors of metabolism provide good illustrations of other important genetic concepts.

## Type of gene action

In the case of citrullinaemia discussed above, and many other inborn errors of metabolism, the normal allele is said to be completely **dominant** to the defective allele, with respect to clinical signs. Another way of expressing this is to say that the defective allele is **recessive** to the normal allele, or that citrullinaemia is a recessive disease.

More generally, an allele is recessive for any trait if its effect with respect to that trait is not evident in the heterozygote. Likewise, an allele is dominant with respect to a particular trait if its effect is the same in heterozygotes as in homozygotes.

Suppose that the trait with which we are concerned is the level of ASS activity, rather than clinical signs. In this case, the normal allele and the defective allele are said to be each **co-dominant** or **incompletely dominant**, because the heterozygote exhibits the effect of both alleles. The terms recessive, dominant, co-dominant and incompletely dominant describe relationships between alleles, or **types of gene action**. From the above example, it is evident that two alleles at one locus can exhibit more than one type of gene action, depending on the trait being considered.

### Genotype and phenotype

It is convenient to introduce two more terms at this stage. The first is **genotype**, which refers to the genetical constitution of an individual at one or more loci. Using the symbol $D$ for the normal allele, and $d$ for the defective allele, the genotype for carriers of citrullinaemia is $Dd$, while affected calves have the genotype $dd$. The other term is **phenotype**, which is an observable trait of an individual. In relation to ASS activity, there are three different phenotypes (normal activity, 50 per cent activity, and zero activity) corresponding exactly to the three respective genotypes ($DD$, $Dd$, and $dd$). In relation to clinical signs, however, a one-to-one relationship between genotype and phenotype does not exist: the same three genotypes give rise to only two phenotypes. $DD$ and $Dd$ animals are normal, while $dd$ animals are affected. Situations in which there is a one-to-one relationship between phenotype and genotype are the exception rather than the rule.

## Sex-limited inheritance

The typical feathering of hens is part of their secondary sexual characteristics, produced by the action of oestrogen. Much of this oestrogen is produced from androgen in the ovaries by the enzyme aromatase. In certain strains of two breeds of chicken, the Sebright Bantam and the Golden Campine, roosters have the same feathering as hens, rather than the typical male form of feathering. This disorder is called henny feathering. It results from a mutation in the aromatase gene, causing the gene to be expressed in the skin of both sexes. In males, this leads to abnormally high levels of oestrogen, which in turn produces henny feathering.

The aromatase gene is autosomal, but the form of inheritance of henny feathering is not what is normally seen with an autosomal mutation, because the phenotype associated with the mutation (female feathering in males) can be seen only in males. This is an example of a **sex-limited** disorder.

Henny feathering is interesting on three counts. First, it illustrates that not all mutations result in loss of activity; some can cause a gene to be switched on in cells in which it is normally inactive. Second, it provides a different illustration of the ideas expressed in the previous section. With respect to aromatase activity in skin, gene action is co-dominant, i.e. heterozygotes have an enzyme activity mid-way between that of the two homozygotes. In this case, however, the activity in the skin of the normal homozygote is zero. With respect to feathering, the mutant is dominant, because heterozygotes produce sufficient enzyme in the skin, and hence sufficient oestrogen, to cause henny feathering. Third, while the mutation gives rise to a phenotype that is seen only in males, the normal expression of the gene is seen only in females. Thus, two alleles at the one locus give rise to the two possible forms of sex-limited inheritance.

## Genetical heterogeneity of disease

Some animals are born with easily extendible and very fragile skin, a condition that is known as Ehlers–Danlos syndrome, dermatosparaxis or cutaneous asthenia. In animals suffering from this disease, severe lacerations result from the slightest scratch that in normal animals would cause only trivial damage. The basic cause of these severe clinical signs is the presence of abnormal type-I collagen in the skin.

Like all collagens, type-I collagen is a protein, and must therefore be the product of a gene. In fact, it is the product of two genes, because a type-I collagen molecule consists of a triple helix of two alpha-1 chains (the product of one gene) and one alpha-2 chain (the product of a separate gene), as shown in Fig. 3.2. As with many polypeptides, the products of the type-I collagen genes are precursors: they contain additional amino acids at each end of the chain, that are not present in the mature molecule. When the two alpha-1 and one alpha-2 chains initially form a triple helix, the resultant molecule (called type-I procollagen) is not functional, and cannot form itself into the cylindrical fibrils that are characteristic of normal connective tissue. In order for this precursor molecule to become fully functional, the surplus amino acids at each end of each chain must be removed, thereby creating a type-I collagen molecule. Not surprisingly, this removal of terminal amino acids is performed by specific enzymes, namely two endopeptidases called procollagen I carboxy-proteinase (PCP-C-I) and procollagen I amino-proteinase (PCP-N-I), as shown in Fig. 3.2. Since each of these enzymes is also the product of a gene, we now have at least four genes involved in the manufacture of mature type-I collagen molecules: two coding for procollagen chains, and at least one for each of the enzymes. (In fact, the enzymes themselves consist of at least two

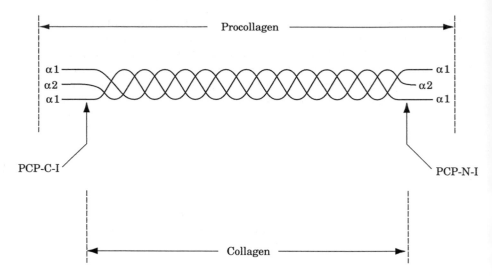

**Fig. 3.2** A procollagen type I molecule, showing the cleavage sites of the endopeptidases PCP-N-I and PCP-C-I.

different polypeptides, and hence are the product of at least two genes, but this need not concern us here.)

Obviously, mutations can occur in any of these genes. For example, in cattle and sheep, mutations have occurred in one of the genes coding for one of the chains of the enzyme PCP-N-I. Animals that are homozygous for such a mutation are deficient in the enzyme, and therefore experience a buildup of partially processed collagen molecules, still having the surplus amino acids at their N-terminal ends. The resultant clinical signs are easily extendible, fragile skin. In contrast, heterozygotes for this mutation do not show any clinical signs, because one-half of the normal concentration of enzyme is sufficient to process all the procollagen molecules. Since heterozygotes are normal, this defect is recessive.

Exactly the same type of abnormal collagen molecule (and hence exactly the same clinical signs) results from a mutation in either one of the procollagen genes, which alters the procollagen molecule so that the cleavage site for the enzyme PCP-N-I is suppressed. In heterozygotes for such a mutation, one-half of all type-I collagen molecules are only partially processed; despite both enzymes being present at normal concentration, only one of them (PCP-C-I) can actually cleave the procollagen. Since heterozygotes for this mutation have only 50 per cent normal type-I collagen molecules, they show the clinical signs of the disorder. In other words, this form of the disorder is dominant.

If a specific set of clinical signs arises from more than one mutation, there is genetical heterogeneity for that disorder.

From the somewhat limited evidence available, it appears that the dominant form of the disorder occurs in horses, cats, dogs, mink, and rabbits. The recessive form definitely occurs in sheep and cattle.

This is an example of genetic heterogeneity *between* species. Although such heterogeneity can cause confusion from time to time, a far greater source of confusion is genetic heterogeneity *within* a species. For example, both forms of the above connective tissue disorder are well documented in humans, and it would be most surprising if both forms of the disorder do not occur within particular species of animals as well.

Genetic heterogeneity of disease is not confined to situations where more than one gene is involved; it also exists if there are two or more different mutations in the one gene. In some human genes, hundreds of different mutations have been detected. Not surprisingly, some of the mutations have a greater clinical effect than others; on average, for example, nonsense mutations and deletions in coding sequences produce more serious clinical signs than mis-sense mutations. In some cases, different mutations within the one gene give rise to different clinical entities. In animals, there is little comparable information. However, in a few cases, there is indirect evidence that the same clinical signs in different populations within a species are due to different mutations. In broiler chickens, for example, sex-linked dwarfism is due to a deletion in the growth-hormone receptor gene, but in Leghorns with the same disorder, there is no evidence of a deletion in this gene.

The above discussion has highlighted two important points, namely that mutations in different genes can give rise to exactly the same clinical entity, and different mutations within the same gene can produce different clinical entities. Both situations represent genetic heterogeneity, but only the former has the potential to cause confusion.

If a set of clinical signs appears to have a genetic basis, but if genetic heterogeneity within a species remains undetected, it may be difficult or even impossible to establish the form of inheritance. Although it is easy to be wise after the event, it is very difficult in practice to ensure that the available data on any syndrome all belong to the one disorder entity and hence are homogeneous. Data are more likely to represent genetic homogeneity if they have been obtained from animals that not only present with the same clinical signs, but which also have the same histopathological and biochemical lesions as well. In addition, data obtained from animals which are related (have at least one ancestor in common) are more likely to be homogeneous than data collected from several unrelated families.

## Type of gene action and type of disease

In the connective tissue disorders described above, two types of gene action have been observed. One disorder is inherited as an autosomal recessive condition and is associated with an enzyme deficiency. The other is inherited as an autosomal dominant condition, and is due to a mutation in one of the genes for type-I collagen.

In general, recessive disorders tend to be due to enzyme deficiencies, while dominant or co-dominant disorders are more likely to be caused by defects in non-enzymatic polypeptides. The reason for this is that enzymes are required in such small quantities that 50 per cent of normal activity (as in heterozygotes) is sufficient for normal functioning. In contrast, if the mutant polypeptide has, for example, a structural role, the structures incorporating that polypeptide will be defective, and the heterozygote may well show some form of the disorder. Similarly, if the polypeptide is a substrate in a particular process or is involved in transport, a decrease by one-half in the production of normal polypeptide, as occurs in heterozygotes, might be expected to cause some clinical signs in the heterozygote, because such polypeptides are also often required in relatively large quantities.

A special comment must be made concerning X-linked diseases, because random X-inactivation has important practical implications. In females that are heterozygous for X-linked disorders, one half of their cells are expected to express the normal allele, while the other half are expected to express the mutant allele. If the gene product normally functions outside the cell, e.g. in the blood or some other body fluid, the result is the same as with heterozygotes for autosomal disorders: the gene product is at one-half the normal concentration. However, if the gene product's normal role is inside the cell, all of those cells expressing only the mutant allele are deficient in the gene product, and the animal may show some clinical signs. In addition, since inactivation is a random process, not all females have exactly one half of each type of cell. In fact, a wide range of proportions of the two cell types can occur, from females having most cells with the normal allele active, to females having most cells with the mutant allele active. Females in the former category may be indistinguishable from females that are homozygous for the normal allele, in terms of concentration of gene product and/or lack of clinical signs. In contrast, those with a high proportion of cells expressing the mutant allele may actually exhibit quite severe clinical signs, resembling males with a mutant X chromosome. Finally, even in cases where the mutant allele is active in only a small proportion of cells, if these cells happen to be the only ones in which the X-linked gene is transcribed and translated, the female may show clinical signs. Obviously, X-inactivation can create substantial complications in inheritance patterns for X-linked disorders, and for biochemical detection of carriers of such disorders.

## Phenocopies

Sometimes the phenotype of a single-gene disorder occurs due to an environmental cause. Such an occurrence is called a **phenocopy**. A good example of a phenocopy is provided by α-mannosidosis, which is a lysosomal storage disease in cats and cattle.

Lysosomes are small membrane-bound organelles found in the cytoplasm.

They are the digestive system of the cell: they contain many enzymes that act in a step-wise manner to break down complex molecules into monomeric units of simple lipids, amino acids, monosaccharides, and nucleotides. If a particular lysosomal enzyme is absent or inactive, the step-wise degradation is halted, with a consequent build-up ('storage') of the material that is normally broken down by that enzyme. In other words, an inborn error of lysosomal catabolism produces a **lysosomal storage disease**. For most lysosomal storage diseases, affected animals are usually normal at birth but fail to grow as rapidly as their contemporaries; in most cases there is a progressive neurological deterioration, caused by the build-up of storage products in nerve cells, producing incoordination and aggression which eventually leads to death, usually before sexual maturity.

In α-mannosidosis, the deficient enzyme is α-mannosidase. In most cases, the deficiency is caused by a mutation in the gene for α-mannosidase, and α-mannosidosis is therefore a single-gene recessive disorder. However, if cattle graze on pasture that contains the legume Darling Pea (*Swainsona* spp.), they often develop α-mannosidosis. The reason for this is that plants in the *Swainsona* genus produce a trihydroxylated indolizidine alkaloid called swainsonine, which inhibits α-mannosidase by binding to it, thereby producing a build-up of exactly the same mannose-rich oligosaccharides that are characteristic of the inherited form of the disorder. A similar compound is produced by plants in the *Astragalus* and *Oxytropis* genera. Indeed, plants within these genera are called locoweed, because of the clinical signs they induce. Not surprisingly, these clinical signs can be induced in any species that grazes on the plants.

By their very nature, it is difficult to distinguish phenocopies from inherited forms of a disorder. All we can do is be aware of the possibility that an individual showing the clinical signs of an inherited disorder may not, in fact, have the genotype usually associated with those clinical signs. Phenocopies, therefore, are another potential cause of complications in inheritance patterns.

## A sample of single-gene disorders

The above discussion has covered the important principles concerning single-gene disorders, using specific examples from domestic animals. Obviously there are many more single-gene disorders than those mentioned above. In fact, the potential total number of single-gene disorders is far greater than the total number of genes: a deficiency in almost any polypeptide is likely to give rise to either embryonic lethality (spontaneous abortion) or clinical signs, and (as we have already seen), different mutations in the same gene can give rise to different sets of clinical signs. Of course, mutations producing embryonic lethals are difficult to detect. However, recalling that the total number of genes is probably somewhere between 50 000 and 100 000, it is evident that the ultimate list of single-gene disorders that will be detected is likely to be very long! At present, only a small fraction of all potential single-gene disorders have been documented in domestic animals.

The increasing use of molecular technology in the investigation of single-gene disorders in animals has already uncovered several interesting examples of different types of mutations.

An example of a mis-sense mutation is provided by canine haemophilia B. This disorder is caused by a substitution of A for G at nucleotide 1477 in the gene for canine factor IX, resulting in the substitution of glutamic acid for glycine at position 379 in the factor-IX molecule (Fig. 3.3). This particular site has been highly conserved throughout evolution—there is a glycine present at this position in factor IX from human, pig, and cattle. Not surprisingly, therefore, this single amino-acid substitution profoundly alters the tertiary structure of the factor-IX molecule, to the extent that no functional factor IX can be detected. Mis-sense mutations are also the cause of bovine leucocyte adhesion deficiency (BLAD), hyperkalaemic periodic paralysis in horses, malignant hyperthermia syndrome in pigs, and a behavioural defect called shaking in dogs (Appendix 3.1).

Nonsense mutations have also occurred. In Afrikander cattle, for example, inherited goitre is due to a nonsense mutation in the thyroglobulin gene. The gene itself is approximately 250 kb long, while the mRNA consists of 8431 bases. The disease is due to a C → T substitution in exon 9, changing a CGA triplet (arginine) to TGA (stop). In Dutch goats, a nonsense mutation in exon 8 of the thyroglobulin gene, changing TAC (tyrosine) to TAG (stop), causes the same disorder. Other disorders caused by nonsense mutations are citrullinaemia in cattle (mentioned earlier), deficiency of uridine monophosphate synthase (DUMPS) in cattle, hypotrophic axonopathy in quail, maple syrup urine disease in cattle, nanomelia in chickens, X-linked nephritis in dogs, and rod–cone dysplasia-1 in dogs (Appendix 3.1).

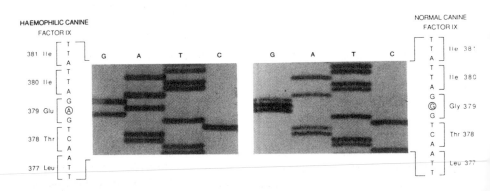

**Fig. 3.3** A small section of sequencing gels showing the substitution of A for G in the gene for factor IX in dogs. The consequent substitution of glutamic acid for glycine results in haemophilia B. When checking the sequences against the genetic code in Table 1.2, note that in this figure they are read from bottom to top.

DUMPS is particularly interesting, because it is an example of an embryonic lethal that has been detected. The enzyme that is deficient in this disorder, namely uridine monophosphate (UMP) synthase, is responsible for converting orotic acid to UMP, which is an essential component of pyrimidine nucleotides. Since nucleotides are required in such vast quantities during embryonic growth, it is not surprising that homozygosity for the nonsense mutation in the UMP synthase gene results in embryonic death around 40 days *in utero*. The practical effect of this disorder is that carrier cows show a higher rate of return to service, because some of their pregnancies end in early natural abortion. Given that returns to service can have so many different causes, it would not have been possible to identify the mutation from reproductive records. How, then, was this embryonic lethal mutation detected initially? The answer is: by chance! As part of a nutrition study at the University of Illinois, the level of orotic acid was determined in the milk of cows in the university herd. Some cows had exceptionally high levels of this acid, and one possible explanation was that they were deficient in UMP synthase. Subsequent biochemical tests showed that these cows had only 50 per cent of the normal activity of this enzyme. Inheritance and molecular studies finally brought the whole story to light.

All of the above point mutations occur in exons (more specifically, in coding sequences within exons). In contrast, it might seem that point mutations occurring in introns do no damage, since introns are excised before translation. However, if a point mutation occurs in the first few bases or in the last few bases of an intron, it is very likely to disrupt the RNA splicing mechanism. Muscular dystrophy in Golden Retriever dogs, for example, is due to a base substitution in the 3' splice-acceptor site of intron 6 of the dystrophin gene (Fig. 3.4). This changes the sequence in the mRNA transcript from the usual AG (see Chapter 1) to GG, which means that the following exon 7 is not recognized as such, and is therefore excised along with intron 6 and intron 7 (Fig. 3.4). The dystrophin gene is one of the largest known; it is approximately 2000 kb long, and its mature mRNA is 14 kb long. The mutation in Golden Retrievers occurs at base 736 of the mRNA, i.e. very early in the gene. Exon 7 actually starts at the third base of a codon, and finishes 119 bases later, at the first base of a codon (Fig. 3.4). In effect, therefore, the deletion of exon 7 introduces a frameshift mutation, so that the remainder of the mRNA transcript contains a garbled message. In this particular case, the frameshift introduces a stop codon in the following exon (Fig. 3.4). The result is a truncated transcript, and no functional polypeptide.

An example of a disorder caused by a mutation at the other end of an intron is riboflavinuria in chickens. In this case, the 5' splice-donor sequence GT (see Chapter 1) in intron 2 of the gene for riboflavin-binding protein becomes AT, resulting in exon 2 being spliced out of the mRNA transcript. In normal chickens, riboflavin-binding protein is synthesized in the liver, and is released into the blood stream, where it binds riboflavin derived from the diet. Riboflavin-binding protein transports its bound riboflavin from the

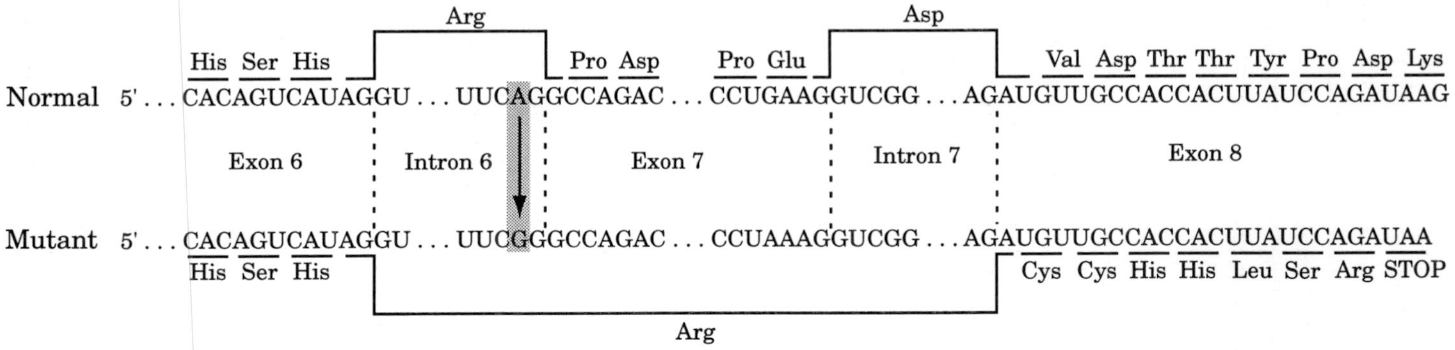

**Fig. 3.4** Part of the base sequence of the normal and mutant dystrophin mRNA transcripts in Golden Retrievers, showing the A → G mutation in the 3' splice-acceptor site of intron 6. The consequent excision of exon 7 from the mRNA creates a frameshift mutation, which produces a stop codon in exon 8. Codons in each mRNA are indicated by lines spanning three adjacent bases.

serum to the yolk of the developing egg, and from the oviduct to the egg white. The deletion of exon 2 causes a deficiency of riboflavin-binding protein, which in turn leads to a deficiency of riboflavin in the developing embryo. This causes embryonic death around day 13, because riboflavin is essential for embryonic development.

Yet another type of mutation is illustrated by henny feathering, which was described earlier in this chapter. This disorder is an example of an insertion mutation. In this particular case, it appears that the terminal repeat sequence (described in Chapter 1) of a retrovirus has been inserted into the 5' promoter region of the aromatase gene. This terminal repeat has a promoter of its own, which causes the aromatase gene to be switched on in atypical places, such as the skin of both sexes, giving rise to the henny-feathering trait in males. The actual peptide produced by the mutant allele is exactly the same as that produced by the normal allele, as we would expect for such a mutation.

Another source of single-gene disorders has recently come to light in humans, and is likely to be discovered in animals in the future. Known as **unstable trinucleotide repeats**, they arise in some genes that contain microsatellites (see Chapter 2) in which the repeat unit is a triplet. Small numbers of the repeat unit appear to be a normal part of the gene, and appear to do no harm, being usually located in an untranslated region. However, for reasons that are not yet understood, these repeats can sometimes rapidly expand in numbers between generations, and as the number of repeat units increases, clinical signs begin to appear, associated with a deficiency of the polypeptide product of the gene. Apparently the expanded number of repeats results in the surrounding DNA becoming methylated, which inactivates the gene (see Chapter 1). As the number of repeat units continues to increase during subsequent generations, the clinical signs become increasingly severe. This increase in the severity of the disease over generations is called **genetic anticipation**. Human diseases caused by unstable trinucleotide repeats include fragile-X syndrome, myotonic dystrophy, spinal and bulbar muscular dystrophy, Huntington's disease, and dentatorubral–pallidoluysian atrophy. Many more are likely to be discovered in the future, both in humans and in animals.

These examples provide an insight into the range of possible mutations that can cause single-gene disorders. There are, of course, many other single-gene disorders. Appendix 3.1 provides a sample of such disorders. Several cases of genetic heterogeneity are present in the table; some of the disorders represent more than one clinical entity (and genetic cause) within a species. The practical aspects of controlling single-gene disorders are discussed in Chapter 11.

## Further reading

### General

Edney, A. T. B. (ed.) (1989). Heredity and disease in dogs and cats—proceedings of a symposium held jointly by BSAVA and BVA Animal Welfare Foundation in liaison with the Kennel Club. *Journal of Small Animal Practice*, **30**, 125–94. (Also relevant to Chapters 6, 7 and 11.)

Hoffman, E. P. and Jaffurs, D. (1993). Disease genetics—an expanding enigma. *Current Biology*, **3**, 456–9.

Womack, J. E. (1992). Veterinary medicine—molecular genetics arrives on the farm. *Nature*, **360**, 108–9.

## Genetical heterogeneity of disease

Beutler, E. (1993). Gaucher disease as a paradigm of current issues regarding single gene mutations of humans. *Proceedings of the National Academy of Sciences, USA*, **90**, 5384–90.

## Reviews of single-gene disorders in humans and mice

Cooper, D. N. and Schmidtke, J. (1993). Diagnosis of human genetic disease using recombinant DNA. Fourth edition. *Human Genetics*, **92**, 211–36.

McKusick, V. A. (1994). *Mendelian inheritance in man*, (11th edn). Johns Hopkins University Press, Baltimore. [The electronic form of this catalogue, Online *Mendelian Inheritance in Man*, (OMIM), is updated continually. A joint search of the human and mouse catalogues can be conducted via the World Wide Web on the Internet at: http://www.informatics.jax.org]

McKusick, V. A. and Amberger, J. S. (1994). The morbid anatomy of the human genome—chromosomal location of mutations causing disease (update 1 December 1993). *Journal of Medical Genetics*, **31**, 265–279.

Searle, A. G., Edwards, J. H., and Hall, J. G. (1994). Mouse homologues of human hereditary disease. *Journal of Medical Genetics*, **31**, 1–19.

## Reviews of single-gene disorders in domestic animals

Alroy, J., Warren, C. D., Raghavan, S. S., and Kolodny, E. H. (1989). Animal models for lysosomal storage diseases—their past and future contribution. *Human Pathology*, **20**, 823–6.

Alroy, J., Orgad, U., Degasperi, R., Richard, R., Warren, C. D., Knowles, K., Thalhammer, J. G., and Raghavan, S. S. (1992). Canine GM1-gangliosidosis—a clinical, morphologic, histochemical, and biochemical comparison of two different models. *American Journal of Pathology*, **140**, 675–89.

Barnett, K. C. (1988). Inherited eye disease in the dog and cat. *Journal of Small Animal Practice*, **29**, 462–75.

Basrur, P. K. and Yadav, B. R. (1990). Genetic diseases of sheep and goats. *Veterinary Clinics of North America—Food Animal Practice*, **6**, 779–802.

Bouw, J. (1991). Genetic defects of the eyes in dogs. *Tijdschrift voor Diergeneeskunde*, **116**, 898–905.

Brinkhous, K. M., Reddick, R. L., Read, M. S., Nichols, T. C., Bellinger, D. A., and Griggs, T. R. (1991). von Willebrand factor and animal models—contributions to gene therapy, thrombotic thrombocytopenic purpura, and coronary artery thrombosis. *Mayo Clinic Proceedings*, **66**, 733–42.

Brooks, M., Dodds, W. J., and Raymond, S. L. (1992). Epidemiologic features of von Willebrand's disease in Doberman-Pinschers, Scottish Terriers, and Shetland

Sheepdogs—260 cases (1984–1988). *Journal of the American Veterinary Medical Association*, **200**, 1123–7.

Catalfamo, J. L. and Dodds, W. J. (1988). Hereditary and acquired thrombopathias. *Veterinary Clinics of North America—Small Animal Practice*, **18**, (1), 185–93.

Clark, R. D. and Stainer, J. R. (ed.) (1983). *Medical and genetic aspects of purebred dogs*. Veterinary Medicine Publishing Company, Edwardsville, Kansas.

Desnick, R. J., Patterson, D. F., and Scarpelli, D. G. (ed.) (1982). *Animal models of inherited metabolic diseases*. Alan R. Liss, New York.

Evans, R. J. (1989). Lysosomal storage diseases in dogs and cats. *Journal of Small Animal Practice*, **30**, 144–150.

Fogh, J. M. and Fogh, I. T. (1988). Inherited coagulation disorders. *Veterinary Clinics of North America—Small Animal Practice*, **18**, (1), 231–43.

Franco, D. A., Lin, T. L., and Leder, J. A. (1992). Bovine congenital erythropoietic porphyria—bovine review article. *Compendium on Continuing Education for the Practicing Veterinarian*, **14**, 822–6.

Healy, P. J. and Dennis, J. A. (1993). Inherited enzyme deficiencies in livestock. *Veterinary Clinics of North America—Food Animal Practice*, **9**, (1), 55–63.

Hoskins, J. D. and Taboada, J. (1992). Congenital defects of the dog. *Compendium on Continuing Education for the Practicing Veterinarian*, **14**, 873–97.

Jesupret, C. (1989). [Hereditary diseases, anomalies of the iris.]. *Pratique Medicale et Chirurgicale de l'Animal de Compagnie*, **24**, 139–41.

Johnson, G. S., Turrentine, M. A., and Kraus, K. H. (1988). Canine von Willebrand's disease. A heterogeneous group of bleeding disorders. *Veterinary Clinics of North America—Small Animal Practice*, **18**, (1), 195–229.

Jolly, R. D., Martinus, R. D., and Palmer, D. N. (1992). Sheep and other animals with ceroid-lipofuscinoses—their relevance to Batten disease. *American Journal of Medical Genetics*, **42**, 609–14.

Jolly, R. D. (1993). Lysosomal storage diseases in livestock. *Veterinary Clinics of North America—Food Animal Practice*, **9**, (1), 41–53.

Leipold, H. W. and Dennis, S. M. (1987). Cause, nature, effect and diagnosis of bovine congenital defects. *Irish Veterinary News*, **9**, 11–19.

Littlewood, J. D. (1989). Inherited bleeding disorders of dogs and cats. *Journal of Small Animal Practice*, **30**, 140–3.

Littlewood, J. D. (1992). Differential diagnosis of haemorrhagic disorders in dogs. *In Practice*, **14**, 172–80.

Meyers, K. M., Wardrop, K. J., and Meinkoth, J. (1992). Canine von Willebrand's disease—pathobiology, diagnosis, and short-term treatment. *Compendium on Continuing Education for the Practicing Veterinarian*, **14**, 13.

Patel, S. C. and Pentchev, P. G. (1989). Genetic defects of lysosomal function in animals. *Annual Review of Nutrition*, **9**, 395–416.

Patterson, D. F., Haskins, M. E., and Jezyk, P. F. (1982). Models of human genetic disease in domestic animals. *Advances in Human Genetics*, **12**, 263–339.

Pidduck, H. (1987). A review of inherited disease in the dog. *The Veterinary Annual*, **27**, 293–311.

Robinson, R. (1987). Genetic defects in cats. *Companion Animal Practice*, **1**, 10–14.

Robinson, R. (1989). Genetic defects in the horse. *Journal of Animal Breeding and Genetics*, **106**, 475–8.

Robinson, R. (1991). Genetic anomalies in dogs. *Canine Practice*, **16**, 29–34.

Robinson, R. (1991). Genetic defects in the pig. *Journal of Animal Breeding and Genetics*, **108**, 61–5.

Rubin, L. F. (1989). *Inherited eye disease in purebred dogs*. Williams and Wilkins, New York.

Scott, D. and Tizard, I. (1993). Primary immunodeficiencies of food animals. *Veterinary Clinics of North America—Food Animal Practice*, **9**, (1), 65–75.

Smith, R. I. E. (1989). Inherited diseases of the canine eye. *Australian Veterinary Practitioner*, **19**, 186–95.

Stades, F. C. (1991). Hereditary eye diseases—diagnostics, therapy and prevention. *Tijdschrift Voor Diergeneeskunde*, **116**, 889–97.

Stefanon, G., Stefanon, B., Stefanon, G., and Dodds, W. J. (1993). Inherited and acquired canine bleeding disorders in northeastern Italy. *Canine Practice*, **18**, 15–23.

Valentine, B. A., Winand, N. J., Pradhan, D., Moise, N. S., Delahunta, A., Kornegay, J. N., and Cooper, B. J. (1992). Canine X-linked muscular dystrophy as an animal model of Duchenne muscular dystrophy—a review. *American Journal of Medical Genetics*, **42**, 352–6.

## Appendix 3.1 A sample of single-gene disorders in animals

Sex-linked inheritance is indicated by X or Z after the species name. A continually updated and expanded version of this table (with references), called Mendelian Inheritance in Animals (MIA), can be accessed on the Internet through the Australian National Genomic Information Service (ANGIS) at the University of Sydney. The World Wide Web address is: http://morgan.angis.su.oz.au. MIA is also available (in a different format) at: http://probe.nalusda.gov

| Name(s) of disorder | Deficiency or abnormal expression | Causative mutation or linked marker | Species |
|---|---|---|---|
| **Disorders with a known molecular defect** | | | |
| C8 deficiency | complement component 8, alpha | mutation at exon/intron junction of alpha gene | rabbit |
| Citrullinaemia | argininosuccinate synthetase (ASS) | nonsense mutation in ASS gene | cattle |
| Congenital adrenal hyperplasia | cytochrome-P450 cholesterol side-chain cleavage enzyme (P450scc) | deletion in P450scc gene | rabbit |
| Deficiency of uridine monophosphate synthase (DUMPS) | uridine monophosphate synthase (UMPS) | nonsense mutation in UMPS gene | cattle |
| Dwarfism, sex-linked | growth-hormone receptor (GHR) | broilers: deletion in GHR gene Leghorns: unknown, but not deletion in GHR gene | chicken(Z) |
| Goitre | thyroglobulin (TG) | cattle and goat: nonsense mutation in TG gene | cattle, goat |
| Haemophilia B | coagulation factor IX | dog: mis-sense mutation in factor-IX gene | cat(X), dog(X) |

**Appendix 3.1** *Continued*

| Name(s) of disorder | Deficiency or abnormal expression | Causative mutation or linked marker | Species |
|---|---|---|---|
| Henny feathering | aromatase | insertion mutation (retrovirus) in the 5' end of aromatase gene has introduced a second promoter that causes expression in skin | chicken |
| Hyperkalaemic periodic paralysis (HYPP) | adult skeletal muscle sodium channel (SMSC) | mis-sense mutation in gene for α subunit of SMSC | horse |
| Hypotrophic axonopathy | neurofilament-L (NF-L) | nonsense mutation in NF-L gene | quail |
| Leucocyte adhesion deficiency (LAD) | beta-2 integrin (CD18) | cattle: mis-sense mutation in CD18 gene | cattle, dog |
| Malignant hyperthermia syndrome (MHS) | calcium-release channel (ryanodine receptor, RyR1) | mis-sense mutation in RyR1 gene | pig |
| Maple syrup urine disease | branched-chain alpha-ketoacid dehydrogenase (BCKDH) complex, which consists of enzymes E1, E2, E3, a kinase, and a phosphatase | nonsense mutation in gene for α subunit of E1 | cattle |
| Muscular dystrophy | dystrophin | dog: point mutation in 3' splice-acceptor site of intron 6 in dystrophin gene causes deletion of 7th exon during mRNA splicing, and introduces a stop codon into exon 8 | cat(X), dog(X) |
| Nanomelia | cartilage proteoglycan core protein (CPCP) | nonsense mutation in CPCP gene | chicken |

| Disorder | Protein / gene | Molecular defect | Species |
|---|---|---|---|
| Nephritis | dog(X): alpha-5 collagen type IV [a5C(IV)] | dog(X): nonsense mutation in exon 35 of a5C(IV) gene | dog(X), dog (autosomal) |
| Riboflavinuria | riboflavin and riboflavin-binding protein (ribBP) in eggs | point mutation in 5′ splice-donor site of intron 2 of ribBP gene causes deletion of 2nd exon during mRNA splicing | chicken |
| Rod–cone dysplasia-1 | beta-subunit of cyclic GMP phosphodiesterase (cGMP-PDE-beta) | nonsense mutation in cGMP-PDE-beta gene | dog |
| Shaking | proteolipid protein (PLP) | mis-sense mutation in the PLP gene | dog(X) |
| **Disorders with a linked marker** | | | |
| Horns (polledness) | | cattle: linked microsatellite marker (15 cM) | cattle, goat, sheep |
| Muscular hypertrophy | | sheep (callipyge gene): linked VNTR marker (20 cM) | cattle, sheep |
| Narcolepsy | | tightly linked (0 cM) to μ immunoglobulin heavy-chain gene | dog |
| Progressive degenerative myeloencephalopathy (Weaver disease) | | linked microsatellite marker (3 cM) | cattle |
| **Disorders with a known deficiency or abnormal expression** | | | |
| Albinism | tyrosinase | | cat, cattle, chicken, dog, rabbit, sheep |
| Analphalipoproteinaemia | high-density lipoprotein deficiency | | chicken(Z) |
| Arginaemia | arginase | | sheep |
| C3 deficiency | complement component 3 | | dog, rabbit |

**Appendix 3.1** *Continued*

| Name(s) of disorder | Deficiency or abnormal expression | Causative mutation or linked marker | Species |
|---|---|---|---|
| Crooked neck dwarf | alpha ryanodine receptor | | chicken |
| Dermatosparaxis, Ehlers–Danlos syndrome, cutaneous asthenia | procollagen | | cat, dog, horse, mink, rabbit |
| Dermatosparaxis, Ehlers–Danlos syndrome, cutaneous asthenia | procollagen I amino-proteinase (PAP) | | cattle, sheep |
| Diplopodia-5 | homeobox proteins GHox-4.6 and GHox-8 | | chicken |
| Dwarfism | thyroxine and tri-iodothyronine | | cat |
| Epidermolysis bullosa, dystrophic | sheep: collagen VII | | cattle, sheep |
| Factor X deficiency | coagulation factor X | | dog |
| Factor XI deficiency | coagulation factor XI | | cattle, dog |
| Factor XII deficiency | coagulation factor XII | | cat, dog |
| Fucosidosis | $\alpha$-fucosidase | | dog |
| Globoid cell leucodystrophy, Krabbe disease | $\beta$-galactocerebrosidase | | cat, dog, sheep |
| Glucocerebroside storage disease, Gaucher's disease | glucocerebrosidase | | dog |
| Glycogen storage disease type II, Pompe disease | $\alpha$-glucosidase | | cat, cattle, dog, quail, sheep |
| Glycogen storage disease, type III | amylo-1,6-glucosidase | | dog |
| Glycogen storage disease, type IV | branching enzyme | | cat |
| Glycogen storage disease, type VII | 6-phosphofructo-1-kinase | | dog |
| $GM_1$ gangliosidosis | $\beta$-galactosidase | | cat, dog, cattle, sheep |
| $GM_2$ gangliosidosis | hexosaminidase A | | cat, dog, pig |
| Glutathione deficiency | gamma-glutamylcysteine synthetase | | sheep |
| Gyrate atrophy retina | ornithine aminotransferase | | cat |
| Haemolytic anaemia VIII | pyruvate kinase | | dog |

| Disease | Protein/Gene | Species |
|---|---|---|
| Haemolytic anaemia, nonspherocytic | phosphofructokinase | dog |
| Haemophilia A | coagulation factor VIII | cat(X), cattle(X), dog(X), horse(X), sheep(X) |
| Hypercoaguable state | protein C | horse |
| Hyperchylomicronaemia (Hyperlipidaemia type 1) | lipoprotein lipase | cat |
| Hypofibrinogenaemia | coagulation factor I | dog, goat |
| Hypoproconvertinaemia | coagulation factor VII | dog |
| Hypoprothrombinaemia | coagulation factor II | dog |
| Intestinal cobalamin malabsorption | intrinsic factor-cobalamin receptor | dog |
| Limbless | homeobox proteins GHox-7 and GHox-8 | chicken |
| Methaemoglobinaemia | NADH-methaemoglobin reductase | dog |
| Mannosidosis, α | α-mannosidase | cat, cattle |
| Mannosidosis, β | β-mannosidase | cattle, goat |
| Mucopolysaccharidosis I, Hurler syndrome | α-L-iduronidase | cat, dog |
| Mucopolysaccharidosis IIID, San-Filippo syndrome type-D | N-acetylglucosamine 6-sulphatase | goat |
| Mucopolysaccharidosis VI, Maroteaux–Lamy syndrome | arylsulphatase B | cat |
| Mucopolysaccharidosis VII, Sly syndrome | β-glucuronidase | dog |
| Myoclonus | glycine/strychnine receptor in spinal cord | cattle, horse |
| Paralytic tremor | myelin | rabbit |
| Porphyria | uroporphyrinogen III cosynthetase | cat, cattle, pig |
| Primary hyperoxaluria type 2 | D-glycerate dehydrogenase and glyoxylate reductase | cat |
| Protoporphyria | ferrochelatase | cattle, chicken |

## Appendix 3.1 Continued

| Name(s) of disorder | Deficiency or abnormal expression | Causative mutation or linked marker | Species |
|---|---|---|---|
| Restricted ovulator | very-low-density-lipoprotein receptor | | chicken |
| Retinal degeneration | rhodopsin | | cat |
| Sphingomyelinosis, Niemann–Pick disease | sphingomyelinase | | cat, dog |
| Spinal muscular atrophy | low molecular weight neurofilament protein subunit | | cattle, dog |
| Spongiform encephalopathy | prion protein | | cat, cattle, goat, kudu, puma, sheep, Rocky Mountain elk |
| Testicular feminization | androgen receptor | | cat(X), cattle(X), horse(X), sheep(X) |
| Tyrosinaemia type II | tyrosine aminotransferase | | dog |
| Vitamin-D-resistant rickets | renal 1-α-hydroxylase | | pig |
| Vitamin-K-dependent blood coagulation factors deficiency | gamma-glutamylcarboxylase | | cat |
| von Willebrand disease | von Willebrand factor | | dog, horse, pig, rabbit |
| **Other single-gene disorders** | | | |
| Achromatosis, partial feather | | | chicken |
| Albinism, imperfect (sex-linked albinism) | | | chicken(Z) |
| Atresia coli | | | cattle |

| Atypical mitotic metaphase | quail |
| Baldness, congenital | chicken(Z) |
| Blastoderm degeneration | chicken |
| Blindness | chicken |
| Blood ring | turkey |
| Bobber | turkey(Z) |
| Carpal subluxation | dog(X) |
| Ceroid lipofuscinosis (Batten's disease) | cat, cattle, dog, goat, sheep |
| Chediak–Higashi syndrome | cat, cattle, fox, killer whale, mink, white tiger |
| Chondrodysplasia (Spider lamb syndrome) | sheep |
| Combined immunodeficiency disease (CID) | horse |
| Congenital loco | turkey |
| Curling of feathers | chicken |
| Deafness | dog |
| Dwarfism, snorter | cattle |
| Dwarfism, pituitary | dog |
| Dyserythropoiesis and dyskeratosis, congenital | cattle |
| Epitheliogenesis imperfecta | cat, cattle, sheep |
| Exostosis, multiple | horse |
| Faded shaker | chicken |
| Fecundity, Inverdale | sheep(X) |
| Frizzling | chicken |
| Hyperbilirubinaemia | sheep |
| Hypotrichosis (hairlessness) | dog, cattle |
| Legg-Calve-Perthes disease | dog |

**Appendix 3.1** *Continued*

| Name(s) of disorder | Deficiency or abnormal expression | Causative mutation or linked marker | Species |
|---|---|---|---|
| Lethal trait A-46 | | | cattle |
| Muscular dystrophy | | | chicken, sheep |
| Myasthenia gravis, congenital | | | dog |
| Myoclonus epilepsy of Lafora (Lafora disease) | | | dog |
| Naked neck | | | chicken |
| Neutropenia, cyclic (cyclic haematopoiesis) | | | dog |
| Orange | | | quail |
| Paroxysm | | | chicken(Z) |
| Persistent Mullerian duct syndrome | | | dog |
| Prenatal lethal | | | chicken(Z) |
| Rod-cone dystrophy | | | cat |
| Scaleless | | | chicken |
| Severe combined immunodeficiency | | | dog(X) |
| Sperm degeneration | | | chicken |
| Spinal myelinopathy, progressive | | | cattle |
| Syndactyly | | | cattle |
| Taillessness | | | cat |
| Tetanic torticollar spasms | | | turkey(Z) |
| Tibial hemimelia | | | cattle |
| Tremor type A III, congenital | | | pig(X) |
| Vertical fibre hide defect | | | cattle |
| Vibrator | | | turkey(Z) |
| White, lethal, overo (Hirschsprung disease) | | | horse |
| Wilson disease | | | dog |
| XX sex reversal | | | dog, goat, llama, pig |

# Chromosomal aberrations

From time to time, mistakes occur in mitosis, in meiosis, or in fertilization, and sometimes these mistakes give rise to aberrant karyotypes. The aim of this chapter is to describe these aberrations, and to discuss the role they play in determining abnormalities in animals.

In many cases, abnormal karyotypes have been observed in healthy and/or highly productive animals. Likewise, many diseased and/or unproductive animals have normal karyotypes. It follows that a normal karyotype is not itself a guarantee of high production and freedom from disease, and neither is an abnormal karyotype certain to indicate a diseased or unproductive animal.

## Abnormal chromosome number

One of the most common abnormalities is the absence of an X chromosome. The lack of just one chromosome is termed **monosomy**, and animals lacking a chromosome are said to be **monosomic** for that chromosome. In the case of females that are monosomic for the X chromosome, their karyotype is written as XO, with the O indicating absence of an X chromosome.

XO individuals have been reported in many domestic species, and also in humans where the condition is called Turner's syndrome. All XO individuals have a more-or-less normal female external phenotype, but are usually sterile.

Another abnormality is the presence of three X chromosomes rather than the normal two. This is an example of **trisomy**, and individuals having an additional chromosome are said to be **trisomic**. In the case of the X chromosome, their karyotype is written as XXX. When examined cytologically, non-dividing cells of X trisomics are seen to contain two Barr bodies, which indicates that only one X chromosome in each cell remains active. Consequently, XXX individuals are less abnormal than XO individuals; they are often fertile. Some of their offspring have normal karyotypes, while others are trisomic.

XO and XXX individuals arise from **non-disjunction**, which is failure of the chromosomes or chromatids to disjoin during meiosis. Since there is normally one disjunction in each stage of meiosis (one during meiosis I and one during meiosis II), as described in Chapter 1, there are two opportunities for non-disjunction during the formation of a germ cell. Non-disjunction occurs in approximately 5 per cent of all meioses, and can involve any of the autosomes or the sex chromosomes. In the latter case, the results differ depending on the sex of the individual in which meiosis is occurring. In females, the results are straightforward: irrespective of when non-disjunction occurs, some of the ova contain two X chromosomes while others contain none. With males, however, four different types of unbalanced sperms can result, depending on whether non-disjunction occurs during meiosis I or meiosis II (Fig. 4.1).

The unbalanced gametes that result from non-disjunction are usually still able to be involved in fertilization, and the possible outcomes are illustrated in Table 4.1. It is evident that XO and XXX individuals can arise from non-disjunction in either sex. It is also evident that many other types of unbalanced karyotypes can result from non-disjunction in one or both parents. In general, karyotypes with a small number of extra chromosomes, and karyotypes that lack a small number of chromosomes, are said to be **aneuploid**, in comparison with those having the normal number, which are said to be **euploid**. Thus monosomics and trisomics are both aneuploids. Some of the other aneuploids shown in Table 4.1 such as O, YO, and YYO, have never been observed, and are assumed to be lethal at an early stage of embryonic development. All the remaining aneuploids in Table 4.1 have been recorded in at least one species of mammal. Among those reported in domestic animals are XXY and XXXY, both of which have a predominantly male phenotype, often associated with underdeveloped male sexual behaviour. Among domestic animals, XXY individuals have been reported in cats, cattle, dogs, pigs, and sheep (Appendix 4.1). They are usually sterile. In humans, the condition is known as Kleinfelter's syndrome.

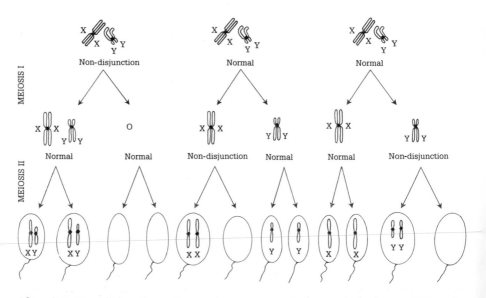

**Fig. 4.1** Non-disjunction of sex chromosomes during meiosis in an XY male. 'Normal' refers to normal disjunction, as illustrated in Fig. 1.4.

**Table 4.1** The zygotes that can theoretically result from all possible combinations of abnormal sperms and eggs, in relation to sex chromsomes

|  |  |  | Sperm |  |  |  |  |  |
|---|---|---|---|---|---|---|---|---|
|  |  |  | Normal |  | Abnormal |  |  |  |
|  |  |  | X | Y | XY | XX | YY | O |
| Eggs | Normal | X | XX | XY | XXY | XXX | XYY | XO |
|  | Abnormal | XX<br>O | XXX<br>XO | XXY<br>YO | XXXY<br>XY | XXXX<br>XX | XXYY<br>YYO | XX<br>O |

As with XO and XXX females, XXY males are generally not recognizable in domestic animals until they are karyotyped. One notable exception is male tortoiseshell cats. In Chapter 1, we saw that tortoiseshell cats are heterozygous at an X-linked coat-colour locus, and since males have only one X chromosome, we would expect all tortoiseshells to be female. But male tortoiseshells do occur from time to time. They are usually sterile, and when examined cytogenetically, a majority of them are found to be XXY in at least a proportion of their cells. The most interesting tortoiseshell males are those that have a normal XY karyotype. Being tortoiseshell, they must have two different types of X chromosome, but each cell appears to have only one X chromosome. The most likely explanation is that XY tortoiseshell males result from the fusion of two male embryos, one carrying an orange allele on its X chromosome, and the other carrying a non-orange allele. Having a normal genome in every cell, these males are fertile. It is possible, therefore, to come across a fertile male tortoiseshell cat. But they constitute only a minority of tortoiseshell males, and are therefore very rare.

One of the most common forms of sex-chromosomal aneuploidy is the occurrence of more than one cell line in an individual, e.g. XY/XXY or XX/XXY/XXYY. The usual cause of these mixtures is non-disjunction during mitosis at an early stage of embryo development. The result is almost invariably some form of sexual abnormality. Since each of the cell lines has come from a single source (the fertilized ovum), the individuals are called **mosaics**.

The general conclusion we can draw from the above discussion is that aneuploidy of sex chromosomes is usually associated with sexual abnormalities.

We have concentrated on sex chromosomes when discussing aneuploidy because most cases of aneuploidy involve these chromosomes. However, aneuploidy of autosomes can also arise from non-disjunction, and some cases have been reported. The best known example in animals is trisomy 18 in cattle, which is associated with extreme brachygnathia in calves which die soon after birth (known as lethal brachygnathia trisomy syndrome or LBTS). Trisomies of several other small autosomes have been reported in cattle, and similar cases have been observed in horses (Appendix 4.1). Autosomal trisomics often have severe abnormalities, resulting in early death. However, some cases have survived to adulthood.

All of the occurrences of autosomal trisomy in domestic animals (and in humans) involve small chromosomes; trisomics for large autosomes, and monosomics for any autosome have not been observed in living animals or humans. The absence of monosomics is somewhat surprising, because non-disjunction gives rise to equal numbers of gametes with an extra chromosome and gametes lacking a chromosome. Evidence in mice indicates that equal numbers of trisomic and monosomic embryos are produced at fertilization, and remain alive at least until the late morula or early blastocyst stage (day 3 in the mouse). Thereafter, the frequency of monosomics relative to trisomics decreases, and no monosomics remain alive beyond days 12–13.

This introduces us to the second major effect of chromosomal abnormalities, namely the loss of embryos prior to birth. Surveys of embryos in animals have shown that approximately 7 per cent of all embryos have chromosomal abnormalities which are rarely, if ever, seen in animals after birth or hatching. Noting that approximately 30 per cent of all conceptions in animals are naturally aborted, we can conclude that around one-quarter of embryonic loss is due to chromosomal abnormalities.

Common among the chromosomal abnormalities seen in early-stage embryos are the presence of just one set of chromosomes (**haploidy**) or the presence of more than two sets (**triploidy**, **tetraploidy**, etc.; collectively called **polyploidy** if there is just one type of ploidy, or **mixoploidy** if there are mixtures of different ploidies). While most of these abnormalities are never seen in living animals after birth or hatching, there are reports of triploid adult chickens. Indeed, in Australia there is a line of chickens which regularly produces around 12 per cent live triploid chickens that survive to adulthood. However, the triploids that survive are only about 50 per cent of those that are hatched. In other words, even in this unusual case where triploids survive to adulthood, polyploidy decreases life expectancy.

The triploid individuals in the Australian line arise from a high frequency of non-disjunction in both meiosis I and meiosis II in the normal (fertile) diploid females of this line. It is interesting to consider the different combinations of sex chromosomes that could occur in triploids. WWW chickens are never seen, even as embryos, because the gametic contribution from any male parent has to contain a Z chromosome. ZWW embryos are seen, but none of these survive to hatching. ZZW chickens are particularly unusual. At hatching, their left gonad is an ovary containing oocytes, while their right gonad is a testis. Soon after hatching, the left gonad begins to develop testicular-like tissue. Externally, these chickens have a normal female appearance until they reach puberty, at which stage they undergo an apparent sex reversal, ending up looking like a normal mature male! By then, both gonads are producing abnormal sperm cells. These sex-reversed birds are still viable, but are sterile. The final category, namely ZZZ, have a normal male phenotype but produce abnormal sperm cells, and are sterile.

Summarizing the results described above, we can conclude that abnormal chromosomal numbers have a relatively high incidence among newly conceived zygotes, but have a relatively low incidence among individuals sampled after birth. Chromosomal abnormalities, therefore, are an important cause of embryonic loss.

## Induced polyploidy in fish

Unlike mammals, many species of fish can happily exist as polyploids. If normal diploid females are subjected to short treatments of heat or cold or pressure, some of their developing ova fail to undergo meiosis II, and therefore remain in a diploid state. When such ova are fertilized with normal (haploid) sperm, triploid offspring result. Because of their unusual chromosome complement, triploid fish are sterile. Their viability, however, is quite good. Their sterility is one of their main attractions; they can devote all of their energies to growth, without being sidetracked by reproduction, which not only reduces growth but also increases mortality in males. And there is some evidence that the extra level of ploidy in itself results in faster growth. However, being sterile, each new generation of triploids has to be produced from diploids, as described above. If triploids really are advantageous from the commercial fishery point of view, it would be of great benefit to be able to produce them without having to go to the trouble of the treatments described above. This can be achieved by first producing tetraploid stock, as follows.

If normal fertilized ova are subjected to the same short treatment as described above, one round of mitosis is suspended, resulting in tetraploid offspring, which are viable and fertile. (The fertility presumably arises from the fact that every chromosome can find a homologue with which to pair.) The attraction of fertile tetraploids is that their 'natural' gamete is diploid, which means that a mating between a tetraploid and a normal diploid produces triploid offspring. And since the tetraploids themselves are fertile, they are self-reproducing. In fish, therefore, polyploidy can be exploited as a means of increasing food production.

## Abnormal chromosome structure

### Reciprocal translocations

In Sweden in 1963, a Swedish Landrace boar served 21 sows and produced an average litter size of 5.6 piglets. In previous pregnancies when mated to other boars, the same sows had an average litter size of 12.7 piglets. The karyotype of this boar was examined, and, as shown in Fig. 4.2, it was found that part of

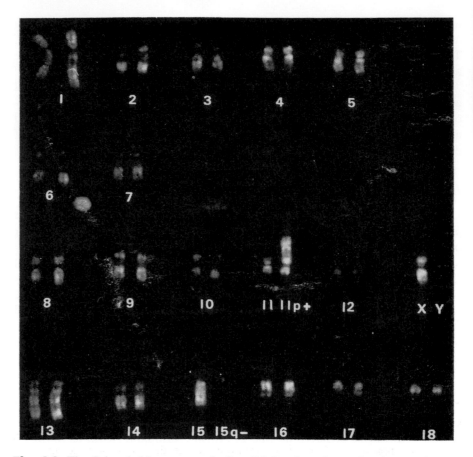

**Fig. 4.2** The Q-banded karyotype of a Swedish Landrace boar, showing a reciprocal translocation between chromosomes 11 and 15, which caused the boar to produce substantially smaller litters than other boars.

one chromosome had been interchanged with part of another, by a process called **reciprocal translocation**. This involves each of two non-homologous chromosomes breaking into two segments, followed by an exchange of segments between the two chromosomes.

In the translocation shown in Fig. 4.2, one chromosome 15 lacks most of its long arm and is therefore written as 15q−. And since the short arm of one chromosome 11 has been extended by the addition of the portion from 15, it is designated 11p+. The translocation is written as t(11p+; 15q−) or rcp(11p+; 15q−). Because only one member of each pair of chromosomes is affected, the individual in Fig. 4.2 is said to be a **translocation heterozygote** or **translocation carrier**.

Many reciprocal translocations have been reported in domestic animals,

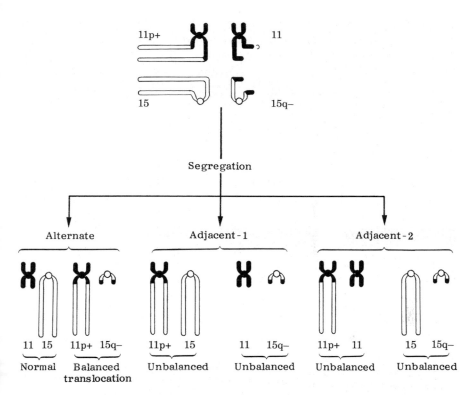

**Fig. 4.3** *Top*: quadrivalent formed by the synapsis of homologous segments of chromosomes 11 and 15 in an animal heterozygous for the reciprocal translocation t(11p+; 15q−). *Bottom*: the six possible outcomes from the quadrivalent, assuming there is no crossing-over between the centromere and the breakpoint, i.e. in interstitial segments.

including some that involve exchanges between three different chromosomes (Appendix 4.1). Animals carrying a reciprocal translocation have a normal phenotype, but show a significant reduction in fertility. The reason for the normal phenotype is that animals with a reciprocal translocation still have a normal complement of chromosomal material; it just happens to have been rearranged. The decrease in fertility arises from the problem faced during meiosis I in these animals. In normal circumstances, as we saw in Chapter 1, pairs of homologous chromosomes synapse to form bivalents. But in animals heterozygous for a reciprocal translocation, as shown in Fig. 4.3, four chromosomal structures have to come together in order to enable all homologous regions to synapse. This combination of four chromosomes is called a **quadrivalent**. There are many possible outcomes of disjunction from a quadrivalent, depending on how close the breakpoints are to the centromeres, and on the type of disjunction. Some of the outcomes are shown in Fig. 4.3; full details are given in Section 4.3.2.1 of *Veterinary genetics*. In summary, we can say that in many cases, at least some unbalanced gametes are produced, containing either one or more additional chromosome segments, or lacking some segments. Most unbalanced gametes are able to function quite well as ova or sperm cells. But when an unbalanced gamete combines with another gamete to form a zygote, that zygote is unbalanced, and dies before term. Thus, unbalanced gametes result in embryonic death. In theory, the resultant reduction in fecundity can range from zero through to 100 per cent, depending on the factors mentioned above. In practice, there is always a substantial reduction in fecundity.

The importance of this reduction in fecundity is that it is an inherited defect: it is passed on from parents to offspring. This is because one-half of the balanced gametes resulting from meiosis contain translocation chromosomes, which, when combined with a normal gamete, result in another translocation heterozygote. Thus, among the offspring produced by a translocation heterozygote, one-half are translocation heterozygotes.

Finally, if two gametes carrying balanced translocation chromosomes unite, a translocation homozygote results, with pairs of chromosomes that are exactly homologous and which consequently form only bivalents during meiosis. Thus, animals that are homozygous for reciprocal translocations produce only balanced gametes and therefore show normal fecundity.

## Tandem translocations

Occasionally there are reports of part of the arm of one chromosome breaking off and joining onto the end of another chromosome. This is called a **tandem translocation**. In domestic animals, this type of translocation is quite a rarity compared with reciprocal translocations. Those that have been reported are listed in Appendix 4.1.

## Centric fusions and fissions

A type of translocation that has generated considerable interest is one in which two acrocentric chromosomes fuse to produce one metacentric chromosome. This is known as a **centric fusion** or **Robertsonian translocation** (Fig. 4.4). It contains all of the genetic material previously present in the two separate chromosomes.

Since centric fusions involve the replacement of two chromosomes by one, it follows that the total number of separate chromosomes in individuals heterozygous for a centric fusion is one less than the normal number (Fig. 4.4). However, unlike monosomics, which also have one less than the normal number of chromosomes, individuals heterozygous for a centric fusion have a complete genome and hence have normal phenotypes. Individuals that are homozygous for a centric fusion have two less than the normal number of chromosomes, but they too have normal phenotypes because they still have a complete genome.

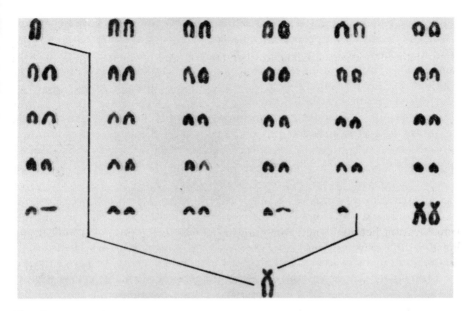

**Fig. 4.4** An unbanded karyotype of a Swedish Red and White cow that is hetero-zygous for a centric fusion translocation between chromosomes 1 and 29.

What is the effect of centric fusions on reproductive ability? Meiosis in individuals heterozygous for a centric fusion is certainly unusual, because three chromosomes have to synapse, forming a **trivalent**, as shown in Fig. 4.5. If the centric-fusion chromosome disjoins from the other two, balanced gametes result. Any other type of disjunction leads to unbalanced gametes which would be expected to lead to aneuploid embryos. In practice, results

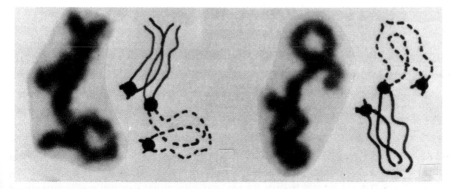

**Fig. 4.5** Two examples of trivalents in meiosis I in rams heterozygous for a centric fusion between chromosomes 9 and 12.

vary substantially. In cattle, most centric fusions have an adverse effect, giving rise to a varying proportion of monosomic and trisomic embryos that fail to survive to term. In sheep, there seems to be no adverse effect. The most likely explanation for this difference is that unbalanced gametes fail to function in sheep, whereas they do function in cattle. It is still an open question as to why this should be so.

Occasionally, a metacentric chromosome splits into two acrocentrics, i.e. there is a **centric fission**, producing an animal having one additional chromosome, but not being trisomic. This has been reported in the donkey (Appendix 4.1).

## Inversions and deletions

As their name suggests, inversions arise when a segment of chromosome becomes inverted following breakage of a chromosome in two positions. If the segment includes the centromere, the inversion is said to be **pericentric**; if the centromere is not included, the inversion is **paracentric**. Deletions arise if, following the breakage of a chromosome in two positions, the segment between the two breakpoints is lost. It is obvious that inversions give rise to the realignment of genes on a chromosome, and deletions result in the loss of genetic material.

Inversions and deletions are the least frequently observed of chromosomal abnormalities in domestic animals, and only isolated cases have been reported (Appendix 4.1). Deletions usually produce serious abnormalities, as the individual is monosomic for the segment of chromosome deleted. In contrast, because inversions involve the rearrangement of existing genes without any loss or addition, individuals carrying inversions usually have a normal phenotype. Furthermore, inversions are not always easy to detect in karyotypes. A chromosome with a paracentric inversion, for example, has exactly the same shape and size as a normal chromosome. It may, however, differ in banding pattern, and as banding techniques become more sophisticated, so too will more inversions be detected.

## Isochromosomes

This type of chromosomal abnormality arises when the centromere of a metacentric chromosome splits transversely (i.e. perpendicular to the chromatids) rather than longitudinally (i.e. parallel to the chromatids), during mitosis or meiosis. This leaves two identical chromatid arms joined to the one centromere, so that each arm contains exactly the same set of genes, in the same centromere-to-telomere order. The resultant structure is called an **isochromosome**. Each transverse split of a centromere gives rise to two isochromosomes (one corresponding to the p arm of the original chromosome, and the other corresponding to the q arm). However, sometimes one of the products of the split is lost, especially if the centromere splits unequally. There have been isolated reports of isochromosomes in animals. For example, an infertile heifer which was a mosaic for sex-chromosome aneuploidy, also had an isochromosome Y in a proportion of her cells.

## *Fragile sites*

If certain substances, such as caffeine or aphidicolin, are added to the cell culture from which karyotypes are being prepared, partial gaps appear at particular sites on some chromosomes. Known as **fragile sites**, these gaps are inherited in a Mendelian manner. In dogs, for example, there are three fragile sites on the X chromosome, at Xp22, Xq21, and Xq27.2. Interestingly, each of these sites corresponds to a fragile site on the human X chromosome. For many years, fragile sites in human chromosomes have been known as sites where chromosomal rearrangements often occur in certain types of cancer, or have been associated with various inherited defects. Some of the fragile sites in pigs correspond to sites where breakage and reunion has occurred in reciprocal translocations. The Xq27.2 fragile site in humans (which is associated with mental retardation) is actually an unstable trinucleotide repeat (described in Chapter 3). It is quite likely that fragile sites in animals will be shown to be due to unstable trinucleotide repeats, and to be associated with various chromosomal aberrations and inherited diseases.

## Chromosomal aberrations in cancer

A wide spectrum of chromosomal aberrations has been recorded in cancerous tissue, including aneuploidy, polyploidy, translocations, centric fusions, deletions, and isochromosomes. In most cases, the abnormalities are a consequence of the lack of control of cell division that is characteristic of cancer cells.

## Evolution of karyotypes

Despite the wide range of chromosome numbers in different species, the total amount of DNA in each cell in all mammals is almost identical. In fact, the evolution of modern mammals has been associated with much rearrangement and shuffling of the same total amount of DNA. One of the most common forms of shuffling appears to have been centric fusion. For example, the metacentric chromosomes (1, 2, and 3) in the domestic sheep appear to be the result of centric fusion of acrocentrics 1 and 3, 2 and 7, and 5 and 10, respectively, of the goat.

Bearing this in mind, it is interesting to compare the total number of chromosome arms in different species. If chromosomal evolution has proceeded largely by the accumulation of centric fusions, we would expect to find that the total number of major chromosome arms (called the **Nombre Fonda-mental** or **NF**) should be fairly constant across species. In many situations, this is indeed so. Within the superfamily Bovoidea, for example, the diploid number varies from 30 to 60, but the NF in all but three cases varies only from 58 to 62.

Furthermore, there is extremely close resemblance in banding patterns within chromosome arms of sheep, goats and cattle. And we have already seen in Chapter 2 that there is considerable similarity in the gene maps between species. In other words, the chromosome structure within arms is also conserved.

## Interspecific hybridization

An appreciation of the differences in karyotype among species is necessary for an understanding of the results of matings between members of different species. These matings are known as interspecific hybridizations. At one extreme, the result is an unsuccessful fertilization which is reflected in a failure of the female parent to conceive. At the other extreme is the produc-tion of viable, fertile offspring. In between are all possible combinations of success and failure. This is exactly what we would expect from the fact that the concept of species is an artificial human contrivance by which we attempt to categorize into discrete units what is in reality a continuum. In most cases, the result of interspecific hybridization is primarily determined by the degree of similarity between the chromosomes of the two species, rather than the degree of physical resemblance.

This last point can sometimes be the source of considerable frustration in attempts to save a species by bringing together animals that come from different areas. Even if the animals closely resemble each other, and thus appear to belong to exactly the same species, it is possible that they differ sufficiently at the chromosome level for there to be only a low chance of a viable, fertile offspring being produced. Other aspects of captive breeding programmes are discussed in Chapter 13.

## Freemartins

As long ago as the first century BC, it was known that most female calves born co-twin to a male are sterile. Such females are called **freemartins**. The same condition has since been recognized in other species, and the term freemartin is now used to describe sterile females born co-twin to a male in any species. In the following discussion, we shall concentrate mainly on cattle, because freemartins occur much more commonly in cattle than in any other species.

If an individual receives cells from another individual, it has two populations of cells, each derived from a different source. Such individuals are said to be **chimeric**. In the case of freemartins, there is a fusion of chorions of the two embryos, and anastomosis of their blood vessels (called **vascular anastomosis**). The result is an exchange of haemopoietic cells which remain active for the remainder of each animal's life. Thus, each member of the twin pair is chimeric for erythrocytes and for leucocytes. This in turn means that each member exhibits its own blood groups (see Chapter 8) plus those of its co-twin. Since chromosomes are readily visible in leucocytes (as described in Chapter 1), it follows that in unlike-sex twins, the two populations of leucocytes are readily distinguishable according to their sex chromosomes: those derived originally from male haemopoietic cells are XY, and those derived originally from female haemopoietic cells are XX. The existence of these two readily observable different populations of leucocytes in unlike-sex twins is called **XX/XY chimerism**. A wide range of proportions of XX leucocytes in unlike-sex twins has been reported, ranging from 1 per cent to 100 per cent, with an average of approximately 50 per cent.

We are accustomed to thinking of the karyotype of leucocytes as indicating the karyotype of all other cells in an individual. But in twins whose chorions were fused, this is not so. Indeed, erythrocytes and leucocytes are the only cells for which there is convincing evidence of chimerism following vascular anastomosis; all other cells in female twins are XX, and all other cells in male twins are XY. Similarly, blood-cell chimerism can cause confusion when genotyping individuals using either biochemical or DNA technologies, because the blood cells may show the genotype of the individual's twin, as well as its own genotype (see Chapter 11). Obviously, if the twins are identical, this presents no problem. But if the twins are not identical (i.e. if they are dizygotic), considerable confusion can result, especially if it is not realized that the individual was born as a twin. Of course, the problem can be avoided by using some tissue other than blood cells.

The final result of vascular anastomosis is homograft tolerance, which is the ability of a co-twin to accept a graft of skin or other tissue from its fellow co-twin without showing any signs of rejection. The practical implication of this phenomenon is that in cattle, where vascular anastomosis is common, skin grafting cannot be used to distinguish between monozygous and dizygous twins.

In females that are born co-twin to a male, the major effects are seen in the gonads and in the reproductive tract. Until day 60 of foetal life in cattle, the female gonads appear to be developing normally. Thereafter, development is 'masculinized' to an extent that varies considerably from female to female. At one extreme, the gonads sometimes develop into apparently normal ovaries that are capable of ovulation. At the other extreme, the gonads sometimes develop into miniature testes. In most cases, the result is that one or both gonads are classified as ovatestes, containing both ovarian and testicular tissue. The external genitalia are usually the same as those for normal females, except for the clitoris, which is often enlarged. Internally, there tends to be repression of the Mullerian duct derivatives (Fallopian tubes, uterus, cervix, and upper portion of the vagina) and over-development of Wolffian duct derivatives (epididymis, vas deferens, and seminal vesicle). Depending on the extent of alteration from normal development, the internal reproductive tract varies from more-or-less normal female to more-or-less normal male; some females have a normal vagina, cervix, and uterus, while at the other extreme, some have a blind vagina together with vasa deferentia and seminal vesicles instead of a cervix and uterus. All intermediate combinations are possible. Unfortunately, the extent of masculinization is not correlated with the proportion of XY leucocytes in the female co-twin.

Vascular anastomosis between unlike-sex twins has little, if any, effect on the structure of male gonads and reproductive tracts; their structure is essentially normal. There is, however, an effect on reproductive ability, with decreased sperm motility and sperm concentration leading to a 10-fold increase in the chance of a bull born co-twin to a female being culled for poor reproductive performance.

The probability of vascular anastomosis occurring between cattle twins is very high, being approximately 90 per cent. Since vascular anastomosis almost invariably leads to sterility of the female in unlike-sex twins, it follows that approximately 90 per cent of all female calves born co-twin to a male are freemartins.

Freemartins have been reported in red deer, goats, pigs, sheep and Rocky Mountain bighorn sheep but in each case, the incidence is much lower than in cattle. In sheep, for example, exchange of cells occurs in only about 1 per cent of twins. In other species such as horses, exchange of cells between embryos is common, but the resultant chimerism does not lead to infertility. The reasons for these differences are not known.

The most effective way to check whether a young female calf born co-twin to a male is likely to be a freemartin, is to search for XX/XY chimerism. Since some freemartins have only a small proportion of XY leucocytes, it is obvious that the efficiency of this diagnosis increases with the number of cells scored from each suspect female. Taking account of the observed distribution of XY leucocytes in freemartins, the general recommendation is to score around 200 cells. Of course, as soon as the first XY cell is spotted, the counting can stop. More recently, molecular techniques have been developed for diagnosis of freemartins. For example, Southern analysis with a cloned fragment from the Y chromosome, or PCR amplification of a segment of the Y chromosome, can be used to detect XY cells.

## Biological basis of sex

We saw in Chapter 1 that sex is inherited in a simple Mendelian manner, determined by the presence or absence of a Y chromosome. Until recently, the way in which the Y chromosome exerts its vital influence was not known. In 1990, however, Andrew Sinclair and colleagues showed that the male-producing effect of the Y chromosome is due to a gene which they called *SRY*, for sex-determining region of the Y chromosome. *SRY* is located on the short arm of the Y chromosome, quite near to the pseudo-autosomal region (described in Chapter 1). The importance of the *SRY* gene is that it appears to provide the initial signal which causes the undifferentiated gonad in an embryo to develop into a testis rather than an ovary. The exact nature of this signal has still to be worked out, but the polypeptide product of the *SRY* gene is a DNA-binding protein, which is consistent with its apparent role as a regulator, being able to start a whole series of developmental steps resulting in the formation of a testis.

While there is still much to be learned about *SRY* and other genes involved in sexual development, the general principle is that female is the 'default' sex. In other words, if the undifferentiated gonad does not receive any message from the *SRY* gene, it develops as an ovary, whose hormones result in female secondary sexual characteristics. If the *SRY* gene does send its message, the undifferentiated gonad develops into a testis, whose hormones result in male secondary sexual characteristics.

## *XX males and XY females*

Occasionally there are reports of phenotypic males with an XX karyotype and phenotypic females with an XY karyotype. In most cases, molecular inspection shows that one of the X chromosomes of XX males has a very small insertion from the Y chromosome (which includes the *SRY* gene). XY females have several possible causes. In some cases, their Y chromosome has a small deletion, including the *SRY* gene. In other cases, they could have a mutant *SRY* allele that results in a deficiency of SRY polypeptide. In either case, in the absence of the message from the *SRY* gene, these individuals develop ovaries, which (as described above) then give rise to female secondary sexual characteristics. Some XY females, however, have a normal *SRY* gene, but lack the receptor for the male hormones (androgens) produced by the testes. This means that the only hormones that can exert any influence on secondary sexual development are the small quantities of female hormones produced by the testes. The result is that these XY individuals develop all the secondary sexual characteristics of females, despite having testes rather than ovaries. This particular defect is called testicular feminization. Since the gene for the androgen receptor is located on the X chromosome, testicular feminization is an X-linked defect. It has been reported in cats, cattle, horses, and sheep, as well as in humans.

## Classification of intersex

It is evident from this chapter that there is a continuing occurrence of **intersex** individuals, i.e. individuals having various mixtures of maleness and femaleness. Several terms are used to classify intersexes. One is **hermaphrodite**. In its broadest sense, this term is synonymous with intersex as just defined. However, it is sometimes used in a narrower sense to indicate the presence of both ovarian and testicular tissue. Such individuals are often called **true hermaphrodites**, to distinguish them from **pseudohermaphrodites**, which are intersexes having either ovarian or testicular tissue, but not both. If only ovarian tissue is present, the intersex is called a **female pseudohermaphrodite**, whereas if only testicular tissue is present, the term male **pseudohermaphrodite** is used.

A very useful way to classify intersex is according to the stage at which the abnormality of sexual development occurs. This gives rise to the following three categories:

1. Chromosomal intersex: animals whose abnormal sexual development is caused by abnormalities in sex chromosomes. It includes all the cases of sex-chromosome abnormalities discussed in this chapter.

2. Gonadal intersex: individuals having either a normal male or a normal female karyotype, but with gonads that do not correspond to the chromosomal sex. Included in this category are XX and XY individuals with ovatestes, XX individuals with testes only, and XY individuals with ovaries only. Freemartins fit into this category because the vast majority of their cells are XX. Also included in this category are cases of XX and XY individuals in which the gonads have failed to develop, a condition called gonadal dysgenesis.

3. Phenotypic intersex: individuals with normal chromosomal and gonadal sex, but with abnormalities in some or all of their reproductive tract and in other sexual characteristics. Testicular feminization fits into this category.

The final word on intersexuality must be left for the case of an intersex rabbit, which started life as a male, siring more than 250 offspring. It then lost interest in mating with females, and instead became pregnant to itself, giving birth to a litter of three males and four females, which it raised quite successfully on its own milk. We can conclude that just about anything is possible in the realm of intersexuality.

## A sample of chromosomal aberrations

Just as with single-gene disorders in Chapter 3, it is possible to draw up a sample list of chromosomal aberrations that have been reported in animals. Such a list is presented in Appendix 4.1. It is not complete, but it does provide an overview of the range of different abnormalities that do occur.

# Further reading

## Chromosomal aberrations

Chastain, C. B. (1992). Pediatric cytogenetics. *Compendium on Continuing Education for the Practicing Veterinarian*, **14**, 333–41.

Cribiu, E. P. (1992). Cytogenetics and pathology in horse. *Recueil de Medecine Veterinaire*, **168**, 1005–10.

Fechheimer, N. S. (1990). The domestic chicken (*Gallus domesticus*) as an organism for the study of chromosomal aberrations. *Journal of Animal Breeding and Genetics*, **S5**, 43–54.

Long, S. E. (1991). Reciprocal translocations in the pig (*Sus scrofa*): a review. *Veterinary Record*, **128**, 275–8.

McFeely, R. A. (1993). Chromosome abnormalities. *Veterinary Clinics of North America—Food Animal Practice*, **9**, (1), 11–22.

Nie, G. J., Momont, H. W., and Buoen, L. (1993). A survey of sex chromosome abnormalities in 204 mares selected for breeding. *Journal of Equine Veterinary Science*, **13**, 456–9.

Popescu, C. P. and Pech, A. (1991). Cattle 1/29 translocation in the world (1964–1990)—a review. *Annales de Zootechnie*, **40**, 271–305.

## Induced polyploidy in fish

Mair, G. C. (1993). Chromosome-set manipulation in Tilapia—techniques, problems and prospects. *Aquaculture*, **111**, 227–44.

Ozoufcostaz, C. and Foresti, F. (1992). Fish cytogenetic research—advances, applications and perspectives. *Netherlands Journal of Zoology*, **42**, 277–90.

Thorgaard, G. H. (1992). Application of genetic technologies to rainbow trout. *Aquaculture*, **100**, 85–97.

## Fragile sites

Yang, M. Y. and Long, S. E. (1993). Folate sensitive common fragile sites in chromosomes of the domestic pig (*Sus scrofa*). *Research in Veterinary Science*, **55**, 231–5.

Stone, D. M. and Stephens, K. E. (1993). Bromodeoxyuridine induces chromosomal fragile sites in the canine genome. *American Journal of Medical Genetics*, **46**, 198–202.

## Cancer

Schnurr, M. W., Carter, R. F., Dube, I. D., Valli, V. E., and Jacobs, R. M. (1994). Nonrandom chromosomal abnormalities in bovine lymphoma. *Leukemia Research*, **18**, 91–9.

## Evolution of karyotypes

Gallagher, D. S. and Womack, J. E. (1992). Chromosome conservation in the bovidae. *Journal of Heredity*, **83**, 287–98.

Robinson, T. J. and Elder, F. F. B. (1993). Cytogenetics—its role in wildlife management and the genetic conservation of mammals. *Biological Conservation*, **63**, 47–51.

## Freemartins

Khan, M. Z. and Foley, G. L. (1994). Retrospective studies on the measurements, karyotyping and pathology of reproductive organs of bovine freemartins. *Journal of Comparative Pathology*, **110**, 25–36.

## Sex determination

Bogan, J. S. and Page, D. C. (1994). Ovary—testis—a mammalian dilemma. *Cell*, **76**, 603–7.

Goodfellow, P. N. and Lovell-Badge, R. (1993). SRY and sex determination in mammals. *Annual Review of Genetics*, **27**, 71–92.

Gustafson, M. L. and Donahoe, P. K. (1994). Male sex determination—current concepts of male sexual differentiation. *Annual Review of Medicine*, **45**, 505–24.

Halverson, J. L. and Dvorak, J. (1993). Genetic control of sex determination in birds and the potential for its manipulation. *Poultry Science*, **72**, 890–6.

Meyers-Wallen, V. N. (1993). Genetics of sexual differentiation and anomalies in dogs and cats. *Journal of Reproduction and Fertility*, **Suppl. 47**, 441–52.

Wachtel, S. S. (ed.) (1993). *Molecular genetics of sex determination*. Academic Press, San Diego.

## Intersex

Frankenhuis, M. T., Smith-Buijs, C. M. C., de Boer, L. E. M., and Kloosterboer, J. W. (1990). A case of combined hermaphroditism and autofertilisation in a domestic rabbit. *Veterinary Record*, **126**, 598–9.

## Appendix 4.1 A sample of chromosomal aberrations in animals

(An updated catalogue is accessible via World Wide Web on the Internet at: http//morgan.angis.su.oz.au/)

**Aneuploidy of sex chromosomes**

| | |
|---|---|
| XO | buffalo, cat, dog, pig, horse, sheep |
| XXX | cattle, dog, horse, buffalo |
| XXY | cat, cattle, dog, pig, sheep |
| XXXY | horse, pig |
| XXXXY | horse |

**Aneuploidy of autosomes**

| | |
|---|---|
| trisomy 12, trisomy 16, trisomy 17, trisomy 18, trisomy 20, trisomy 22, trisomy 23, trisomy 24 | cattle |

# **Appendix 4.1** *Continued*

---

| | |
|---|---|
| trisomy 23, trisomy 26, trisomy 28, trisomy 30 | horse |

**Ploidy**
| | |
|---|---|
| triploidy | chicken |

**Translocation, reciprocal**
| | |
|---|---|
| 1/8/9, 8/13, 8/15, 10/11, 20/24, Y/17 | cattle |
| 1/4, Z/1, Z/microchromosome | chicken |
| 1/3 | horse |
| 1/6, 1/7, 1/8, 1/11, 1/14, 1/15, 1/16, 1/17, 2/4, 2/4/15, 2/14, 3/7, 4/13, 4/14, 5/8, 5/14, 5/15, 6/14, 6/15, 7/11, 7/12, 7/13, 7/17, 8/14, 9/11, 11/15, 13/14, 13/17, 14/15, 15/16, 16/17, X/13, X/14 | pig |
| 1/20, 13/20, 23/24 | sheep |

**Translocation, tandem**
| | |
|---|---|
| 1/16, 1/18, X/23 | cattle |
| X/15 | horse |

**Translocation, centric fusions**
| | |
|---|---|
| 23/24 | blue fox |
| 1/4, 1/21, 1/23, 1/26, 1/28, 1/29, 2/4, 3/27, 4/4, 4/8, 5/18, 5/23, 5/26, 6/28, 7/12, 7/21, 8/9, 9/23, 11/21, 11/22, 13/21, 14/20, 14/21, 14/28, 15/25, 16/18, 21/27, 27/29 | cattle |
| 1/31, 13/23, 21/33 | dog |
| 6/15 | goat |
| 1/20, 6/26, 7/25, 8/11 | sheep |
| 13/17 | pig |

**Centric fission**
| | |
|---|---|
| 3 | donkey |

**Deletion**
| | |
|---|---|
| X | horse |

**Insertion**
| | |
|---|---|
| 16 | cattle |

**Inversion, paracentric**
| | |
|---|---|
| 8 | pig |

**Inversion, pericentric**
| | |
|---|---|
| 14, X | cattle |
| 2 | chicken |

**Isochromosome**
| | |
|---|---|
| Y | cattle |

**Sex reversal**
| | |
|---|---|
| XX male | dog, goat, horse, llama, pig |
| XY female | cat, cattle, horse, sheep |

---

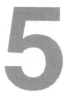

# 5 Single genes in populations

Most single-gene disorders are rare and consequently are not cause for great concern. Occasionally, however, a disorder due to a single gene reaches a high frequency among the animals belonging to one or a few breeders, or sometimes within a breed as a whole. The economic consequences of such an increase in frequency are sometimes quite severe, and breeders often ask how the disorder can be decreased in frequency, if not eliminated. In order to give useful advice, we need to know more than just simple Mendelian genetics; we must also understand the way in which genes behave within a herd or flock or kennel or cattery, or within a breed as a whole. In other words, we need to understand the basic principles of population genetics. The aim of this chapter is to explain those basic principles.

## Gene and genotype frequencies

Haemoglobin in sheep exists in two different forms (HbA and HbB), which are the products of two different alleles, $A$ and $B$, at an autosomal locus. With two different haemoglobin alleles, there are three different possible genotypes ($AA$, $AB$, and $BB$), each of which produces a distinctive protein electrophoretic pattern, as shown in Fig. 5.1. Thus for each genotype there is a distinguishable phenotype. Blood samples were taken from a flock of 175 sheep, and after electrophoresis to determine haemoglobin type for each sheep, it was found that the numbers of the genotypes were 91, 28, and 56 for $AA$, $AB$, and $BB$ respectively. Given this information, it is possible to

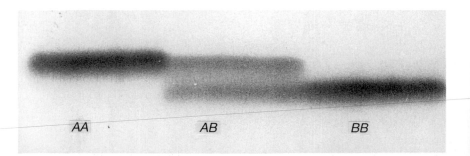

AA          AB          BB

**Fig. 5.1** The electrophoretic patterns, or phenotypes, corresponding to the three different haemoglobin genotypes in Merino sheep.

calculate the proportions of each genotype in the sample. These proportions are called **genotype frequencies**. For this particular example, they turn out to be 91/175 = 0.52 for $AA$, 28/175 = 0.16 for $AB$, and 56/175 = 0.32 for $BB$.

It is also possible to calculate the proportions, i.e. frequencies, of each allele in the sample. By convention, the term 'gene' is used instead of 'allele' in population genetics, when referring to frequencies. The proportions of each allele are therefore called **gene frequencies**.

Since all of the genes in the $AA$ animals are $A$, and half the genes in $AB$ animals are $A$, it follows that the gene frequency of $A$ is the frequency of the $AA$ genotype plus half the frequency of the $AB$ genotype, which equals 0.52 + ½(0.16) = 0.6. Similarly, the gene frequency of $B$ is 0.32 + ½(0.16) = 0.4.

## Random mating

Random mating for a particular trait or locus occurs when the choice of a mating partner is independent of the genotype or phenotype for that trait or locus. Since the breeding of domestic animals is largely under the control of humans, who often decide, for example, to select only a small proportion of individuals to be parents of the next generation, it might be thought that the concept of random mating is largely irrelevant to domestic animals. However, even though selection can be quite intense, mating is usually at random for all traits and loci, *among those animals that have been selected*. In fact, in production species such as cattle, sheep and pigs, it is usually impractical to arrange any other type of mating. And even with companion animals, in deciding which animals to mate to which, humans base their decision on only a relatively small number of traits such as coat colour or various aspects of conformation.

For those traits that are taken into account by humans when matings are being planned, mating is often not random. For most other traits, however, mating is usually at random.

In most situations, for example, mating is at random with respect to blood groups, because these are usually not known. For many single-gene disorders, too, mating among animals that survive to reproductive age is random, because for many such disorders, the different genotypes among survivors all give rise to the same phenotype. Thus the concept of random mating is very important in populations of domestic animals.

## The Hardy–Weinberg law

The Hardy–Weinberg law is a remarkable theory that is extremely useful in enabling us to understand what happens to gene frequencies and genotype frequencies in real populations. The law can be derived by observing what happens to gene and genotype frequencies in any population of animals that goes through one generation of random mating (see *Veterinary genetics*, Section 5.4.1 and Appendix A5.1). When this is done, the following conclusions become evident:

*In a random mating population in which there is no selection, mutation, migration, or genetic drift,*
  *(1) genotype frequencies in offspring are determined solely by gene frequencies in parents, such that*
     *(a) the frequency of homozygotes equals the square of the relevant gene frequency;*
     *(b) the frequency of heterozygotes equals twice the product of the relevant gene frequencies;*
  *(2) gene frequencies and genotype frequencies remain constant from one generation to the next.*

These statements are known as the **Hardy–Weinberg law**. The practical implications of the law are best seen if we express its main conclusions in simple algebra. We can do this by considering just two genes at a locus (e.g. *A* and *B* from the sheep haemoglobin example), and writing their frequencies as *p* and *q*. These frequencies can each have any value from zero to one, providing that the combined frequency of the two genes is one, i.e. $p + q = 1$. The first part of the law says that irrespective of the genotype frequencies in the parents, one generation of random mating results in genotype frequencies of $p^2$, $2pq$, and $q^2$ for *AA*, *AB*, and *BB*, respectively. The second part of the law says that if we worked through another generation (and another and another, etc.), we would discover that *p* and *q* remain the same, and that the genotype frequencies remain the same, namely $p^2$, $2pq$, and $q^2$. These are known as the **Hardy–Weinberg frequencies**.

Some of the assumptions require explanation. The assumption of no selection means that each genotype has an equal opportunity to contribute offspring, and each offspring has an equal opportunity to survive until it has an opportunity to mate. The assumption of no migration means that genes do not enter the population from outside—the population is closed. Genetic drift refers to changes in gene frequency that are due to chance (see later in this chapter). The assumption of no genetic drift means that the number of parents is sufficiently large, and the number of offspring is sufficiently large, that chance fluctuations in gene frequency are negligible.

The part of the Hardy–Weinberg law that makes a specific prediction about the relationship between gene and genotype frequencies is often tested by comparing the observed numbers of each genotype in a population, with the numbers expected if the genotypes occur in Hardy–Weinberg frequencies. Despite the large number of assumptions in the law, it turns out that most populations have Hardy–Weinberg frequencies of genotypes. In other words, despite the fact that selection, migration, mutation, and genetic drift are known to occur in almost all populations, Hardy–Weinberg frequencies of genotypes are usually observed. How can this be? The answer is that the test for Hardy–Weinberg frequencies cannot detect mutation, and it fails to detect many cases of selection, migration, and genetic drift. As we shall see below, this is a very fortunate situation, because it means that for most populations, we can safely assume that Hardy–Weinberg frequencies exist, which in turn enables us to draw conclusions that have very important practical implications.

## The special case for recessives

The Hardy–Weinberg law applies irrespective of the type of gene action at the locus in question. In fact, so long as there is no selection, the type of gene action at a locus has no effect on the frequency of genes or genotypes. For example, it is clear from the second part of the Hardy–Weinberg law that recessive traits will neither decrease nor increase in frequency from one generation to the next, unless selection, mutation, migration, or genetic drift acts in such a way as to alter the frequency of the recessive gene. In fact, recessive traits can have a frequency anywhere in the range zero to one, depending solely on the frequency of the recessive gene.

Let us now examine the recessive case more closely, using coat colour in Angus cattle as an example. The typical black coat colour seen in Angus cattle is due to a dominant allele $B$, while the red coat colour seen occasionally in the same breed is due to homozygosity for a recessive allele $b$. Because there are two alleles at this locus in Angus cattle, there are three genotypes ($BB$, $Bb$, and $bb$). However, because $B$ is completely dominant to $b$, the genotypes $BB$ and $Bb$ have exactly the same phenotype, namely black. In general, for traits determined by dominant and recessive alleles, it is not possible to deduce the genotype of all animals simply from their phenotype. We cannot, therefore, calculate gene frequencies as in the case where all genotypes are identifiable. We can, however, distinguish red ($bb$) from black ($B-$, where the dash indicates either $B$ or $b$). In order to estimate gene frequencies, we make use of the general principle discussed in the previous section, namely that for the majority of loci, most populations have Hardy–Weinberg frequencies of genotypes, which means that the genotypes at a single locus with two alleles are in the proportions $p^2$, $2pq$, and $q^2$. Applying this to the case of red versus black in Angus cattle, and letting $q$ be the frequency of $b$, we have the following situation:

| Genotype | $BB$ | $Bb$ | $bb$ |
|---|---|---|---|
| Phenotype | Black | Black | Red |
| Frequency | $p^2$ | $2pq$ | $q^2$ |

It is obvious that the frequency of red Angus equals $q^2$, which is the square of the gene frequency of $b$. The gene frequency of $b$ can therefore be estimated as the square-root of the frequency of red calves.

For example, the frequency of red calves in pedigree Angus herds in the USA is approximately 5 per 1000. Assuming Hardy–Weinberg frequencies, the estimate of the gene frequency of $b$ is $\sqrt{(0.005)} = 0.07$. And since the only other allele at this locus is $B$, its frequency must be $1 - 0.07 = 0.93$.

We can now make one more interesting calculation. Since $p = 0.93$ and $q = 0.07$, it follows that the frequency of heterozygotes or carriers, which is $2pq$, equals $2 \times 0.93 \times 0.07 = 0.13$. Thus 13 per cent of Angus calves born in the USA are carriers of red. What proportion of black Angus are carriers? The answer is $2pq/(p^2 + 2pq)$, which equals $0.13/(0.86 + 0.13) = 0.13/0.99$, which equals 0.13.

This is a surprisingly high figure, but it is typical of the situation for all rare recessive traits, namely that the frequency of carriers is much higher than the frequency of the recessive trait itself.

Another example of a simple recessive trait is yellow coat colour in Labrador dogs, which is recessive to black. Since many dog breeders prefer yellow to black, the frequency of the yellow genotype ($ee$) is quite high in many populations. In one Australian population, for example, the frequency of yellow is approximately 64 per cent. Assuming Hardy–Weinberg frequencies, the gene frequency of $e$ in Australian Labradors must be $\sqrt{(0.64)} = 0.8$, which means that the frequency of the dominant allele must be only 0.2. This is a good illustration of the fact that recessive genes and recessive traits can be much higher in frequency than dominant genes and dominant traits.

## Extensions to the Hardy–Weinberg law

### Multiple alleles

There are three different forms of glucose 6-phosphate dehydrogenase (G6PD) in horses, corresponding to three alleles, $D$, $F$, and $S$ at the G6PD locus. Of course, any one horse can have at the most only two different alleles. But in a large sample of horses, all three alleles are likely to be found, and the frequency of each allele can be estimated.

If $p$, $q$, and $r$ represent the frequencies of the three alleles, the expected frequencies of the respective homozygotes are $p^2$, $q^2$, and $r^2$, and the respective heterozygotes have expected frequencies of $2pq$, $2qr$, and $2pr$. Using exactly the same principle, this prediction can be extended to any number of alleles at a locus.

### X-linked genes

As we saw in Chapter 1, X-linked genes have a different pattern of inheritance compared with autosomal genes. To understand the implications of this, consider the X-linked coat colour locus in cats, for which each genotype in each sex has a distinguishable phenotype. Many population surveys have been conducted on cats in many countries, and the results for X-linked coat colour from two such surveys are shown in Table 5.1.

**Table 5.1**  Combined results of two surveys taken in Iceland of X-linked coat colour in cats, together with calculations of gene frequencies in males and females

| Sex | Female | | | | Male | | |
|---|---|---|---|---|---|---|---|
| Phenotype | Non-orange | Tortoiseshell | Orange | Total | Non-orange | Orange | Total |
| Genotype | $oo$ | $Oo$ | $OO$ | | $o$ | $O$ | |
| Numbers | 117 | 53 | 3 | 173 | 149 | 28 | 177 |

Gene frequency of $o$ in females $= (2 \times 117 + 53)/(2 \times 173) = 0.83$
Gene frequency of $O$ in females $= (2 \times 3 + 53)/(2 \times 173) = 0.17$
Gene frequency of $o$ in males $= 149/177 = 0.84$
Gene frequency of $O$ in males $= 28/177 = 0.16$

Because males have only one X chromosome, they have only one gene (i.e. they are **hemizygous**) at all X-linked loci. This means that the frequency of each phenotype in males equals the frequency of the respective gene, so that the calculation of gene frequencies in males is very straightforward. In females, where there are three genotypes, gene frequencies can be calculated from first principles. It is evident from Table 5.1 that the gene frequencies in males and females are essentially the same, with average values of 0.835 for $o$ and 0.165 for $O$. Since the existence of the three genotypes in females is analogous to the general case for autosomal genes discussed earlier, it is tempting to see whether the female genotypes occur in Hardy—Weinberg frequencies. Using the average gene frequencies, expected genotype frequencies are $(0.835)^2$, 2 $\times 0.835 \times 0.165$, and $(0.165)^2$ for $oo$, $Oo$, and $OO$ respectively. With a total of 173 females in the sample in Table 5.1, this gives expected numbers of 120.6, 47.7, and 4.7, which agree very closely with the observed numbers of 117, 53, and 3 respectively. Thus the female genotypes occur in Hardy—Weinberg frequencies.

These results are typical of those obtained with X-linked genes, which means that it is usually safe to assume that X-linked gene frequencies are the same in males and females, and that X-linked female genotypes occur in Hardy—Weinberg frequencies. What are the practical implications of this conclusion? The most important implication is that X-linked traits are expected to occur with different frequencies in males and females. This is most relevant to X-linked recessive traits, for which the frequency of the trait in males ($q$) is expected to be much higher than the frequency of the trait in females ($q^2$). Notice that the square of $q$ is much smaller than $q$ because $q$ is always less than one. For example, if an X-linked recessive condition occurs with a frequency of 10 per cent in males ($q = 0.1$), its expected frequency in females is 1 per cent ($q^2 = (0.1)^2 = 0.01$).

Similar types of predictions can be made for any trait that is seen only in animals homozygous or hemizygous for an X-linked allele. For all such traits, the frequency in males (either $p$ or $q$) is greater than the frequency of the same trait in females (either $p^2$ or $q^2$ respectively). This simple observation can be used to great effect to make some money from a small bet: if, for example, the frequency of the $O$ gene is around 0.2, the expected frequency of orange males is 0.2, whereas the expected frequency of orange females is $(0.2)^2 = 0.04$. Thus the odds are 5:1 that the next orange cat you see will be a male. It is left to the reader to verify that the lower the gene frequency, the greater the odds.

## Selection and mutation

Selection acts on phenotypes, and occurs whenever some phenotypes have a greater opportunity to contribute offspring to the next generation than do other phenotypes. Selection may act at any stage during the life cycle of an animal from conception to mating.

Selection most commonly occurs through differential viability and/or differential reproductive ability, with reproductive ability including factors such as mating ability, fecundity and fertility. For convenience we shall refer to the combined effect of viability and reproductive ability as **fitness**. If selection occurs as a result of decisions made by humans it is called **artificial selection**, while in all other situations it is called **natural selection**. In either case, the principles by which selection operates are exactly the same. Although selection acts on phenotypes, we are mainly interested in its effect on genotypes and through them, on gene frequencies. Because of this interest, we often talk about selection acting on genotypes and on genes. Whenever we do this, however, we must remember that selection really acts only on individual animals according to their phenotype. The extent to which this affects genotypes and hence genes, depends on the extent to which particular phenotypes are associated with particular genotypes. In order to understand how selection works in practice, we shall start by considering the population of Labrador dogs mentioned earlier. Let us write the frequencies of the $E$ and $e$ genes as $p$ and $q$, respectively.

### Selection against a dominant

We have already noted that many Labrador breeders tend to favour yellow coat colour. This means that there is selection in favour of the recessive phenotype, which is the same thing as saying there is selection against the dominant phenotype. Let us represent this selection by saying that, relative to the fitness of genotype $ee$, the fitness of genotypes $EE$ and $Ee$ is reduced by a proportion $s$, where $s$ is called the **selection coefficient**. The so-called **relative fitnesses** of the three genotypes are then $1 - s$, $1 - s$, and 1 for $EE$, $Ee$, and $ee$

respectively. To obtain the genotype contributions after selection, we multiply the genotype frequency prior to selection (which will be the Hardy–Weinberg frequency) by the relative fitness:

|  | Genotype | | | |
| --- | --- | --- | --- | --- |
|  | $EE$ | $Ee$ | $ee$ | Total |
| Frequency prior to selection | $p^2$ | $2pq$ | $q^2$ | 1 |
| Relative fitness | $1 - s$ | $1 - s$ | 1 | |
| Proportion after selection | $p^2(1 - s)$ | $2pq(1 - s)$ | $q^2$ | $1 - sp(2 - p)$ |

What is the frequency of the $E$ gene after selection? Using exactly the same approach as earlier, this is the frequency of the $EE$ genotype plus ½ the frequency of the $Ee$ genotype, which is $p^2(1 - s) + ½ × 2pq(1 - s)$, all divided by the new total, namely $1 - sp(2 - p)$.

Now that we have an expression for the gene frequency after selection, we can calculate the change in gene frequency due to selection, $\Delta p$, which must equal the new gene frequency minus the previous gene frequency, which was simply $p$. When this expression is written out and simplified (as shown in *Veterinary Genetics*, Appendix A5.4.1), we end up with $\Delta p = - sp(1 - p)^2/\{1 - sp(2 - p)\}$. Among other things, this expression shows us that the change in gene frequency resulting from selection against a dominant phenotype depends on just two factors: the strength of selection (measured as $s$) and the gene frequency before selection. By substituting various values for these two parameters into the above equation, it can be seen that selection against a dominant phenotype can lead to quite substantial decreases in the frequency of the dominant gene. With strong selection, the gene is soon eliminated from the population. In the extreme case where selection is complete, i.e. no $EE$ or $Ee$ animals are able to contribute genes to the next generation, then $s = 1$, and the above expression reduces to $\Delta p = - p$, which means that the gene frequency after just one generation of selection will be zero. In other words, the $E$ gene will be eliminated from the population in just one generation, which is, of course, exactly what we would expect, since in this extreme situation, no $E$ genes are passed on to the next generation.

## Selection/mutation balance for a dominant

With the black gene removed from the population, we might expect that black dogs would never appear again, unless the gene for black was introduced from another population by migration. However, mutation occurs from time to time at all loci, and the effect of mutation in the present context is to alter occasionally a yellow gene, $e$, to a black gene, $E$.

We thus have two forces opposing each other: mutation is occasionally introducing dominant genes into the population, and selection is removing them. The result of these two opposing forces is that an equilibrium is reached, at which stage the number of mutant genes entering the population is the same as the number removed by selection, and the frequency of the dominant gene remains stable from generation to generation. This is called a **selection/mutation balance**. The smaller the effect of the dominant gene on fitness (the weaker selection is against it), the higher is the equilibrium frequency. Similarly, the greater the mutation rate, the greater is the equilibrium frequency. In fact, if $\mu$ is the mutation rate, then, as shown in Appendix A5.4.2 of *Veterinary genetics*, the frequency of a dominant gene at a mutation/selection balance is $\mu/s$, and the corresponding frequency of the dominant phenotype is $2\mu/s$.

To get some feel for what these expressions mean, consider a dominant trait that is subjected to only weak selection, say, $s = 0.05$; and let us take a common value for the mutation rate, say $\mu = 10^{-6} = 0.000001$. This gives the equilibrium gene frequency as 0.00002, and the corresponding phenotypic frequency as 0.00004, or 4 per 100 000, which is quite a low frequency. We can conclude that only very weak selection against a dominant gene is required to keep that gene at a very low frequency.

## Selection against a recessive

Suppose now that the Labrador breeders tend to favour black instead of yellow. In this case we have selection against the recessive gene for yellow, and selection in favour of the dominant gene for black.

Let us examine the effects of this type of selection for the general case, again using symbols.

Our approach is exactly the same as that taken in the previous section, except that now the relative fitnesses are 1, 1, and $1 - s$ for the three genotypes *EE*, *Ee*, and *ee* respectively. Readers are urged to work through one generation of this type of selection for themselves, and to check their results against those given in Appendix A5.4.3 of *Veterinary genetics*. It should be possible to show that the change of frequency of a recessive gene following one generation of selection against a recessive trait is $\Delta q = - sq^2(1 - q)/(1 - sq^2)$. Study of this equation shows that while selection against a recessive is effective at reducing gene frequency if the initial frequency is quite high, this type of selection becomes very ineffective at lower frequencies. In other words, selection against a recessive gene is a very inefficient means of removing that gene from a population. The reason for the decreasing effectiveness of selection against a recessive gene is that as the frequency of the gene decreases, an increasing proportion of recessive genes are 'hidden' from the effects of selection by occurring in heterozygotes. It follows, therefore, that selection against a recessive gene would be much more effective if heterozygotes could be detected.

If all heterozygotes were detected and then not used for breeding, all recessive genes would be removed from the population at once, and the frequency of the recessive gene would fall to zero. However, in practice there is no need to go to this extreme. As we shall see in Chapter 11, in order to eliminate recessive disorders from a population, all that has to be done is to prevent heterozygotes mating with other heterozygotes. This is the reason why so much research effort is being devoted to detection of heterozygotes in relation to recessive disorders. Notice that there is no requirement to destroy heterozygotes once detected. In fact, they could still be used for breeding, provided that no two heterozygotes were ever mated together. In this way, although the recessive gene remains in the population, the abnormality or disease that it causes never occurs, because homozygotes for the recessive gene never occur.

## Selection/mutation balance for a recessive

Even if we are successful in removing a recessive gene from the population or at least preventing its appearance in homozygotes, we still have to contend with the effect of mutation, which, slowly but consistently, is adding new recessive genes to the population.

If we are detecting heterozygotes and not using them for breeding, we are in essentially the same situation as with complete selection against a dominant gene ($s = 1$): each new recessive gene entering the population is immediately removed, and a selection/mutation balance is reached at which the frequency of the recessive gene equals the mutation rate. However, because homozygotes never occur in this situation, the frequency of the recessive trait at this selection/mutation balance is zero: affected animals never appear.

If we are detecting heterozygotes and then using them for breeding but avoiding matings between heterozygotes, there is no selection operating against the recessive gene. In this case, the frequency of the recessive gene will increase very gradually at a rate determined solely by the mutation rate, which is usually so low that we would be unlikely to detect an appreciable increase in frequency during a period of, say, 100 years, even in species with short intervals between generations. The final case that we must consider is the conventional scheme of selection against a recessive gene, where heterozygotes are not detected. As shown in Appendix A5.4.4 of *Veterinary genetics*, it turns out that the equilibrium frequency of a recessive gene under these circumstances is $\sqrt{(\mu/s)}$, and the corresponding equilibrium frequency of the recessive phenotype is $\mu/s$. It is left to the reader to verify that even with weak selection against a recessive gene, the equilibrium frequency resulting from a selection/mutation balance is very low.

## Selection favouring heterozygotes

We saw in previous sections that the effect of selection against a dominant gene or against a recessive gene is to reduce the frequency of that gene to a relatively low level, at which stage a balance between mutation and selection maintains an equilibrium. Selection favouring heterozygotes also results in an equilibrium, but of a rather different type. In the extreme case, where no homozygotes pass on their genes, the only parents are heterozygotes, in which case both genes are maintained in the population at a frequency of 0.5. In less extreme circumstances, where both homozygotes have only a partially reduced fitness, the results are exactly the same so long as both homozygotes have equal fitness. Thus, even if both homozygotes have only a 1 per cent reduction of fitness, selection is still acting equally against each gene and maintains an equilibrium gene frequency of 0.5. However, if one homozygote has a lower fitness than the other, selection is less intense against the gene whose homozygote has the highest fitness.

It turns out, as shown in Appendix A5.4.5 of *Veterinary genetics*, that if $s_1$ is the selection coefficient against one homozygote, say $A_1A_1$, and $s_2$ is the selection coefficient against the other homozygote, say $A_2A_2$, the equilibrium frequency of the $A_2$ gene is $s_1/(s_1 + s_2)$.

If for example, one homozygote is only 10 per cent less fit than the heterozygote ($s_1 = 0.10$), while the other one is lethal (100 per cent less fit; $s_2 = 1.00$), the equilibrium frequency of the lethal gene is $0.10/(0.10 + 1.00) = 0.09$. Thus, if heterozygotes for a lethal gene are slightly more fit than homozygotes for the normal gene, the result is an equilibrium frequency much higher than that expected under a selection/mutation balance with a recessive lethal gene. Although definite proof is usually lacking, selection favouring heterozygotes is often suggested as a reason for recessive lethal traits reaching unusually high frequencies. In many situations, it is certainly the most plausible explanation available, and sometimes data are available to back it up. Syndactyly or fusion of digits in Holstein–Friesian cattle, for example, is an effectively lethal recessive trait for which there is some evidence of selection favouring heterozygotes. In this case, there is a suggestion that heterozygotes produce higher milk and butterfat yields and thus have a higher fitness as a result of artificial selection. In a similar manner, it appears that carriers of the lethal recessive genes for DUMPS and for weaver syndrome in cattle may be favoured by artificial selection for milk traits. In pigs, carriers of the recessive gene for malignant hyperthermia (see Chapter 9) have been favoured by selection for leanness; and there is some evidence that horses carrying the dominant gene for hyperkalaemic periodic paralysis tend to be favoured by judges in the show ring.

When carriers of defective genes are consistently favoured by artificial selection, one explanation is that the gene has a favourable effect on the trait that is being selected, in addition to its negative effect on viability or reproductive ability. The term **pleiotropy** is used to describe situations where a gene affects two or more seemingly unconnected traits. Alternatively, the defective gene could be closely linked to a gene that affects the trait being selected. In either case, the defective gene provides an opportunity for investigating the genetic basis of the desirable trait.

*Selection against heterozygotes*

Neonatal diarrhoea in piglets is of considerable economic importance. It is often caused by strains of *Escherichia coli* bacteria having a cell-surface antigen called K88, which combines with a receptor on the wall of a piglet's intestines, enabling the bacteria to attach themselves to the intestine. Once attached, they proliferate, releasing enterotoxins and thus producing di-arrhoea which can lead to very high mortality. Some strains of *E. coli* lack the K88 antigen (they are said to be K88-negative) and cannot therefore attach themselves to the intestinal mucosa. Being thus unable to proliferate and release enterotoxins, such strains are non-virulent. Certain piglets, however, are not susceptible even to K88-positive bacteria, and it has been found that they lack the appropriate receptor for K88, thus preventing the attachment and subsequent proliferation of bacteria. Lack of the K88 receptor (and hence resistance to the K88-positive bacteria) is due to homozygosity for a recessive gene called *s*. Piglets having the receptor and therefore being sus-ceptible are either homozygous for a dominant gene *S* or are heterozygous.

Since K88-positive *E. coli* are fairly common, and since the susceptibility gene is dominant, we might expect that the susceptibility gene would be maintained at a very low frequency by a selection/mutation balance. How-ever, in four English herds examined in one survey, the frequency of the dominant gene in three herds was much greater than 0.5, and in the other herd it was around 0.4. The most satisfactory explanation for these un-expectedly high frequencies involves a fascinating combination of basic principles from immunology and population genetics.

Consider a population into which the resistance gene *s* has been introduced only recently by mutation and/or migration, and suppose that a build-up of K88-positive bacteria occurs. Because nearly all animals are susceptible, there is very strong selection against the dominant susceptibility gene, i.e. in favour of the recessive resistance gene. At the same time, however, the susceptible sows mount an immune response to the K88-positive bacteria, supplying antibodies to K88 via their colostrum to all their piglets. These antibodies are sufficient to prevent diarrhoea, and so selection against the dominant susceptibility gene becomes less intense not long after it com-menced. Thus, the previously expected rapid elimination of the dominant gene does not occur. Suppose that it has, however, been reduced in frequency from 1.0 to, say, 0.7, which means that $(1 - 0.7)^2 = (0.3)^2 = 0.09$ of all sows are now homozygous for the resistance gene. These sows certainly carry the K88-positive bacteria, but because attachment does not occur, they never develop antibodies to K88 and hence they provide no protection to their piglets. This is of no consequence to their *ss* piglets because they are naturally resistant anyway. However, not all offspring of *ss* sows are *ss*; some of the *ss* sows mate with *Ss* or *SS* boars and consequently produce some or all *Ss* piglets, all of which are susceptible. These heterozygous piglets get the worst of both worlds; they have a receptor for K88, and they fail to receive antibody from their *ss* female parent.

Thus we have selection against heterozygotes, with both homozygotes having equal and normal fitness, in the case of *SS* because of antibodies received from the sow, and in the case of *ss* because of lack of a receptor for K88. Selection against heterozygotes in this situation is only partial, because only those born to *ss* sows are likely to be affected by diarrhoea. What are the likely effects of selection against heterozygotes?

A moment's reflection indicates that for every heterozygote eliminated from a population, an equal number of both genes is removed, which has a greater effect on the less common gene. Consider, for example, a herd of 100 pigs which has Hardy–Weinberg genotype frequencies corresponding to gene frequencies of 0.7 and 0.3 prior to selection. The numbers of the genotypes are 49 *SS*, 42 *Ss*, and 9 *ss*. Suppose that ten heterozygotes die from neonatal *E. coli* diarrhoea, leaving 49 *SS*, 32 *Ss*, and 9 *ss* in a total of 90 pigs after selection. The gene frequencies are now $(2 \times 49 + 32)/(2 \times 90) = 0.72$ for *S* and $1 - 0.72 = 0.28$ for *s*, which represents a reduction in frequency of the less common gene.

In general, if homozygotes have equal fitness, selection against heterozygotes results in a decrease in frequency of the less frequent gene. Thus, the gene that was at a frequency of less than 0.5 when selection against heterozygotes commenced, gradually decreases in frequency so long as such selection continues.

In the piglet case, selection against heterozygotes ceases when the pathogenic *E. coli* disappear, leaving the frequency of the *s* gene at whatever level it had reached at that time. With the next outbreak of neonatal *E. coli* diarrhoea, the cycle of events described above recommences. If the *s* gene had increased in frequency to more than 0.5 before selection against heterozygotes became effective, such selection would increase its frequency even further. If it were less than 0.5, it would decrease in frequency towards its former low level. If a large number of herds were surveyed, it might be expected that the *s* gene would be at a low frequency in some and at a high frequency in others. Results of the very limited surveys reported to date are consistent with this prediction.

## Genetic drift and the founder effect

There is another reason why deleterious and even lethal conditions can reach quite high frequencies in certain populations. It is called **genetic drift**, which, as we saw earlier in this chapter, refers to changes in gene frequency due entirely to chance. These changes result from the sampling of finite numbers of genes that is inevitable in all finite populations. Because these changes in gene frequency are entirely due to chance, their direction is random and is completely outside the control of humans. Since all populations are finite, it follows that genetic drift occurs in all populations. However, the larger the population size, the smaller is the magnitude of genetic drift.

The most extreme case of genetic drift in domestic animals can be illustrated by imagining that only one male and one female are chosen to be parents of the next generation. Consider a single locus with two alleles $A$ and $B$. Irrespective of what the frequency of $A$ was in the generation from which the parents were chosen, its frequency in the actual parents must be either 0.00 (if both parents happen to be homozygous for $B$), 0.25 (if one parent is $AB$ and the other is $BB$), 0.50 (if the parents are $AB$ and $AB$, or $AA$ and $BB$), 0.75 ($AA$ and $AB$), or 1.00 (both parents homozygous for $A$). Suppose that the frequency of $A$ was, say, 0.1 in the population from which the parents were chosen, and suppose that the parents were chosen at random, and happened to be $AA$ and $AB$. In this case, the gene frequency has changed from 0.1 to 0.75, a change of 0.65, which is very large and which is due entirely to chance or sampling. Since the gene frequency in the parents is now 0.75, it follows that the gene frequency in the offspring of these parents will also be 0.75, unless selection, mutation, or migration causes a further change. If only one male and one female are chosen at random from the offspring generation, to be parents of the next generation, exactly the same situation applies: the gene frequency in the next generation will be either zero, 0.25, 0.50, 0.75, or one. If it reaches zero, the gene is **lost** forever, or until mutation recreates it. If the frequency reaches one, the gene is said to have been **fixed** in the population, and all other genes at that locus have been lost.

The **founder effect** is a special case of genetic drift, referring to situations where a small number of individuals move to a new site, and commence (found) a new population. Even if the new population rapidly expands in numbers, and soon has a large number of parents in each generation, the gene frequencies will be a reflection of the frequencies in the founders, rather than in the population from which the founders came. The reason for this is that, in the absence of selection, mutation, and migration, the gene frequencies remain at whatever level they were when the population was started. Thus a population that is founded by just one male and one female can have a very different set of gene frequencies to that from which the founding parents were chosen.

The founder effect is an example of a **population bottleneck**, which is a situation in which the number of parents in a population becomes very small for one or more generations. As illustrated above, a population emerging from a bottleneck may be very different from the population that existed before the bottleneck.

## Genetic distance

Irrespective of how many animals are used to found a new population, the old and the new populations increasingly differ from each other as time passes:

mutation introduces unique alleles into each population, and the frequencies of all alleles at all loci change randomly (i.e. genetic drift occurs) in each population. The longer the time since any two populations diverged, the greater is the difference in their gene frequencies. The extent to which two populations differ in their gene frequencies is called the **genetic distance** between them. If we estimate the frequencies of alleles at a number of loci in a set of populations (e.g. breeds of cattle from different parts of the world), the genetic distance between all pairs of populations can be estimated from the gene-frequency data. An evolutionary tree (a **phylogenetic tree**) can then be drawn, in which the length of the branches separating any two populations is proportional to the genetic distance between them.

Microsatellites are an ideal source of data for calculating genetic distances, because they are so polymorphic and are located throughout the genome. In addition, it is also possible to deduce phylogenies from the divergence in sequences of amino acids in proteins or of bases in genes, between breeds and/or species.

Fascinating pictures of the evolution of breeds and species are emerging. Apart from their inherent interest, these studies provide a guide to genetic diversity within and between species, which in turn provides a foundation for decisions about which populations are most in need of conservation (see Chapter 18).

## Further reading

*Books*

Christiansen, F. B. and Feldman, M. W. (1986). *Population genetics*. Blackwell Scientific Publications, Oxford.

Crow, J. F. (1987). *Basic concepts in population, quantitative, and evolutionary genetics*. Freeman, New York.

Doolittle, D. P. (1987). *Population genetics: basic principles*. Springer-Verlag, Berlin.

Falconer, D. S. (1989). *An introduction to quantitative genetics*, (3rd edn). Longman Chesire, London.

Hartl, D. L. (1988). *A primer of population genetics*, (2nd edn). Sinauer Associates, Sunderland, Massachusetts.

Hartl, D. L. and Clark, A. G. (1989). *Principles of population genetics*, (2nd edn). Sinauer Associates, Sunderland, Massachusetts.

Hedrick, P. W. (1985). *Genetics of populations*. Jones and Bartlett, Boston.

Smith, J. M. (1989). *Evolutionary genetics*. Oxford University Press, Oxford.

Smith, J. M. (1993). *The theory of evolution*, (4th edn). Cambridge University Press, Cambridge.

*Bottlenecks*

Hoelzel, A. R., Halley, J., O'Brien, S. J., Campagna, C., Arnbom, T., Leboeuf, B., Ralls, K., and Dover, G. A. (1993). Elephant seal genetic variation and the use of simulation models to investigate historical population bottlenecks. *Journal of Heredity*, **84**, 443–9.

## *Genetic distance/phylogeny*

Lake, J. A. (1994). Reconstructing evolutionary trees from DNA and protein sequences—paralinear distances. *Proceedings of the National Academy of Sciences USA*, **91**, 1455–9.

Loftus, R. T., MacHugh, D. E., Bradley, D. G., Sharp, P. M., and Cunningham, E. P. (1994). Evidence for two independent domestications of cattle. *Proceedings of the National Academy of Sciences USA*, **91**, 2757–61.

Stanley, H. F., Kadwell, M., and Wheeler, J. C. (1994). Molecular evolution of the family Camelidae—a mitochondrial DNA study. *Proceedings of the Royal Society of London Series B*, **256**, 1–6.

Taberlet, P. and Bouvet, J. (1994). Mitochondrial DNA polymorphism, phylogeography, and conservation genetics of the brown bear *Ursus arctos* in Europe. *Proceedings of the Royal Society of London Series B*, **255**, 195–200.

# Familial disorders not due to a single gene

Many important disorders are familial—they 'run in families', which means that the incidence among relatives of affected animals is greater than the incidence in the population to which they belong. If a disorder is familial, it may be due to shared environment or to shared genes, or to a combination of shared environment and shared genes.

With single-gene disorders of the type discussed in previous chapters, there is no difficulty in determining why they are familial: it is because of shared genes. There are, however, many familial disorders that do not fit into any of the categories of single-gene inheritance.

The aim of this chapter is to explain what is known about such disorders.

## Liability and threshold

For reasons that will soon become evident, it is convenient to think of each animal as having a certain **liability** to a disorder, where liability refers to the combined effect of all factors, both environmental and genetic, that render an animal more or less likely to develop that disorder.

It must be clearly understood that the term 'environment' is used here and throughout this book in its widest possible sense, literally meaning non-genetic. Thus, an environmental factor is any factor that cannot be attributed to the action of genes.

Liability is a continuous variable that could, in principle, be measured on a continuous scale, in the same manner as we measure a trait such as body weight. But in this chapter we are discussing discontinuous traits in which there are often only two classes: affected and normal. We can accommodate all-or-none traits on a continuous scale by using the concept of **threshold**, which is a certain level of liability above which all animals develop the disorder, and below which all animals are normal.

Although the aim of this chapter is to explain the inheritance of disorders not due to single genes, the easiest way to introduce the important concepts is to start by considering a single-gene disorder. With an autosomal recessive disorder, for example, the position of the three genotypes can be represented on an arbitrary scale of liability as shown in Fig. 6.1.

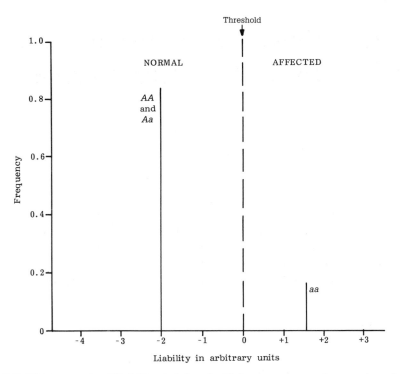

**Fig. 6.1** The concepts of liability and threshold for an autosomal, recessive, single-gene disorder.

## Incomplete penetrance

Malignant hyperthermia syndrome (MHS) is characterized by a progressive increase in body temperature, muscle rigidity, and respiratory and metabolic acidosis, leading rapidly to death. It occurs in certain pigs if they are subjected to mild stress such as loading and/or transport. Affected pigs are homozygous for a mis-sense mutation in the gene for a calcium-release channel (see Appendix 3.1 and Chapter 9); MHS is a single-gene, autosomal, recessive disorder. A standard test for assessing the clinical phenotype in relation to MHS is to expose pigs to halothane vapour breathed through a tight-fitting mask. Susceptible pigs (reactors) usually show signs of stiffening in hindquarter muscles after 2 minutes, but if the mask is removed as soon as this happens, the majority of reactors show a complete recovery in 5 minutes. If there is no stiffening after 3 minutes of exposure to halothane, the animal is classed as a non-reactor, and is regarded as being resistant to MHS. The practical problems involved in administering halothane to pigs inevitably lead to variation in the efficiency of the test, even from pig to pig within a single test batch. It is to be expected, therefore, that the halothane test could produce the occasional false positive and false negative result. In other words, phenotypic classification may not be completely accurate.

For example, when a major research organisation commenced halothane testing, the probability of misclassifying a reactor as a non-reactor was as high as 25 per cent. One year later, by which time the operators had gained experience, the probability of misclassification had been substantially reduced.

But even with this improvement in accuracy, there were still some problems with interpreting results of particular matings. For example, among the offspring of affected × affected matings in one survey, 98 per cent were classified as affected (reactors).

With results like this, the only way to explain the inheritance of MHS in terms of a recessive gene is to say that all the offspring of affected × affected matings are actually homozygous for the recessive gene, but that only 98 per cent of them show the effect of the gene.

Results such as this have led to use of the term **penetrance**, which is the proportion of animals with a particular genotype that exhibit the phenotype normally associated with that genotype. As an example, the above results indicate a penetrance of the homozygous recessive genotype of 98 per cent. If penetrance is less than 100 per cent, it is said to be **incomplete**. In relation to liability, the existence of incomplete penetrance means that animals with the same genotype (*aa*) can have different liabilities; those with MHS have a liability on the affected side of the threshold, and those that are not affected have a liability somewhere on the other side of the threshold. Possible causes for this difference in liability include various non-genetic (environmental) factors, such as the skill and experience of operators conducting the test, and age at the time of testing (younger pigs are more likely to be misclassified). There is also some evidence that alleles at other (unknown) loci also affect the chances of an animal being classified as MHS after the standard halothane test.

## The multifactorial model

We shall start this section by considering one of the best known familial disorders, namely hip dysplasia in dogs. In the past, this disorder was thought by some veterinarians and breeders to be due to a single, autosomal, recessive gene. In several different studies of hip dysplasia in German Shepherd dogs, the results of affected × affected matings have been an average of 86 per cent affected offspring. Similar matings of affected × affected Labradors have produced an average of 63 per cent affected offspring.

If we used the same arguments as used previously for MHS in pigs, we could attribute hip dysplasia to a recessive gene (*a*) with 86 per cent penetrance in German Shepherds and 63 per cent penetrance in Labradors. In the latter case, for example, we would then have 63 per cent of *aa* Labradors with a

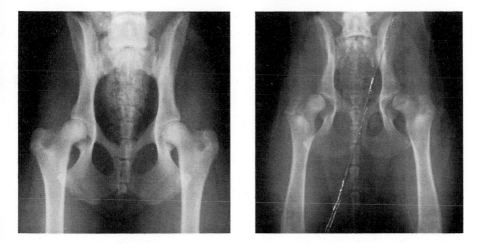

**Fig. 6.2** Radiographs of (*left*) normal canine hip joints, and (*right*) hips showing bilateral coxofemoral subluxation due to joint instability or laxity, which is the earliest sign of canine hip dysplasia.

liability sufficiently high to place them on the affected side of the threshold and 37 per cent with a liability sufficiently low to place them on the normal side. As with MHS in pigs, we could ask: what factors are likely to be responsible for this difference in liability among *aa* animals?

Since hip dysplasia is usually diagnosed by subjective evaluation of a radiograph (Fig. 6.2) or by palpation, misclassification is one factor. In addition, level of feeding, dietary electrolyte balance, and extent of exercise during early growth have been shown to affect an animal's liability to hip dysplasia. The difference in liability could also be partly due to the action of alleles at other loci that in various ways determine the way in which the hip joint develops.

The situation is now like that shown in Fig. 6.3, where there is a bell-shaped or Normal distribution of liability values for *aa* animals. Animals that are overfed and overexercised, and happen to have alleles at other loci tending to produce ill-fitting hip joints, have a relatively high liability. Animals with only some of these predisposing factors are more common than those with all the predisposing factors, which accounts for the increasing frequency of animals with liabilities closer to the mid-point of the distribution. A similar trend is expected on the other side of the mid-point: animals given the most favourable diet and most appropriate exercise regime, and who also happen to have alleles at other loci that tend to produce sound hip joints, have much lower liabilities. But such animals are less common than those with only some of these factors operating to decrease liability.

The important point to understand is that any animal having a liability less than the threshold value, for whatever combination of environmental and genetic factors, will not have hip dysplasia.

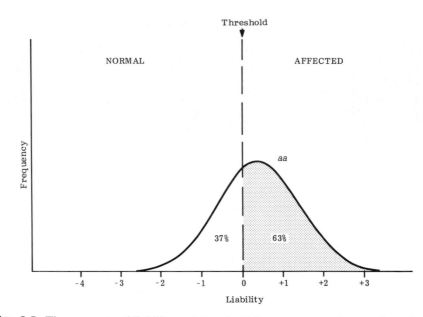

**Fig. 6.3** The concepts of liability and threshold for an autosomal, recessive, single-gene disorder where the homozygote recessive genotype (*aa*) has incomplete penetrance, in this particular case at a level of 63 per cent.

When a trait is determined by the combined effect of many factors, both environmental and genetic, it is said to be **multifactorial**. In general, if there is a large departure from the expectations of single-gene inheritance, it is more sensible to describe the disorder as being multifactorial than to talk in terms of a single locus with incomplete penetrance.

In order to understand the relationship between these two methods of describing the inheritance of an all-or-none trait, we shall expand the concepts illustrated in Fig. 6.3. If alleles at other loci and/or environmental factors produce a Normal distribution of liability for *aa* homozygotes as in Fig. 6.3, it is reasonable to expect a similar distribution in liability for genotypes *AA* and *Aa*, as shown in Fig. 6.4. And if dominance is incomplete (i.e. the average liability of heterozygotes is in between the average liability of the homozygotes), there is a considerable overlap of the distributions of liability among the three genotypes, leading to an overall distribution of liability (solid line in Fig. 6.4) approaching that of a single Normal distribution, which is the distribution expected for a multifactorial disorder.

In the above discussion, we started by considering hip dysplasia as a single-gene disorder with incomplete penetrance, and finished by describing it as multifactorial. Which of these descriptions or models is the most appropriate? It should be obvious that the latter model is more appropriate than the former. Indeed, there are so many non-genetic factors contributing to liability to hip dysplasia, and there is such a wide departure from single-gene inheri-

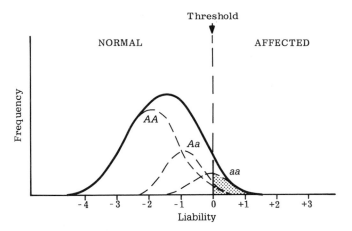

**Fig. 6.4** The similarity between a single-gene model with incomplete penetrance and incomplete dominance (dotted lines), and a multifactorial model (solid line). The solid line represents the total frequency of animals with a particular liability, and is obtained by summing the frequency of the three genotypes from the single-gene model.

tance, that it is rather pointless to describe the inheritance of hip dysplasia in terms of a single locus with incomplete penetrance.

One virtue of the multifactorial model is that it enables a simple estimate to be made of the relative importance of genetic and environmental factors as contributors to the aetiology of a disorder. This is done by estimating a parameter called **heritability**, which for present purposes is the proportion of total variation in a trait that can be attributed to variation in genetic factors.

In the present case, the trait is liability. Variation in liability refers to the differences among animals in liability to a particular disorder. Heritability of liability, then, is the proportion of differences in liability that are due to genetic differences among animals.

The majority of familial disorders have an intermediate heritability, which indicates that both environmental and genetic factors contribute to their aetiology.

## More than one threshold

Congenital heart disease occurs in many forms, the most important of which are familial in humans and in animals. In an extensive and very thorough set of analyses conducted by Don Patterson and colleagues, the inheritance of congenital heart disease in dogs has been clearly demonstrated to be compatible with a multifactorial model.

The most common congenital heart disease is patent ductus arteriosus (PDA), resulting from defective closure of the ductus arteriosus.

Like many other disorders that are compatible with the multifactorial model, defective closure of the ductus arteriosus is a graded phenomenon, with increasing severity corresponding to increasing liability.

This is clearly indicated in the results of various matings among Poodles, which produced some normal offspring, others with partial closure (called ductus diverticulum or DD), and others with PDA. The presence of these three grades can be represented in the multifactorial model by two thresholds, as illustrated in Fig. 6.5a. In this case, the PDA × PDA matings produced 66 per cent of offspring with PDA, 17 per cent with DD, and 17 per cent normal offspring.

An even better understanding of the multifactorial model can be obtained from other types of matings, the results of which are also given in Fig. 6.5.

From a practical point of view, the difference in incidence of affected offspring from the two types of matings involving normal dogs is particularly important: normal dogs that are closely related to affected dogs (Fig. 6.5b) produce more than three times the incidence of affected offspring, and more than four times the incidence of severely affected offspring, when compared with normal dogs that are unrelated to affected dogs (Fig. 6.5c).

In general, the tendency for normal animals to throw affected offspring and the severity of the disorder among their affected offspring, depends on how closely the normal animal is genetically related to an affected animal.

This important conclusion is a direct consequence of the multifactorial model.

Another relatively common form of congenital heart disease, conotruncal septum defects (CSD) in Keeshonds, clearly illustrates another important implication of the multifactorial model, namely that the frequency and severity of the disorder will be greatest among relatives of more severely affected animals.

Conotruncal septum defects are particularly useful in this context, as they can be divided into four different grades of increasing severity, as illustrated in Fig. 6.6. If CSD were due to a single gene, the existence of more than one grade of defect would be said to indicate **variable expressivity** of that gene. But the possible causes of variable expressivity are the same as those for incomplete penetrance: environmental factors, alleles at other loci, or a combination of both. In general, therefore, single-gene disorders with variable expressivity can be more usefully regarded as being multifactorial.

From an extensive set of matings among Keeshonds with various grades of CSD, the overall incidence of CSD and the incidence of each grade of CSD in offspring was determined for various mating types, according to the average CSD grade of parents. The results for overall CSD incidence and for incidence of the most severe form (grade 3) are shown in Fig. 6.7. It is evident that the overall frequency of CSD and the frequency of grade 3 are almost directly proportional to the average severity in parents. These results are entirely consistent with the multifactorial model, in which frequency and severity in relatives of affected animals are expected to increase as liability increases.

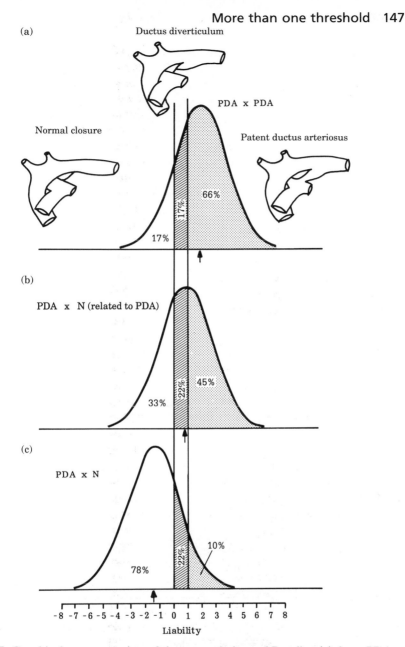

**Fig. 6.5** Graphical representation of three populations of Poodles (a) from PDA × PDA matings; (b) from PDA × normal matings, where the normal parent has a close relative that is affected, e.g. parent or offspring or full-brother or full-sister; (c) from PDA × normal matings, where the normal parent has no close relatives that are affected. The position of the distributions relative to the thresholds is determined solely by the incidence of each grade of defect.

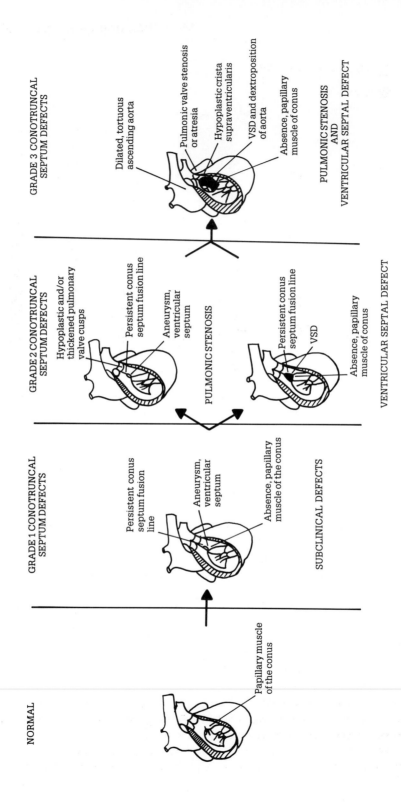

**Fig. 6.6** A graded series of defects of the conotruncal septum in Keeshond dogs.

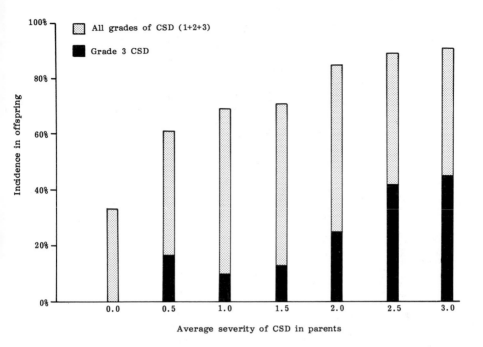

**Fig. 6.7** Overall incidence of conotruncal septum defects or CSD (grades 1, 2, and 3) and incidence of grade 3 CSD in offspring, as a function of average severity of CSD in parents.

## Some final points

### *Heritability*

Since the concept of heritability was introduced when the multifactorial model was introduced, it might be thought that heritability is a valid concept only in relation to multifactorial traits. But this is not so: it is, in fact, an equally valid parameter for any trait (including disorders) determined by a single locus.

As introduced earlier in this chapter, heritability is 100 per cent for all traits determined by a single locus, because all the differences in phenotype between animals in relation to those traits are due to different genotypes at the locus in question. When heritability is defined in this sense, we refer to it as **heritability in the broad sense** or the **degree of genetic determination**.

There is, however, another sense in which the term heritability is used. Known as **heritability in the narrow sense**, it expresses the extent to which phenotypes are transmitted from parents to offspring. In other words, it expresses the extent to which offspring resemble their parents, or in more general terms, the extent to which relatives resemble each other.

Because we are most interested in understanding and predicting how traits are transmitted from one generation to the next, narrow-sense heritability is much more useful than broad-sense heritability. In fact, whenever we see the word 'heritability' on its own, we can take it to mean narrow-sense heritability, unless otherwise stated.

Estimating heritability involves using statistical techniques to estimate the extent to which relatives resemble each other for the trait of interest, compared with unrelated animals. The actual methodology is not a simple business, and a description of the methods is beyond the scope of this book. Table 6.1 lists

**Table 6.1** Representative values of heritability of liability, expressed as a percentage. Since there is considerable variation in actual estimates, values have been rounded to the nearest 5 per cent

| | |
|---|---|
| **Cattle** | |
| Bloat | 10 |
| Cystic ovaries | 10 |
| Displaced abomasum | 10 |
| Foot problems | 10 |
| Ketosis | 20 |
| Leg problems | 10 |
| Metritis | 5 |
| Milk fever | 40 |
| Retained placenta | 5 |
| | |
| **Chicken** | |
| Tibial dyschondroplasia | 45 |
| | |
| **Dog** | |
| Calcified intervertebral discs | 20 |
| Elbow osteochondrosis | 50 |
| Hip dysplasia | 35 |
| | |
| **Duck** | |
| Chronic interstitial nephropathy | 45 |
| | |
| **Horse** | |
| Osteochondrosis in the tibiotarsal joint | 50 |
| Bony fragments in the palmar plantar portion of the metacarpophalangeal and metatarsophalangeal joints | 20 |
| | |
| **Pig** | |
| Cryptorchidism | 55 |
| Hernia | 50 |
| | |
| **Turkey** | |
| Tibial dyschondroplasia | 15 |

some representative values for heritability of liability for a range of disorders in domestic animals. The practical importance of this table is that if the heritability of liability is greater than zero, it is possible to decrease the incidence of the disorder by selection; and the higher the heritability, the greater the response to selection. The use of selection to control inherited disorders is discussed in Chapter 11.

## Penetrance and expressivity

We have seen in this chapter that the concepts of incomplete penetrance and to a lesser extent variable expressivity are often invoked to explain any departure from simple single-gene inheritance. In many circumstances, this is an entirely useful and valid approach. However, with a little ingenuity, most data on most disorders can be made to fit a single-gene model by choosing the appropriate values of penetrance for each genotype, by postulating a certain amount of incomplete dominance and if necessary by invoking variable expressivity as well. But having done this, are we any the wiser? The disadvantage of continuing to think in terms of a single-gene model if the data clearly do not fit a single-gene model, is that we continue to think in terms of carriers of a single gene, and we are therefore inclined to believe that if we can eradicate that gene, the disorder will disappear. This approach will lead to great disappointment for breeders. On the other hand, by regarding such disorders as multifactorial, we can forget about detecting carriers or removing a gene from a population, and concentrate instead on more fruitful tasks. For such disorders, our willingness to use an affected animal in any mating will depend solely on the severity of its own disorder and on its relationship to other defective animals. We will not waste our time searching for Mendelian ratios. Instead, we will simply proceed with various matings, using as our guide the incidence of affected animals achieved in previous matings of that type.

In addition, by thinking in terms of the multifactorial model for such disorders, we will avoid the common misconception that if the inheritance of a disorder is not compatible with simple dominant or simple recessive inheritance, its mode of inheritance is not known. In fact, the mode of inheritance is known, and appropriate breeding plans for the reduction in incidence of a particular disorder can easily be drawn up and put into practice on the basis of that understanding (as explained in Chapter 11).

## Future resolution of multiple factors

A major aim of research into multifactorial disorders is to identify the important factors, both environmental and genetic, that determine liability. Considerable progress has been made in this area, especially in regard to environmental factors. Much more progress can be expected in the future. On the genetic side, for example, much effort is being devoted to searching for single genes that make a major contribution to variation in liability. This is done by analysing the occurrence of the disorder in families (called **complex segregation analysis**; see Chapter 7). Unfortunately, this is an inexact science, and some claims of single genes having been identified will not stand the test of time. However, as described in Chapter 7, the methods of analysis are being improved rapidly, and the search will be much more effective in the future. Increasingly, members of families in which a disorder occurs are being genotyped for DNA markers, enabling **linkage analysis** to be conducted between the markers and the disorder phenotype. This leads to the identification of DNA markers that are associated with the disorder, and ultimately to the identification of genes that play important roles in determining liability to the disorder (see Chapter 11).

It is important to note that the discovery of a single gene or even several genes that contribute to variation in liability for a disorder does not invalidate the multifactorial concept, and does not remove the need for control programmes based on the multifactorial model. However, knowledge of DNA markers associated with liability, and of genes that contribute to liability, can be used to increase the effectiveness of control programmes.

## Recurrence risks

On many occasions in this chapter, we have spoken about the percentage of affected offspring resulting from a certain type of mating. These percentages are called **recurrence risks**, because they give an indication of the risk of a particular disorder recurring (i.e. occurring again), should that type of mating be repeated. The recurrence risks presented in this chapter are called **empirical recurrence risks**, because they have been obtained by observing results of actual matings. Empirical recurrence risks can be very useful in planning and conducting breeding programmes aimed at reducing the frequency of certain disorders. For example, the figures for incidence of CSD shown in Fig. 6.7, which are really empirical recurrence risks, clearly show that the frequency of all grades of CSD will be decreased most rapidly by breeding only from parents that have no signs of CSD. If this is not possible, for example because the incidence of CSD is very high in a certain population of dogs, the empirical recurrence risks in Fig. 6.7 indicate that breeders should aim for matings in which the average severity of CSD is as low as possible.

There are, however, limitations to empirical recurrence risks, e.g. they cannot indicate the risk for a type of mating from which no offspring records are currently available.

These disadvantages can be overcome by using **theoretical recurrence risks**, which are predictions arising directly from either a single-gene model or a multifactorial model, whichever is appropriate. Because they are predicted from the model, theoretical recurrence risks can be calculated for any imaginable type of mating, whether or not such matings have ever occurred before. In the simplest cases, theoretical recurrence risks equal segregation ratios for single-gene models, and, for the multifactorial model, they can be calculated from the population incidence and heritability. In most cases, however, the calculation of theoretical recurrence risks involves complications that are beyond the scope of this book, and should be left to people with experience in this area.

## Further reading

### General

Falconer, D. S. (1989). *Introduction to quantitative genetics*, (3rd edn), Chapter 18. Longman, London.
Patterson, D. F., Haskins, M. E., Jezyk, P. F., Giger, U., Meyers-Wallen, V. N., Aguirre, G., Fyfe, J. C., and Wolfe, J. H. (1988). Research on genetic diseases: reciprocal benefits to animals and man. *Journal of the American Veterinary Medical Association*, **193**, 1131–44.

### Hip dysplasia

Brass, W. (1989). Hip dysplasia in dogs. *Journal of Small Animal Practice*, **30**, 166–70.
Rettenmaier, J. L. and Constantinescu, G. M. (1991). Canine hip dysplasia. *Compendium on Continuing Education for the Practicing Veterinarian*, **13**, 643–54.

### Congenital heart disease

Darke, P. G. G. (1989). Congenital heart disease in dogs and cats. *Journal of Small Animal Practice*, **30**, 599.
Patterson, D. F. (1989). Hereditary congenital heart defects in dogs. *Journal of Small Animal Practice*, **30**, 153–65.

# 7

# Is it inherited?

'Is it inherited?' is a common question asked in relation to a wide range of disorders. Unfortunately, the answer for the majority of disorders is 'we don't know', because insufficient data have been collected and analysed to enable a decision to be made.

The situation will gradually improve as more studies are conducted. In order to conduct such studies, an understanding is required of Mendelian inheritance (Chapter 1), population genetics (Chapter 5), the multifactorial model (Chapter 6) and elementary statistics. The aim of this chapter is to show how knowledge in these areas can be put to practical use in investigating the mode of inheritance of a disorder.

It is important that such studies be conducted, not only from the immediate veterinary point of view, but also because medical researchers are increasingly on the lookout for inherited diseases of animals that could serve as models of human disease.

## General evidence for a genetic aetiology

If genes make any contribution to the aetiology of a disorder, then, as discussed in Chapter 6, it follows that there will be a positive relationship between the chance of an individual being affected and the extent to which that individual has genes in common with affected individuals.

The most important practical implication of this relationship is seen in families and breeds. Members of the same family have more genes in common than members of different families, and members of the same breed have more genes in common than members of different breeds. If the incidence of a disorder is higher in some families than in others within a breed, or if the incidence is higher in some breeds than in others, one possible explanation is that there is a genetic contribution to the aetiology of the disorder.

Of course, evidence of variation in incidence between families and/or between breeds does not constitute proof of a genetic contribution to aetiology, because environmental factors common to members of a family and/or common to members of a breed may be sufficient to account for the observed variation in incidence. The first step, then, in attempting to disentangle environmental causes from genetic causes, is to remove or allow for the effects of environmental factors. This can be done only after a detailed investigation of all environmental factors that are thought likely to affect the occurrence of the disorder. The trouble with this approach is that the investigator often has no prior indication as to which factors should be examined: each one that comes to mind as being possibly important must be investigated, in order to determine which ones (if any) are important.

In many cases, variation between breeds and variation within breeds are directly related. Malignant hyperthermia syndrome (MHS; see Chapters 6 and 9), for example, has a completely genetic aetiology within pig breeds, in each of which it is due to homozygosity for a recessive allele. There is also considerable variation in incidence between breeds, from well over 50 per cent in the Pietrain breed down to less than 5 per cent in Large Whites, and this between-breed variation can be explained in terms of different frequencies of the recessive allele in the different breeds.

But such a relationship need not necessarily exist. In fact, the existence of a genetic contribution to aetiology within each of several breeds does not necessarily indicate that there is a genetic difference between breeds.

To continue with MHS as an example, it is evident that if the recessive allele occurs with the same frequency in two breeds, there will be no variation between those two breeds but there will still be considerable variation within each breed.

The final piece of general evidence suggesting a genetic contribution to aetiology is when the same or a very similar disorder is definitely inherited in another species of animal, or in humans. Single-gene disorders of the type discussed in Chapter 3 illustrate this point particularly well, and so too do inherited coat colours and patterns, which are described in Chapter 12. Of course there are exceptions to the rule, and we must be on the lookout continually for them; but the general principle holds very well. We can go one step further with X-linked loci, and predict quite confidently that if a particular locus is X-linked in one species of mammal, it will be X-linked in all species of mammals.

## The four types of simple, Mendelian inheritance

If a disorder is still familial, after removing or allowing for all conceivable environmental factors, the next step is to determine if the available data correspond in general terms to any of the four simple, Mendelian types of inheritance: autosomal dominant, autosomal recessive, X-linked dominant, and X-linked recessive.

Drawing on a knowledge of Mendelian inheritance (Chapter 1) and of population genetics (Chapter 5), it is possible to assemble a list of criteria that, taken together, suggest a particular form of inheritance. The relevant criteria for each type of inheritance are summarized below.

## Autosomal dominant

(1) The disorder is transmitted from generation to generation without skipping any generations.
(2) Every affected offspring has at least one affected parent, except in the case of a new mutant.
(3) Normal offspring from affected parents produce only normal offspring when mated to normals, and the same is true for all their descendants.
(4) Approximately equal numbers of males and females are affected.
(5) If the disorder is rare but not lethal, most matings producing affected offspring will be normal × affected (*aa* × *Aa*), in which case the expectation is that one-half of each sex among the offspring will be affected. Thus the segregation frequency is ½.*
(6) If the disorder is lethal, it will be very rare, occurring sporadically with an incidence equal to twice the mutation rate.

## Autosomal recessive

(1) The disorder may skip generations.
(2) All offspring of two affected parents are affected.
(3) Approximately equal numbers of males and females are affected.
(4) If the disorder is rare:
   (i)   most affected individuals will have both parents normal;
   (ii)  most matings producing affected offspring will be *Bb* × *Bb*, for which the segregation frequency is ¼;*
   (iii) carriers (*Bb*) will usually mate with homozygous normals (*BB*), producing one-half carriers among their offspring; if, then, a carrier sire is mated to his own daughters, or to the daughters of another carrier sire, it follows that one-half of such matings will be *Bb* × *Bb*, in which case the segregation frequency is ½ × ¼ = ⅛;
   (iv)  matings between an affected animal and an unrelated normal animal usually produce only normal offspring;
   (v)   affected × normal matings that do produce affected offspring must be *bb* × *Bb*, in which case the segregation frequency is ½;*
   (vi)  the average genetic relationship between normal parents of affected individuals is greater than between normal parents that have not produced affected individuals. (The reason for this is that the greater the genetic relationship between two individuals, the more likely they are to be carrying the same mutant gene; see Chapter 13.)

## X-linked dominant

(1) Affected males when mated to normal females transmit the disorder to all their daughters but to none of their sons.

---

* See later in this chapter for a discussion of a bias that arises in data collected from such matings.

(2) Unless the disorder is very common, affected females when mated to normal males transmit the disorder to an average of one-half of their sons and one-half of their daughters.

(3) If the disorder is rare, its incidence in females is approximately twice that in males, in the general population.

(4) Every affected offspring has at least one affected parent, except in the case of a new mutant.

## X-linked recessive

(1) The disorder may skip generations.

(2) All offspring of two affected parents are affected.

(3) Incidence is lower in females than in males, with the incidence of the disorder in females being approximately the square of the incidence in males, in the general population.

(4) If the disorder is rare:
  (i)   most affected individuals are males, and result from matings among normal parents;
  (ii)  most matings producing affected offspring will be $X^D X^d \times X^D Y$, for which the segregation frequency is zero in females and ½ in males;*
  (iii) affected males when mated with normal unrelated females transmit the disorder to none of their offspring, but all of their daughters are carriers;
  (iv)  affected females when mated with normal males transmit the disorder to all their male offspring but to none of their female offspring. All female offspring, however, are carriers.

## Studying and analysing the data

### Pedigrees

In many cases, it is convenient to start by drawing pedigrees or family trees. Pedigrees are most informative if drawn in a standard format, using symbols illustrated in Fig. 7.1a. An example of a pedigree is given in Fig. 7.1b, in this case for hereditary multiple exostosis in a family of horses. Constructing pedigrees in this manner can be helpful in providing an initial impression of how a particular disorder is transmitted from one generation to the next. From Fig. 7.1b, for example, it is evident that males and females are affected in approximately equal proportions (six males and five females in generation IV), that matings of affected × affected can produce normal females, and that matings of affected × unrelated normals give rise to quite high proportions of affected offspring. The second observation above is not compatible with either form of X-linked inheritance or with autosomal recessive inheritance, but all three observations are compatible with autosomal dominance. Having

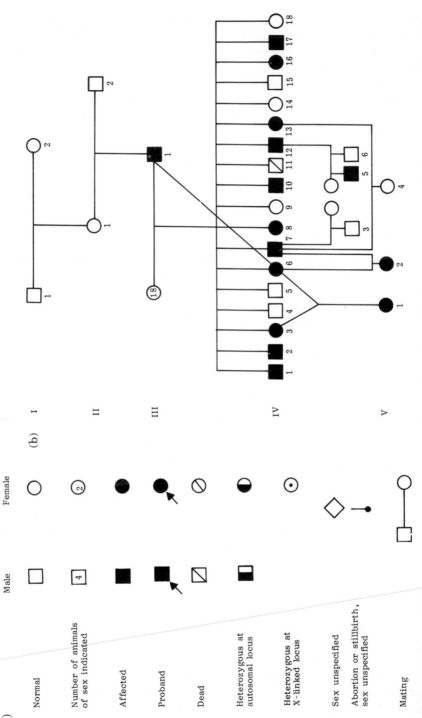

**Fig. 7.1** (a) The symbols used in pedigrees. A **proband** is an affected individual through whom the family came to the notice of the investigator. (b) A pedigree showing the pattern of inheritance of multiple exostosis in horses.

examined a pedigree such as the one shown in Fig. 7.1b, a tentative conclusion could be drawn that the disorder in question, namely multiple exostosis in horses, is an autosomal dominant condition, assuming that III-1 is a new mutant. This conclusion could then be tested on further data.

The problems associated with drawing a pedigree are firstly that it is a time-consuming task, and secondly that in the case of animals, the occurrence of matings between close relatives often results in a large number of inter-crossing lines that are difficult to interpret. Despite these disadvantages, pedigrees can be quite useful, and are often drawn during the initial stages of investigation into the inheritance of a disorder. Fortunately, several software packages are now available for this purpose (sources are listed in Further reading).

## Segregation analysis

If the data on a particular disorder appear to correspond in general terms to one of the four sets of criteria outlined above, the next step is to determine more specifically whether the data are compatible with the respective simple Mendelian mode of inheritance. This is done by means of a segregation analysis. If specifically planned matings can be arranged, it is a simple matter to test agreement with a particular mode of inheritance, by comparing the expected segregation frequencies, which can be obtained from Tables 1.3 and 1.4 in Chapter 1, with those observed. For example, if the disorder is thought to be autosomal recessive, all normal individuals that have produced one or more affected offspring must be carriers. If matings among such known carriers are specifically arranged, we expect one-quarter of all offspring to be affected with the disorder, i.e. the expected segregation frequency is 0.25.

In many situations, however, it is not possible to arrange matings among known carriers and to observe all resultant offspring. Instead, it is much more usual for matings to come to the notice of the investigator after the event, and then only if an affected offspring is produced. This immediately introduces a bias into the data, because those carrier × carrier matings that by chance do not produce any affected offspring are automatically excluded from the data. The result is that even if the defect is really due to an autosomal recessive allele, a segregation frequency greater than 0.25 is expected. This is because all the affected offspring have been included in the data, but not all of the normal offspring.

The existence of this bias was recognized as long ago as 1912, and since then many different methods of segregation analysis have been developed in order to cater for it. A worked example of the best method is given in Appendix 7.1 of *Veterinary Genetics*.

Although the simplest forms of segregation analysis are themselves quite straightforward, in practice there are often considerable difficulties encountered by investigators attempting to determine whether a disorder is Mendelian. For example, it is quite commonly found that while some of the available observations agree very closely with the general criteria for a certain type of inheritance, others are incompatible. Misclassification of phenotypes, as discussed in Chapter 6, is one possible reason. So too are the occurrence of new mutations, and variation in the age of animals when a disorder phenotype becomes visible (i.e. variable age of onset). In addition, complications can arise from sex-limited inheritance, genetic heterogeneity, X-inactivation, phenocopies, genetic anticipation associated with unstable trinucleotide repeats (all discussed in Chapter 3), and genomic imprinting (Chapter 1). In the case of imprinting, for example, carriers of a defective recessive allele show the defect if their normal allele has been inactivated. Another potential source of complication is if the disorder results from a mutation in mitochondrial DNA, because mitochondria are inherited from females but never from males.

Complex methods of segregation analysis have been developed to allow for apparently exceptional animals (called **sporadic cases**) and for other complications. The problem is that as more and more complicating factors are accommodated into segregation analysis, the methods of analysis become more and more complex, and the results become more and more open to debate. In fact, we often reach the stage described in Chapter 6, where the claim of single-gene inheritance has to be qualified in so many ways that it would be more fruitful to think of the disorder as being multifactorial; in many cases, claims of a single gene being primarily responsible do not stand up to close scrutiny.

In circumstances such as these, the aim of segregation analysis should change from simply testing for single-gene inheritance, to testing for the presence of one or more genes making a relatively large contribution to the variation in liability of a multifactorial disorder. A new method of performing such analyses is based on a statistical technique called Markov chain Monte Carlo (MCMC), which utilizes stochastic simulations to estimate parameters. It appears to be more powerful than other methods, and shows considerable promise. In some cases, complex segregation analysis has detected the presence of a single gene of relatively large effect that has subsequently been identified at the molecular level.

As mentioned in Chapter 6, with more and more mapped DNA markers becoming available in domestic species, complex segregation analyses on disorder phenotypes alone are being replaced by linkage analyses conducted jointly on disorder phenotypes and DNA-marker genotypes. The MCMC approach also shows considerable promise in this area. In the end, joint phenotype/marker analyses will lead to the identification of many genes that contribute to disorders (see Chapter 11).

# Further reading

## Reviews

Huston, K. (1993). Heritability and diagnosis of congenital abnormalities in food animals. *Veterinary Clinics of North America—Food Animal Practice*, **9**, (1), 1–9.

Patterson, D. F., Aguirre, G. A., Fyfe, J. C., Giger, U., Green, P. L., Haskens, M. E., Jezyk, P. F., and Meyers-Wallen, V. N. (1989). Is this a genetic disease? *Journal of Small Animal Practice*, **30**, 127–39.

Pidduck, H. (1985). Is this disease inherited? A discussion paper with some guidelines for canine conditions. *Journal of Small Animal Practice*, **26**, 279–91.

Thrusfield, M. (1988). Is it hereditary? *Journal of Small Animal Practice*, **29**, 603–9, 667–78, 719–26.

## Pedigree software

Curtis, D. (1990). A program to draw pedigrees using LINKAGE or LINKSYS data files. *Annals of Human Genetics*, **54**, 365–7.

Fenger, K. and Sorensen, S. A. (1986). ADOXI-PLOT: a computer program for plotting pedigrees illustrating autosomal dominant and X-linked inheritance. *Computer Methods and Programs in Biomedicine*, **23**, 47–52.

Kahn, C. E. (1990). Family Structure—a general program for displaying complex pedigree data. *Computer Methods and Programs in Biomedicine*, **33**, 9–11.

Newton, C. M. (1993). An interactive graphics system for real-time investigation and multivariate data portrayal for complex pedigree data systems. *Computers and Biomedical Research*, **26**, 327–43.

## Segregation and linkage analysis

Elston, R. C. (1992). Segregation and linkage analysis. *Animal Genetics*, **23**, 59–62.

Knott, S. A., Haley, C. S., and Thompson, R. (1992). Methods of segregation analysis for animal breeding data. *Heredity*, **68**, 299–311, 313–20.

Morton, N. E. (1993). Genetic epidemiology. *Annual Review of Genetics*, **27**, 523–38.

Thomas, D. C. and Cortessis, V. (1992). A Gibbs sampling approach to linkage analysis. *Human Heredity*, **42**, 63–76.

**Immunogenetics**

If a foreign substance enters an animal or sometimes even if it just touches the animal's skin, that animal automatically and unconsciously responds to the 'attack' by attempting to inactivate or destroy the foreign substance. Such a response is called an **immune response**, and the protection it provides is called **immunity**. There are two main types of immune response, each of which is brought about primarily by the action of a different type of **lymphocyte** (a type of white blood cell). Lymphocytes originate in the bone marrow stem cells. Those that migrate to the thymus become **T lymphocytes** (often called T cells), while those that migrate to the Bursa of Fabricius in chickens, or remain in the bone marrow in mammals, become **B lymphocytes** (B cells).

In one type of immune response (the **humoral** immune response), B cells mature into plasma cells, which produce large quantities of **antibody**(*anti*-foreign *body*) against the foreign substance, which is called an **antigen** (*anti*body-*gen*erating). The maturation of B cells into plasma cells, and their subsequent production of antibody, is triggered by the presence of antigen. There is an almost infinite range of potential antigens, including viruses, bacteria, foreign molecules of any kind, and blood cells from other animals. If the foreign substance is a cell or a particle of reasonable size, the antibody produced against it is usually directed against specific structures on the surface of the cell or particle. In such cases, the term antigen is applied to the surface structure itself rather than to the whole cell or particle. Despite the huge potential number of different possible antigens, the animal under attack soon produces a quantity of antibody that is specifically directed against the antigen concerned, and the antibody binds with the antigen to form an antigen–antibody complex. The result is agglutination (in which the antigen–antibody complex gives rise to clumps of inactivated cells or particles), or precipitation (clumping of soluble antigens) or cell death (in which the antigen–antibody complex gives rise to a cascading series of reactions that lead to cell lysis). The protection that arises from the production of antibodies is called **humoral immunity**.

The other type of immune response (**cell-mediated** immune response) occurs when T cells, after stimulation by antigen, develop into various types of mature T cells, including cytotoxic T cells (which are directly responsible for the death of viral-infected cells or foreign cells), helper T cells and suppressor T cells (which help or hinder the action of B cells and other T cells), and T cells that give rise to lymphokines, which are soluble factors that can greatly enhance the destructive action of other white blood cells such as macrophages.

The general area of knowledge concerned with the genetic basis of immunity is called **immunogenetics**. The aim of this chapter is to review those aspects of immunogenetics that are most relevant to animals.

## Antibodies

Antibodies are protein molecules that belong to a class of proteins called **immunoglobulins**. The basic immunoglobulin molecule consists of four chains of amino acids, two identical light (L) chains and two identical heavy (H) chains, joined by di-sulphide bonds. Each chain consists of a variable (V) region and a constant (C) region, with the variable regions, as their name implies, differing from one antibody to the next. The constant regions, on the other hand, are usually the same in a large number of different antibodies. The main features of an antibody molecule are illustrated in Fig. 8.1.

Being polypeptides, antibodies are obviously the product of genes. In fact, light and heavy chains are produced from different clusters of genes; for

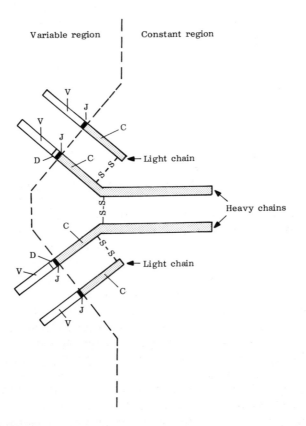

**Fig. 8.1** The main features of an antibody molecule.

heavy chains there is one cluster, and for light chains there are two clusters ($\kappa$ and $\lambda$, only one of which is switched on in any cell). All three clusters are very similar but are located on different chromosomes; they probably arose from the duplication and subsequent translocation of a single ancestral cluster.

As soon as an animal becomes immunocompetent, i.e. becomes capable of producing antibodies, and before being challenged by any antigen, it produces more than one million ($10^6$) different antibodies. Each different antibody is produced by a different clone of B lymphocyte, i.e. a particular clone produces only one type of light chain and one type of heavy chain. How does this huge diversity of antibodies arise?

We shall start by considering the heavy chain. The key to its diversity is that its variable region consists of three segments, namely V, D, and J, and that the heavy-chain gene cluster contains several hundred (around 300) V genes, 12 D genes and four J genes. Since only one of each type of gene contributes to any particular heavy chain, the total possible number of different heavy chains is $300 \times 12 \times 4 = 14\,400$. The light-chain gene clusters have a similar structure, except that they lack the D genes. Thus the total possible number of different light chains is $300 \times 4 = 1200$. Recalling that an antibody molecule comprises one type of heavy chain and one type of light chain, it follows that a total of $14\,400 \times 1200 = 1.728 \times 10^7$ different antibody molecules could be produced, which is sufficient to explain the observed antibody diversity. In fact, not all of the potential combinations occur, but there are other sources of additional diversity (variable recombination between the V and J genes, and somatic mutation), which increase the diversity.

## Red-cell antigens

Red-cell antigens are antigens occurring on the surface of red blood cells. They have been extensively studied in domestic animals for many decades. Most of the antigens are glycoproteins, which exist in different forms corresponding to different sequences of sugars attached to a polypeptide chain. Since the addition of sugars is performed by enzymes, which are the products of genes, it follows that different red-cell antigens are inherited as if they were actually the products of genes themselves. All the red-cell antigens arising from alleles at a single locus belong to the same blood-group system. There are many different blood-group systems (each corresponding to a different locus) in each species of domestic animal. They are usually identified by different letters or combinations of letters of the alphabet. There is a huge range in the number of alleles identified for different systems, from two to several hundred.

Antibodies against most red-cell blood groups are produced only following a challenge with the appropriate antigen. The exceptions to this are the J system in cattle and the AB system in cats. In these systems, antibodies to antigens not carried by an animal occur 'naturally' in that animal, without any obvious challenge. For example, anti-A antibody occurs in almost all cats that have the B antigen. Apart from these exceptions, animals do not normally carry antibodies to red-blood-cell antigens, unless they have been specifically challenged with the appropriate foreign red blood cells.

Since animals do not normally carry antibodies to red-blood-cell antigens, it has been assumed that blood transfusions in animals can be conducted quite safely with any available blood, and that there is normally no need for blood typing before transfusion. However, transfusion with randomly-chosen, un-typed blood may lead to an immediate transfusion reaction if, unbeknown to the practitioner, the recipient has been transfused previously with blood containing the same antigens. Even if this does not occur, it is likely that a random, untyped transfusion will sensitize the recipient to subsequent trans-fusions, or to the blood cells of the recipient's future offspring, if the recipient is a female (see below). Thus, whenever possible, it is advisable to obtain blood for transfusion from donors who have been typed as being compatible or negative for red-blood-cell antigens that are known to evoke strong anti-body responses.

The most clinically important antigens are A in dogs, B in cats, $A_a$ and $Q_a$ in horses, and A, F, and some B antigens in cattle. If untyped donors must be used, a simple cross-match should be conducted, in which a drop of plasma from the recipient is mixed on a slide with a drop of red-cell suspension from the donor. If agglutination occurs, it would be wise to find another donor. However, since this cross-match test is not always effective, a lack of aggluti-nation does not guarantee that a transfusion reaction will not occur. Thus, care should be taken during transfusions, even if the cross-match test is negative.

## Neonatal isoerythrolysis

Occasionally new-born foals that appear perfectly normal at birth, become weak and dull within 24 hours of birth, and develop acute anaemia, jaundice and haemoglobinuria. Their heart and respiratory rates become elevated, and they usually die within a few days. This disease is known as neonatal isoerythrolysis, NI, or haemolytic disease of the newborn. Judging from the above clinical signs, NI is associated with destruction of red blood cells. Why should this happen?

In the case of horses, the answer lies in feto-maternal haemorrhage that occurs sometimes during pregnancy or birth, releasing red blood cells from the fetus into its dam's blood circulation. Consider the A blood-group system, which happens to be the most important in relation to NI, and consider the $A_a$ antigen within that system. Suppose that the fetus has inherited the $A_a$ antigen from its sire, i.e. both sire and fetus are positive for $A_a$ (written as $A_a+$). Suppose also that the dam lacks the $A_a$ antigen (written as $A_a-$). When the cells from the fetus enter the dam, she recognizes antigen $A_a$ as non-self, because she does not have that antigen. She therefore produces anti-$A_a$ antibodies in her serum. These anti-$A_a$ antibodies are transferred along with all other antibodies into the dam's colostrum, which the foal drinks. The reason for the clinical signs of NI should now be evident. The anti-$A_a$ antibodies are absorbed through the foal's gut and pass into its blood stream, where they rapidly destroy all cells with $A_a$ antigen on their surface.

Not all blood-group systems give rise to this problem. Indeed, only the A and Q systems are regularly implicated in horses, with the former being the most important. However, it seems that all donkeys exhibit a red-cell antigen that is absent in horses, which means that all mule fetuses carried in mares are at risk of NI. Fortunately, NI is rare in the first-born of any mare, because the initial immune response is usually too slow to cause any trouble; the mare has not yet been sensitized. If challenged a second time, however, the mare quickly mounts an immune response which gives rise to NI.

There are certain actions that can be taken to alleviate NI. Treatment of affected foals involves either transfusion with whole blood from a suitable donor, or transfusion of washed red blood cells from the dam. The main requirement is that the cells given to the affected foal must not carry any antigens that are carried by the sire but not the dam of the foal, as it is these antigens against which the dam has produced antibodies. Thus the sire is *not* a suitable donor. In contrast, the dam could be a suitable donor, because none of the antibodies that the foal obtained from her colostrum will be directed against her own cells. But her serum contains the offending antibodies, produced by her against the foal's antigens inherited from its sire. Consequently, if the dam's cells are to be used for transfusion, they must first be washed with sterile saline, with the aim of removing all plasma and hence all offending antibody.

NI in foals can be prevented very simply by not allowing the foal access to its dam's colostrum for the first 24–36 hours, until protein molecules are no longer absorbed by the foal's small intestine. Such action should be taken only if the foal is known to be at risk. This can be determined by screening for the presence of antibody to the foal's cells, in the pregnant mare's serum at 4 weeks, 2 weeks, and 1 week prior to the expected parturition date. The cells used in this screening test can be from the sire of the foal or from a panel of horses known to be positive for antigens involved in NI. However, because NI occurs with a frequency of less than 1 per cent, this would be a very wasteful procedure if done on all mares. A more efficient procedure would be to blood-type all mares, and then to screen during the last 4 weeks of pregnancy only those that are $A_a$ negative, i.e. that lack antigen $A_a$. The reason for concentrating solely on $A_a$ is that antibodies to this antigen are thought to be the cause of more than 80 per cent of all cases of NI in horses. At the very minimum, all mares that are thought to have previously produced an NI foal should be screened. If this is not possible, all subsequent foals of such mares should be given colostrum from a source other than their dam, as a precaution against NI.

NI is best known in horses, but has been reported in cats, dogs, cattle, and pigs as well. In the case of cattle and pigs, its cause was traced to the use of blood-based vaccines against babesiosis (tick fever) and anaplasmosis in cattle, and against swine fever (hog cholera) in pigs. These cases of NI have now been largely overcome by phasing out blood-based vaccines.

In the case of naturally occurring NI, it is worth noting that the genetical effect in all species is selection against heterozygotes. This is because the only situation in which the fetus has an antigen not carried by the dam is if the fetus inherited a different antigen from its sire, and must therefore be heterozygous.

## The major histocompatibility complex (MHC)

It is common knowledge that organ and tissue transplants and skin grafts are usually rejected by the recipient. It is also well known that the chance of rejection is considerably reduced if the donor is a close relative of the recipient. Obviously, there is a genetic basis to transplant rejection. In fact, rejection is the result of an immune response determined by naturally occurring cell-surface antigens.

There are many loci whose gene products play a role in compatibility between tissue (**histocompatibility**), and hence in rejection of foreign tissue. But there is one group of tightly-linked loci that plays a much more important role than any of the others. Because of its major role, this group of loci is called the **major histocompatibility complex** (MHC). All domestic species have an MHC. In mammals, the MHC is approximately 3500 kb (approximately 3.5 cM) long, and includes many genes. For ease of description, the MHC is divided into three regions, as shown in Fig. 8.2.

The class I region contains several genes, each of which codes for a polypeptide which combines with another polypeptide called $\beta_2$-microglobulin (encoded by a locus on another chromosome) to form a molecule called **class I histoglobulin** (*histo* because of the role in histocompatibility, and *globulin* because of the molecule's resemblance to immunoglobulins). The class II region contains genes that encode two different types of polypeptide ($\alpha$ and $\beta$ chains) which unite to form a **class II histoglobulin** molecule. As shown in Fig. 8.2, both classes of histoglobulin are expressed on the cell surface. Class I histoglobulins are expressed on almost all nucleated cells, while class II histoglobulins have a limited distribution, occurring mainly on B lymphocytes, macrophages, and dendritic cells. The class II region also contains genes whose polypeptides are involved with the processing of foreign antigen. Some of them are called TAP genes (for *t*ransporter *a*ssociated with antigen *p*rocessing). The class III region contains a mixture of genes having a wide range of functions, only some of which are involved in the immune response. The genes C2, C4A, and C4B encode polypeptides which are components of complement (a set of molecules that form an amplifying cascade of enzymatic activations following the formation of a complex between an antigen and an antibody, resulting in fracture of the cell wall and cell death).

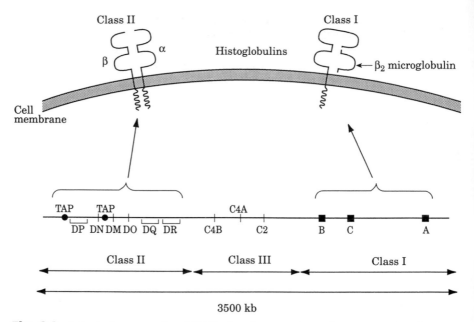

**Fig. 8.2** A typical mammalian MHC, showing representative genes, plus the gene products.

The total number of genes identified within the MHC is more than 100, and the number is steadily growing. Some of these are not functional, either because they have been inactivated by mutation (called **pseudogenes**) or because they are actually a DNA copy of the mature mRNA from a functional gene (called **processed pseudogenes**, as explained in Chapter 2). Many others are only poorly understood at present. For our purposes, we need to concentrate on only a relatively small number of MHC genes.

Within the class I region it is sufficient to consider just three functional genes, namely A, B, and C. The class II region is slightly more complex. The naming of the class II genes arises from the fact that the class II region is also called the D region. For ease of description it is divided into three main subregions: DP, DQ, and DR. Each of these subregions contains at least two functional genes; one encoding an $\alpha$ chain (called the DPA, DQA, and DRA genes), and the other encoding a $\beta$ chain (called the DPB, DQB, and DRB genes). In addition, there are at least three other regions (DM, DN, and DO). The DM region encodes an $\alpha$ chain and a $\beta$ chain, which combine to form a class II-like molecule that is involved in antigen processing. The DN region contains a gene for an $\alpha$ chain (the DNA gene!), and the DO region contains a gene for a $\beta$ chain (the DOB gene).

In chickens, the MHC is the B blood group system, which was originally identified in terms of antigens on the surface of red blood cells. It has a class-I region (called B-F) and a class-II region (B-L), but there is no intervening

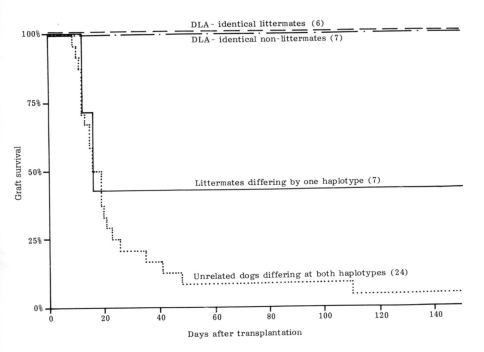

**Fig. 8.3** Survival of kidney transplants in dogs. Numbers in brackets are the numbers of recipients in each group, excluding four recipients that died from causes other than rejection.

class-III region. Instead, there is an adjacent B-G region, which encodes uniquely avian molecules that are expressed primarily on red blood cells.

As stated above, the MHC is the major determinant of tissue rejection. Its importance is illustrated in Fig. 8.3, which shows the results of a series of kidney transplantations in dogs. When the donor and recipient were MHC-identical (i.e. they each had two haplotypes in common), transplantation was 100 per cent successful. If they had only one haplotype in common, transplantation was approximately 50 per cent successful, and if they had no haplotype in common, the success rate was close to zero. Not all transplantation studies have shown such clear-cut effects of the MHC as those in Fig. 8.3. For example, the results for MHC-identical non-littermates are often not as good as those for MHC-identical littermates, confirming that there are other loci that play a role in determining histocompatibility. However, there can be no doubt about the importance of the MHC.

Although initial interest in the MHC arose from its role in tissue rejection, it has since become clear that the MHC plays a vital role in the immune response to pathogens and parasites. In fact, the MHC is the engine room of the immune response to disease. How does it perform this important role? Basically, it does so by enabling T cells to identify anything that is non-self (foreign). How does this occur? By a histoglobulin 'presenting' to T cells a small peptide fragment of the pathogen or parasite. The fragment is held within a groove (called the **peptide binding region**, PBR, or **antigen binding site**, ABS) of the histoglobulin. The T cells recognize the foreign peptide as non-self only if it is presented in the context of self, i.e. only if it is presented by a histoglobulin which the T cells recognize as self. This phenomenon is called MHC restriction. Once they have recognized the peptide as being foreign, the T cells activate either a cell-mediated immune response (if the foreign peptide has come from inside a host cell) or an antibody-mediated immune response (if it came from elsewhere).

## Determining phenotype and genotype at the MHC

In order to investigate the role of the MHC in immunity to disease, it is necessary to be able to identify which histoglobulins are present in any individual. Also, in view of the integral role of the MHC in tissue rejection, it is important to determine the extent to which any potential pair of donor and recipient differ in histoglobulins. Consequently, methods for determining the phenotype (and the genotype) at each MHC locus, have been developed.

The first method, which is still in use, utilizes sera containing polyclonal antibodies which distinguish between histoglobulins. The procedure is called **tissue typing**. It identifies the phenotype (tissue type) corresponding to certain alleles.

More recently, molecular technology has enabled genotypes to be determined directly, right down to the level of nucleotide sequence. As more and more MHC alleles were sequenced, it became evident that differences between alleles do not occur randomly; in fact, almost all of the differences between class I alleles occur within just two small exons (exons 2 and 3), and for class II alleles, the differences occur primarily within a single small exon (exon 2). This is just the situation that is tailor-made for PCR: if primers are chosen from either side of the segment in which the allelic differences occur, the amplified DNA contains the very sequences in which the alleles differ. The alleles can then be identified by RFLP analysis or by dot blotting with allele-specific oligos (as described in Chapter 2). In some cases, alleles can be identified indirectly by association with microsatellite alleles in neighbouring introns. Increasingly, MHC genotypes are being determined by allele-specific amplification or by automated cycle sequencing (also described in Chapter 2).

## MHC polymorphism

One of the most striking features of the MHC to emerge from phenotyping and genotyping thousands of individuals in many species is its extreme polymorphism: there are many alleles at most loci. In humans, for example, there are at least 41 alleles at the A locus, 61 at the B locus, 18 at the C locus, and 60 at one of the DRB loci.

A consequence of this polymorphism is that almost every individual has a unique MHC genotype; the chance of any two individuals chosen at random having the same set of MHC alleles is exceedingly small. Obviously, this makes it very difficult to find a suitable donor for tissue transplantation.

Because MHC loci are so closely linked, the set of alleles (one per locus) that happen to be on a particular chromosome are usually inherited as a single unit called a **haplotype**. The word is a combination of *hap*loid and geno*type*, which indicates its meaning: it refers to the 'genotype' of a single chromosome. Since chromosomes occur in pairs, each animal has two MHC haplotypes, one inherited from its dam, and the other inherited from its sire. If a cross-over occurs within the MHC during meiosis, two new haplotypes are formed. But because the MHC loci are so closely linked, crossing-over within the MHC is not common. Thus, haplotypes are usually passed from parents to offspring in exactly the same form for many generations. In fact, for as long as crossing-over does not occur within the MHC, each haplotype is inherited as if it were an allele at a single locus. Because of the extensive polymorphism within the MHC, the two members of a mating pair are usually each heterozygous for different MHC haplotypes. Consequently, there are usually four different haplotypes in the gametes produced by any pair of parents. By working through Fig. 8.4, it can be seen that this results in only four different

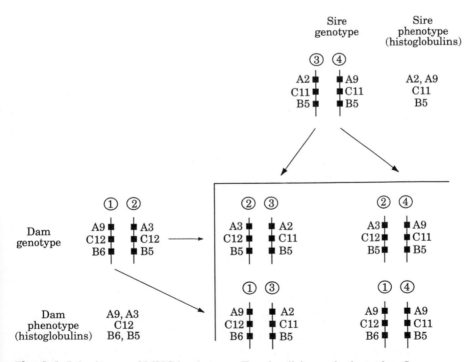

**Fig. 8.4** Inheritance of MHC haplotypes. For simplicity, only three class-I genes are shown. Haplotype numbers are shown in circles.

combinations of haplotypes in the offspring from a particular mating (called full-sibs), with all combinations occurring in equal frequency, namely ¼. It follows that despite the immense polymorphism at the MHC, the chance that any two full-sibs have the same set of MHC genes is $¼ × ¼ = 1/16$ (if we neglect the low chance of crossing-over). Also, for any individual, there is a chance of ¼ that any one of its full-sibs has the same set of MHC genes as it does. Thus, full-sibs are a very useful potential source of tissue for transplantation.

## The adaptive significance of MHC polymorphism

We saw earlier that most of the allelic variation within MHC genes occurs within just one or two exons. In fact, most of the variation is confined to 57 triplets within exons 2 and 3 in class I genes, 19 or 20 triplets in exon 2 of class II α-chain genes, and 15 or 16 triplets in exon 2 of class II β-chain genes. Interestingly, these are the triplets that encode the peptide binding region (PBR) of histoglobulins. Furthermore, comparisons of the differences in sequence between alleles have shown that the rate of silent mutations (sometimes called synonymous base substitutions) is much slower than the rate of mis-sense mutations (non-synonymous base substitutions) in the triplets of the PBR, whereas exactly the opposite is true in non-PBR triplets. These results have been interpreted as indicating that natural selection favours the widest possible range of different amino-acid sequences in the PBR, but at the same time, positively discriminates against amino-acid substitutions in other regions of histoglobulins. It should be evident that this fits in perfectly with the different role of the PBR compared with the rest of the histoglobulin molecule: the PBR needs to be as variable as possible, so as to maximize the number of different foreign peptide fragments that can be presented to T cells. In contrast, the remainder of the histoglobulin has a constant role, irrespective of which peptide is being presented; its job is to anchor itself to the cell membrane, and to provide various forms of physical attachment by which T cells can interrogate the PBR region.

## Associations between the MHC and disease

Given the picture presented above, is there evidence that certain histoglobulins are able to present certain pathogens more effectively than others, and so bring about a more effective immune response? In other words, is there any evidence for association between certain histoglobulins and certain diseases?

At the molecular level, there is convincing evidence of differences between histoglobulins in their ability to present foreign peptides. And at the organismal level, there definitely are some well-documented examples of MHC/disease associations. However, most of these are in humans, most are involved with susceptibility rather than with resistance, and many involve diseases of an autoimmune nature. In domestic animals, despite a huge number of studies and many apparent associations, there are only a few that can withstand close scrutiny. The most convincing evidence to date has been obtained from poultry, in which the association between the $B^{21}$ histoglobulin and susceptibility to Marek's disease is very solidly established.

It seems likely that much progress will be made in the area of MHC/disease associations in the next few years, now that PCR technology enables accurate genotyping right down to the level of base sequence. Among other things, this technology will enable much broader and more sensible questions to be asked about the role of the MHC in determining resistance to disease. We might discover, for example, that the important thing is not to have a particular set of histoglobulins, but to be as heterozygous as possible at as many loci as possible, with the actual identity of histoglobulins being of secondary import- ance. If this is so, the aim which some people have of identifying the 'best' histoglobulins and then making populations homozygous for them, may be the wrong approach.

## Other MHC associations

In view of the MHC's important role in immunity, it seems likely that it also holds the key to the design of effective vaccines. In particular, the effective- ness of a vaccine depends on the extent to which histoglobulins can present the protective components of the vaccine to T cells. With PCR genotyping enabling MHC alleles to be distinguished down to the level of base sequence, there is great scope for vaccine manufacturers to collaborate with immuno- geneticists so as to ensure that commercial vaccines have the greatest chance of success. This is likely to be a very active area of future research.

In addition to transplantation and immunity, the MHC appears to play some role in choice of mate and in reproductive success. For example, some intriguing data from experiments with mice show that when given a choice between mating partners, both males and females tend to choose partners from whom they differ the most in terms of histoglobulins, i.e. there is a tendency for mates to be chosen on the basis of histo*in*compatibility. Further- more, there is evidence suggesting that the discrimination between different MHC phenotypes is based on odours.

In relation to reproductive success, there is tantalizing evidence from humans that couples with a history of recurrent spontaneous abortion (RSA) are more similar in their histoglobulins, i.e. are more histocompatible, than fertile control couples. In addition, among embryos that survive to full term, those which are most histocompatible with their mothers tend to have the lightest birth weights. Some people argue that this is essentially a genetic phenomenon, reflecting the effects of increased homozygosity for defective alleles at loci located in the MHC (but not yet identified) which are involved in early embryonic development. Others favour the suggestion that successful implantation and pregnancy actually require a controlled immune response, which in turn requires the mother to recognize, and respond in a controlled manner to, the non-self embryonic histoglobulins—those which are the products of the MHC alleles inherited from the father. The RSA association with histoincompatibility could be explained on the basis that the greater the MHC similarity between father and mother, the smaller the chance that the mother will be able to mount the controlled immune response that is necessary for successful pregnancy.

The importance of the MHC in mate choice and reproductive success remains an open question at present, especially in relation to domestic animals. However, given the supreme importance of reproductive ability in domestic animals, the possible role of the MHC should be fully investigated, especially now that PCR technology enables such detailed and accurate genotyping.

Finally, mention must be made of the many studies which have investigated associations between the MHC and production traits of domestic animals. The main rationale for these studies has been the argument that if the MHC does have an influence on disease resistance, there may be a consequential effect on production—healthier animals are expected to be more productive. As with the disease association studies, there are many claims of association between MHC and production traits, but on close examination, most turn out to be more apparent than real; and none of the real associations has been sufficiently strong to justify their use in practical breeding programmes. While PCR genotyping is certain to increase the power of MHC/production association studies in the future, it seems likely that the most fruitful areas of future MHC research in domestic animals will involve the immune response directly, rather than the possible indirect effects of MHC associations with production traits.

## Further reading

### Antibodies

Gellert, M. (1992). V(D)J recombination gets a break. *Trends in Genetics*, **8**, 408–12.
Lieber, M. R. (1992). The mechanism of V(D)J recombination—a balance of diversity, specificity, and stability. *Cell*, **70**, 873–6.
Schatz, D. G., Oettinger, M. A., and Schlissel, M. S. (1992). V(D)J recombination—molecular biology and regulation. *Annual Review of Immunology*, **10**, 359–83.

### Red-cell antigens/transfusions

Bell, K. (1983). The blood groups of domestic mammals. In *Red blood cells of domestic mammals*, (ed. N. S. Agar and P. G. Board), pp. 133–64. Elsevier, Amsterdam.
Bruckler, J., Schreiber, W., Blobel, K., and Blobel, H. (1992). Group incompatibilities in horses particularly in neonatal icterus. *Monatshefte für Veterinarmedizin*, **47**, 653–5.

Dodds, W. J. (1992). Hemopet—a national non-profit animal blood bank program. *Canine Practice*, **17**, (6), 12–16.

Giger, U., Bucheler, J., Callan, M. B., Casal, M., and Griotwenk, M. (1993). Feline neonatal isoerythrolysis and transfusion reactions. *Kleintierpraxis*, **38**, 715.

Kerl, M. E. and Hohenhaus, A. E. (1993). Packed red blood cell transfusions in dogs—131 cases (1989). *Journal of the American Veterinary Medical Association*, **202**, 1495–9.

Lutz, P. and Dzik, W. H. (1992). Molecular biology of red cell blood group genes. *Transfusion*, 32, 467–83.

McClure, J. J., Koch, C., and Traubdargatz, J. (1994). Characterization of a red blood cell antigen in donkeys and mules associated with neonatal isoerythrolysis. *Animal Genetics*, **25**, 119–20.

Norsworthy, G. D. (1992). Clinical aspects of feline blood transfusions. *Compendium on Continuing Education for the Practicing Veterinarian*, **14**, 469–75.

Slappendel, R. J. (1992). Blood transfusions in the dog and cat. *Tijdschrift voor Diergeneeskunde*, **117**, (S1), S16–S18.

Stone, E., Badner, D., and Cotter, S. M. (1992). Trends in transfusion medicine in dogs at a veterinary school clinic—315 cases (1986-1989). *Journal of the American Veterinary Medical Association*, **200**, 1000–4.

Vankan, D. M. and Bell, K. (1993). Caprine blood groups. *Biochemical Genetics*, **31**, 7–18, 19–28.

Williamson, L. (1993). Highlights of blood transfusion in horses. *Compendium on Continuing Education for the Practicing Veterinarian*, **15**, 267–9.

## MHC, general

Barber, L. D. and Parham, P. (1993). Peptide binding to major histocompatibility complex molecules. *Annual Review of Cell Biology*, **9**, 163–206.

Brown, J. L. and Eklund, A. (1994). Kin recognition and the major histocompatibility complex—an integrative review. *American Naturalist*, **143**, 435–61.

Chicz, R. M. and Urban, R. G. (1994). Analysis of MHC-presented peptides— applications in autoimmunity and vaccine development. *Immunology Today*, **15**, 155–60.

Germain, R. N. and Margulies, D. H. (1993). The biochemistry and cell biology of antigen processing and presentation. *Annual Review of Immunology*, **11**, 403–50.

Gill, T. J. (1992). Influence of MHC and MHC-linked genes on reproduction. *American Journal of Human Genetics*, **50**, 1–5.

Janeway, C. A. (1993). How the immune system recognizes invaders. *Scientific American*, **269**, (3), 72–9.

Klein, J., Satta, Y., Ohuigin, C., and Takahata, N. (1993). The molecular descent of the major histocompatibility complex. *Annual Review of Immunology*, **11**, 269–95.

Kronenberg, M., Brines, R., and Kaufman, J. (1994). MHC evolution—a long term investment in defense. *Immunology Today*, **15**, 4–6.

McMichael, A. (1993). HLA and disease. In *Advancement of veterinary science*, The Bicentenary Symposium Series, Vol. 1, (ed. A.R. Mitchell), pp. 11–24. CAB International, Wallingford, England.

Pescovitz, M. D. (1992). Organ acceptance and rejection. *Current Opinion in Immunology*, **4**, 577–81.

Potts, W. K. and Wakeland, E. K. (1993). Evolution of MHC genetic diversity—a tale of incest, pestilence and sexual preference. *Trends in Genetics*, **9**, 408–12.

Stern, L. J., Brown, J. H., Jardetzky, T. S., Gorga, J. C., Urban, R. G., Strominger, J. L., and Wiley, D. C. (1994). Crystal structure of the human class II MHC protein HLA-DR1 complexed with an influenza virus peptide. *Nature*, **368**, 215–21.

Yamazaki, K., Beauchamp, G. K., Shen, F. W., Bard, J., and Boyse, E. A. (1994). Discrimination of odortypes determined by the major histocompatibility complex among outbred mice. *Proceedings of the National Academy of Sciences, USA*, **91**, 3735–8.

## MHC, domestic animals

Bacon, L. D. and Witter, R. L. (1994). B-haplotype influence on the relative efficacy of Marek's disease vaccines in commercial chickens. *Poultry Science*, **73**, 481–7.

Burnett, R. C., Derose, S. A., and Storb, R. (1994). A simple restriction fragment-length polymorphism assay for MHC class II gene testing of dog families. *Transplantation*, **57**, 280–2.

Emara, M. G. and Nestor, K. E. (1993). The turkey major histocompatibility complex—characterization by mixed lymphocyte, graft-versus-host splenomegaly, and skin graft reactions. *Poultry Science*, **72**, 60–6.

Garber, T. L., Hughes, A. L., Letvin, N. L., Templeton, J. W., and Watkins, D. I. (1993). Sequence and evolution of cattle MHC class-I cDNAs—concerted evolution has not taken place in cattle. *Immunogenetics*, **38**, 11–20.

McGuire, T. C., Tumas, D. B., Byrne, K. M., Hines, M. T., Leib, S. R., Brassfield, A. L., et al. (1994). Major histocompatibility complex-restricted CD8(+) cytotoxic T lymphocytes from horses with equine infectious anemia virus recognize env and GAG/Pr proteins. *Journal of Virology*, **68**, 1459–67.

Meijssen, M. A. C., Heineman, E., Debruin, R. W. F., Wolvekamp, M. C. J., Marquet, R. L., and Molenaar, J. C. (1993). Long-term survival of DLA-matched segmental small-bowel allografts in dogs. *Transplantation*, **56**, 1062–6.

Ono, H., Ohuigin, C., Vincek, V., and Klein, J. (1993). Exon–intron organization of fish major histocompatibility complex class-II B-genes. *Immunogenetics*, **38**, 223–34.

Plachy, J., Pink, J. R. L., and Hala, K. (1992). Biology of the chicken MHC (B-complex). *Critical Reviews in Immunology*, **12**, 47–79.

Sander, J. E. (1993). The major histocompatibility complex and its role in poultry production. *World's Poultry Science Journal*, **49**, 132–8.

Schat, K. A., Taylor, R. L., and Briles, W. E. (1994). Resistance to Marek's disease in chickens with recombinant haplotypes of the major histocompatibility-(B) complex. *Poultry Science*, **73**, 502–8.

Schwaiger, F. W., Weyers, E., Buitkamp, J., Ede, A. J., Crawford, A., and Epplen, J. T. (1994). Interdependent MHC-DRB exon-plus-intron evolution in artiodactyls. *Molecular Biology and Evolution*, **11**, 239–49.

# Pharmacogenetics 9

Given the vast array of different biochemical pathways that are involved in reactions to drugs, there are obviously many genes which affect drug metabolism. The aim of this chapter is to provide an overview of current knowledge of the genetic control of drug metabolism.

## Genetic polymorphisms affecting drug metabolism

One of the most important sets of genes concerned with drug metabolism is the cytochrome-P450 gene family. The number of different functional P450 genes in a species is at least 60 and could be greater than 200. The products of these genes are haem-containing enzymes called mono-oxygenases, which are in the first line of 'defence' against 'foreign' chemicals, performing many different biochemical functions including hydroxylation, dehalogenation, dealkylation, deamination, and reduction, as a necessary first step in detoxification.

While there is still much to be learnt about these enzymes, especially in domestic animals, there is already substantial evidence of considerable polymorphism at many of the P450 genes, giving rise to marked differences in reaction to a range of drugs including debrisoquin, sparteine, dextrometorphan, tricyclic antidepressants, opioids, beta-adrenergic receptor antagonists, mephenytoin, mephobarbital, hexobarbital, and diazepam. Mutant forms of P450 enzymes inhibit the metabolism of these drugs, resulting in adverse drug reactions, including presentation with extreme side effects.

Another well documented polymorphism in drug metabolism concerns the locus for the enzyme N-acetyltransferase (NAT), which is involved in numerous acetylation reactions. Faulty alleles at this locus result in substantially slower deactivation of a wide range of drugs including isoniazid, sulphamethazine and several other sulphonamides, hydralazine, procainamide, dapsone, para-aminobenzoic acid, phenelzine, and aminoglutethimide; as well as substances such as clonazepam, nitrazepam, benzidine, 2-amino-fluorene, beta-naphthylamine, and even caffeine! Once again, the clinical importance of the mutant alleles arises from the side effects induced by failure to deactivate the chemical.

## Genetics and anaesthesia

One of the best understood cases of the genetic basis of drug response in animals concerns reaction to the anaesthetic halothane in pigs, which, as described in Chapter 6, has been used as a test for malignant hyperthermia syndrome (MHS). Reactors usually show signs of stiffening in the hind quarters after 2 minutes exposure to halothane, associated with rapid hyperthermia which soon leads to death if halothane is not removed. Reaction to halothane is due to homozygosity for a recessive allele, which is usually given the symbol *hal* or *n*.

Apart from its obvious importance in relation to MHS, *hal* is also important because there is a very strong association between adverse reaction to halothane and the economically important set of traits known as porcine stress syndrome (PSS), which is characterized by sudden death after only a minor stress, and by pale, soft, exudative (PSE) meat. In contrast to these undesirable features, *hal* also has a substantial advantage: it increases yield of lean meat. (As mentioned in Chapter 5, this appears to be another example of selection favouring heterozygotes, which explains why *hal* has remained at relatively high frequencies in many populations throughout the world.) Opinion is divided as to whether its advantages outweigh its disadvantages. In any case, because of its obvious importance, tens of thousands of pigs were halothane-tested throughout the world each year during the 1980s, and the halothane locus was the subject of a huge international research effort. In 1991, a major breakthrough occurred when a Canadian research team led by David MacLennan reported the isolation and cloning of the halothane gene in pigs. Furthermore, by comparing the nucleotide sequence of the two alleles (normal and *hal*), MacLennan and colleagues showed that *hal* differed from the normal allele by 18 nucleotide substitutions. However, only one of these nucleotide substitutions creates an amino acid substitution; the remainder are silent mutations. This means that all of the adverse effects of the *hal* allele (MHS, PSS, and PSE), plus its advantageous effects, are due to the simplest of all possible mutations, namely a single base substitution. This occurs at the 1843rd nucleotide (where C is replaced by T), which causes an amino-acid substitution (arginine is replaced by cysteine) at the 615th position in the polypeptide chain.

The polypeptide product of the halothane gene has the unlikely name of ryanodine receptor, because it was first identified as a protein that happens to bind very strongly to a plant alkaloid called ryanodine. It is actually a calcium release channel (CRC) in the sarcoplasmic reticulum of skeletal muscle, allowing calcium ions to flow into the surrounding muscle tissue, resulting in muscle contraction.

The CRC molecule is extremely large, consisting of a single chain of approximately 5000 amino acids, which obviously means that the total coding sequence of the gene is approximately 15 000 bases long. This makes the single base-substitution difference between the normal and *hal* allele all the more remarkable; the two alternative forms of the polypeptide differ by only one amino acid in a chain of 5000 amino acids! This simple difference occurs at a position in the polypeptide which has a critical influence on calcium flow, which in turn gives rise to all of the effects (both advantageous and disadvantageous) of the halothane gene.

The cloning of the CRC gene has enabled extensive DNA testing to be conducted in populations around the world. Initial indications are that the same mutation is responsible for all cases of MHS in pigs. In humans, the situation is not so straightforward; in some families the same mutation as in pigs is associated with MHS, but in other families, MHS segregates independently from the CRC gene, indicating that there are other genes involved in MHS. Given this genetic heterogeneity in humans, we should not be surprised if sometime in the future we find cases of MHS in pigs which are not associated with the CRC gene.

## Warfarin resistance

Warfarin is an anticoagulant that is used extensively in medicine; it is also used as a rodent poison.

Only five years after its introduction as a rodenticide in Britain, resistant rats were detected in the field. Nine years later (in 1967, when estimates first became available), the frequency of resistance rats was nearly 50 per cent in areas in which warfarin was used regularly, and it seemed that this frequency would continue to increase. However, the frequency of resistant rats has remained at an intermediate level ever since. What has caused this apparently stable intermediate equilibrium?

The answer lies in an understanding of the blood coagulation process. In simple terms, coagulation is a complex cascade of biochemical reactions involving various clotting factors. Some of these factors, namely the proteins II, VII, IX, and X, require vitamin K for their activation. Specifically, vitamin K is a co-factor for the carboxylation phase of activation, in which certain glutamic-acid amino acids in the clotting-factor polypeptides are converted to gamma-carboxyglutamic acid (called Gla) by the enzyme γ-glutamylcarboxylase. This carboxylation enables the clotting factors to bind calcium ions, which in turn enables the factors to attach themselves to phospholipids on the surface of platelets. This is how blood clotting is initiated. By the time each vitamin K molecule has completed its carboxylation task, it has become vitamin K epoxide, which is then reduced by the enzyme epoxide reductase back to its original form, in readiness for the next round of carboxylation. The process of carboxylation followed by reduction is called the vitamin-K cycle.

Warfarin has a structure very similar to vitamin K, and therefore binds to epoxide reductase, preventing it from recycling the vitamin K epoxide. The result is a buildup of vitamin K epoxide, a deficiency of vitamin K, and hence a deficiency of clotting factors.

There are several different forms of inherited resistance to warfarin in rodents. One of the best understood involves an autosomal recessive allele, R, which codes for a slightly different form of epoxide reductase which has a lower affinity for warfarin. But since vitamin K and warfarin have such a similar molecular structure, the mutant form of epoxide reductase also has a lower affinity for vitamin K. The practical consequence of this is that animals homozygous for the resistant allele have a 20-fold higher requirement for vitamin K in their diet, to compensate for the lower affinity of the enzyme produced by this allele. If this increased demand can not be met, homozygotes for the resistant allele suffer from the same bleeding disorders as those induced by warfarin in susceptible animals, namely disorders due to deficiencies in the vitamin-K-dependent blood clotting factors.

Several studies of the relative fitnesses of each genotype resulting from the action of these factors have been conducted. Using the results from two such studies in Britain, the following somewhat simplified account illustrates the main aspects of the warfarin story.

Because *RR* homozygotes have a higher requirement for vitamin K than heterozygotes (*RS*, where *S* is the susceptible, wild-type allele), the genotype *RR* has the lowest relative fitness in the absence of warfarin, with the *RS* genotype having a fitness somewhere between the two homozygotes, e.g. 0.46, 0.77, and 1.00 for *RR*, *RS*, and *SS* respectively. From Chapter 5, it should be evident that the result of this set of relative fitnesses is that the *R* allele is either removed from the population, or is maintained at a low frequency by a selection-mutation balance.

When warfarin is introduced, both *RS* heterozygotes and *RR* homozygotes are equally resistant. But *RR* homozygotes still have a lower fitness because of their greater requirement for vitamin K. And *SS* homozygotes have a lower fitness than *RS* heterozygotes because they are susceptible to warfarin. In the presence of warfarin, therefore, there is heterozygote superiority for fitness. In one study, the relative fitnesses in the presence of warfarin were 0.37, 1.00, and 0.68 for *RR*, *RS*, and *SS* respectively. It is left to the reader to verify, using the concepts discussed in Chapter 5, that the expected consequence of this change in relative fitness is an increase in the frequency of the *R* allele to a new equilibrium of 0.34, which corresponds to a frequency of resistant rats of approximately 0.56 at birth in any generation.

This is a classic example of a stable polymorphism. Allowing for the likely deaths of at least some of the *RR* rats due to vitamin K deficiency, and for their apparently smaller body size and consequent lack of social dominance, the above account is an adequate explanation for the observed frequency of resistant rats. It is also an adequate explanation for the gradual decrease in the frequency of resistant rats observed in areas where warfarin use has been discouraged after previous extensive use.

The warfarin story is perhaps the most dramatic example of the practical implications of genetic variation in response to drugs. Although the use of warfarin as a rodenticide is only indirectly relevant to the use of it or any other drug in domestic animals or in humans, the warfarin story does emphasize that differences between individuals do exist in relation to drug response, and that these differences are sometimes under genetic control.

Not surprisingly, the effect of warfarin can be mimicked by mutations at any of the loci encoding the enzymes involved in the vitamin-K cycle. For example, a familial deficiency of all of the vitamin-K-dependent clotting factors (II, VII, IX, and X), reported in Devon Rex cats, appears to be due to a mutation in the locus for γ-glutamylcarboxylase (Appendix 3.1).

## Multifactorial pharmacogenetics

In the examples described above, alleles at a single locus have a large effect on the metabolism of a particular drug. This is illustrated in Fig. 9.1. However, Fig. 9.1 also shows that there is substantial variation *within* each of the two groups. This variation is analogous to that seen in Chapter 6, when we discussed liability to defects and diseases: it is multifactorial, by which we mean that it is due to a combination of an unknown number of non-genetic factors plus an unknown number of genes.

If there is no single gene of large effect involved in the metabolism of a certain drug, the resultant distribution of drug concentration in a population following a standard dose of the drug is the well known unimodal bell-shaped Normal distribution (Fig. 9.2). At one extreme, the concentration may be so high as to produce a toxic effect. At the other extreme, the concentration may be so low that the drug is ineffective. This variability in response to a standard dose of certain drugs has obvious practical implications. Since there is usually

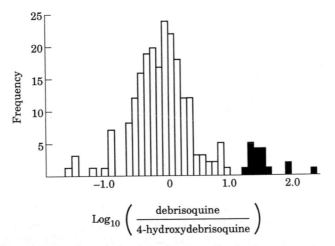

$$\text{Log}_{10}\left(\frac{\text{debrisoquine}}{\text{4-hydroxydebrisoquine}}\right)$$

**Fig. 9.1** The concentration of the drug debrisoquine in the urine of members of a population, after administration of a standard dose of the drug. Concentration is expressed as log of the ratio of the percentage dose excreted as debrisoquine to the percentage dose excreted as 4-hydroxydebrisoquine. Black bars indicate homozygotes for a poor metabolizer allele; white bars are homozygotes for the normal allele, or are heterozygotes.

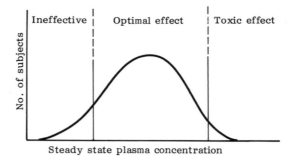

**Fig. 9.2** The continuous distribution of drug concentration resulting from the action of many genes and many non-genetic factors.

no way of knowing, before administering the drug, where a particular individual lies in the overall distribution, there is little that can be done in terms of predetermining the appropriate dose for a particular individual. It is important to remember, however, that there is variability between individuals in response to most drugs, and that this may lead occasionally to toxic or ineffective results from a standard dose of the drug.

Eventually, molecular biology and gene mapping will lead to the identification of all the genes that affect the metabolism of any drug, including those with small as well as large effects.

*Facial eczema in sheep*

A somewhat unusual situation that could be classed as multifactorial pharmacogenetics concerns the disease facial eczema in sheep, which is caused by the fungal toxin sporidesmin. This chemical is produced by members of the *Pithomyces* genus, which live on the dead litter at the base of many pastures in the North Island of New Zealand. The exact biochemistry of this disease is not yet known, but there is substantial evidence for multifactorial variation in response to the toxin: some animals are not affected at all, others are affected at a subclinical level which can cause substantial loss of production, and others show severe clinical signs including photosensitivity and tissue damage, sometimes resulting in death. The heritability of response to the toxin is around 40 per cent, which tells us that there are many genetic differences between individuals in their ability to cope with the toxin. Consistent with this heritability, selection for increased resistance to a standard dose of the toxin has resulted in a dramatic decrease in the incidence of the disease, from around 65 per cent down to around 20 per cent in only 6 years.

# Further reading

Doehmer, J., Goeptar, A. R., and Vermeulen, N. P. E. (1993). Cytochromes P450 and drug resistance. *Cytotechnology*, **12**, 357–66.

Gonzalez, F. J. and Idle, J. R. (1994). Pharmacogenetic phenotyping and genotyping—present status and future potential. *Clinical Pharmacokinetics*, **26**, 59–70.

Kalow, W. (ed.) (1992). *Pharmacogenetics of drug metabolism*. Pergamon, Oxford.

Kalow, W. (1993). Pharmacogenetics—its biologic roots and the medical challenge. *Clinical Pharmacology and Therapeutics*, **54**, 235–41.

MacLennan, D. H. (1992). The genetic basis of malignant hyperthermia. *Trends in Pharmacological Sciences*, **13**, 330–4.

Meyer, U. A. (1994). Pharmacogenetics—the slow, the rapid, and the ultrarapid. *Proceedings of the National Academy of Sciences*, **91**, 1983–4.

Myllymaki, A. (1995). Anticoagulant resistance in Europe: appraisal of the data from the 1992 EPPO questionnaire. *Pesticide Science*, **43**, 69–72.

Oguri, K., Yamada, H., and Yoshimura, H. (1994). Regiochemistry of cytochrome P450 isozymes. *Annual Review of Pharmacology and Toxicology*, **34**, 251–79.

# 10 Hosts, parasites, and pathogens

'. . . can we doubt that individuals having any advantage,
however slight, over others, would have the best chance of
surviving and of procreating their kind?'

(Darwin, 1859)

Parasites and pathogens exert a profound influence on animal health and
production throughout the world. It is therefore very important that we
understand as much as possible about them. Even more importantly, we must
understand the implications of attempts by humans to bring them under
control.

The aim of this chapter is to provide such an understanding. We shall start
by considering host–pathogen interactions, and shall then discuss the genetic
basis of resistance in hosts and in parasites and pathogens. We shall finish up
with some illustrations of ways in which attempts are now being made to
combat parasites and pathogens.

## Host–pathogen interactions

In this section, we shall consider three very different examples of interaction
between hosts and parasites or pathogens, with the aim of providing an
indication of the variety of ways in which such interactions occur.

### Myxomatosis in rabbits

In 1859 a homesick Englishman, who had grown a little tired of seeing
nothing but kangaroos on his property near Geelong in Australia, imported
some rabbits from England. He thought it would improve the hunting. Little
did he know that this innocent importation would give rise to a plague of
rabbits so serious that it would threaten the very existence of the pastoral
industries in Australia.

Nothing done by humans had much effect on the rabbit population until the
CSIRO released a virulent strain of the myxoma virus into the rabbit population in 1950. Having never before been exposed to the virus, the rabbits were
very susceptible; their liability to myxomatosis was very high—almost 100 per
cent of infected rabbits died. The combination of susceptible host and virulent
pathogen assured the scheme of initial success; myxomatosis spread very

rapidly, and rabbits died by the thousands. But the very success of the scheme in its early days ensured that it could not be a success in the longer term. The CSIRO appreciated this because they realized that the death of large numbers of rabbits imposed very strong natural selection for resistance in the host, and also very strong natural selection for avirulence in the pathogen.

If there had been no genetic variation for liability to myxomatosis in the rabbit population, this very strong natural selection would have had no effect. But there was genetic variation (the heritability of liability to myxomatosis is around 35 per cent), and those animals with genes for low liability had a greater chance of surviving to reproduce and hence to pass on their 'resistance' genes to their offspring. Similarly, had there been no genetic variation in the virus and had there been no mechanisms for new variation to be generated in the virus, virulence would not have changed. But either there was genetic variation in the virus, or (as seems more likely) new variation was created by mutation. And as soon as a mutant occurred that decreased the virulence, the rabbits infected with the less virulent virus stayed alive longer and thus enabled more 'offspring' of the less-virulent strain to be produced.

It is not surprising, therefore, that strains of rabbits emerged with varying degrees of increased resistance to the virus, and strains of virus emerged with varying degrees of decreased virulence.

New, virulent strains of virus were developed in the laboratory and were released, with considerable effectiveness in the period immediately following their release. But once again, the very success of the new strain of virus imposed very strong natural selection for decreased virulence in the virus and increased resistance in the host, with the result that fewer and fewer rabbits died.

In a situation like this, there is obviously a very dynamic interaction between host and pathogen. Humans can and do tamper with this interaction from time to time, but their ability to exert a lasting effect in the direction they desire is limited by biological realities of which we all should be very much aware.

That is not to say that the myxomatosis programme should never have been launched by the CSIRO; on the contrary, the programme has been very successful and continues to play a major role in rabbit control. It is simply to say that in order to avoid disappointment, the limitations imposed by biological realities should be appreciated before such a programme is commenced.

The host–pathogen interaction exemplified by the rabbit and the myxoma virus is a typical one. We shall now discuss an example of host–pathogen interaction that is just as important but which is somewhat less typical. Indeed, in this particular example, there is debate about the nature of the pathogen.

## Prion diseases

There is a class of diseases called spongiform encephalopathies, which are fatal neurological diseases that have been known for many years in sheep and goats (where the disease is called scrapie), and in humans (where the diseases are kuru disease, Creutzfeldt–Jacob disease, and Gerstmann–Straussler–Scheinker syndrome). There is still much controversy about the nature of the infectious agent that causes these diseases. However, it seems likely that it is a modified form of a protein encoded by a gene in the host. The name given to this infectious protein particle is **prion**.

The host gene is called the prion protein (*PrP*) gene, which is a normal part of the genome of mammals and chickens. Its polypeptide product, called $PrP^C$, is a naturally occurring protein attached to the outer surface of neurones, and, to a lesser extent, of lymphocytes and other cells. The actual infectious agent, called $PrP^{Sc}$, appears to be a modified form of $PrP^C$, but it still has the same amino acid sequence. One of the more favoured theories for the spread of infection is that when $PrP^{Sc}$ molecules enter a previously uninfected host, they convert the naturally occurring $PrP^C$ molecules, produced by the host *PrP* gene, into infectious particles, which ultimately cause clinical signs in that animal, and which also can spread to other animals, both horizontally (by infection) and vertically (via maternal transmission).

In sheep, the incubation period following infection with the scrapie agent is classed as either short (100–500 days before clinical signs appear) or long (more than 900 days), and this variation in incubation time is controlled by two alleles at a locus called *Sip* (scrapie *i*ncubation *p*eriod). The allele for short incubation period (*sA*) is, in effect, an allele for susceptibility to scrapie; and the allele for long incubation period (*pA*) is an allele for resistance (delayed expression). Interestingly, there is strong circumstantial evidence that the *Sip* locus is, in fact, the *PrP* locus.

This intriguing and unusual example of host–pathogen interaction has puzzled scientists for decades, but in 1986 prion diseases became a major international public-health issue when cattle in Britain developed a completely new disease called bovine spongiform encephalopathy (BSE or mad cow disease). The cause of this new disease is now generally thought to have been the transfer of the scrapie agent from sheep to cattle, via the feeding of sheep offal to cattle. Although the scrapie agent certainly causes fatality in cattle, it does not appear to be infectious in cattle, nor is it capable of moving from cattle to any other hitherto uninfected species. Thus, initial fears that it could be spread to humans simply by eating sheep or cattle meat seem to be unfounded.

The occurrence of BSE has given a new impetus to research into prion diseases, as has the recent discovery of a similar disease in cats and in various captive non-domestic animals such as the Greater Kudu, the cheetah, and the puma. Much will be learnt about this most unusual type of host–pathogen interaction in the years ahead.

Another very important aspect of prion diseases is the challenge that they pose to quarantine authorities in countries that are free from such diseases, such as Australia and New Zealand. How long, for example, should the quarantine period be for a disease whose incubation time may be longer than the lifespan of the host?

This and other questions concerning a disease which is both infectious and inherited will continue to puzzle veterinarians for some time into the future.

## African trypanosomiasis

African trypanosomiasis is the most important of all animal diseases in Africa. It kills many thousands of cattle each year, and decreases production in hundreds of thousands of other cattle suffering chronic infection. In addition to cattle, the disease occurs in sheep, goats, camels, horses, pigs, various wildlife species, and in humans, where it is known as sleeping sickness. It is caused by various species of protozoa called trypanosomes that are transmitted primarily via the tsetse fly.

The most interesting feature of trypanosome infection is that it is characterized by regular fluctuations in the number of trypanosomes in the infected host, ranging from virtually zero to approximately 1500 per ml of blood. The reason for these regular fluctuations is a phenomenon called **antigenic variation**, which is the occurrence of a sequence of different antigenic variants all arising from the single population of pathogens that originally entered the host.

Trypanosomes are encapsulated by a glycoprotein coat, and the antigenic determinant of this coat is the protein portion, which consists of a single chain of approximately 600 amino acids. Being a single chain of amino acids, the antigenic determinant of a trypanosome is obviously the product of a gene in the trypanosome.

When a population of trypanosomes enters a host, all members of that population exhibit a basic antigen, which is one of the frequently occurring antigen types. The host mounts a strong immune response, producing antibodies directed against this basic antigen. Consequently, most of the trypanosomes that originally entered the host are destroyed. But by this time, some trypanosomes have 'switched off' the gene for the basic antigen, and have 'turned on' a gene for another antigen, which differs by many amino acids from the basic antigen. Trypanosomes carrying this second antigen multiply rapidly until the host's immune-response system produces antibodies to this second antigen, by which stage some trypanosomes are now producing yet another different antigen that the host has not previously encountered. And so the regular fluctuations in number of trypanosomes continue for many cycles, with the pathogen regularly 'changing its spots' in order to keep one step ahead of the host's immune-response system.

The trypanosome genome contains more than 100 genes that each code for a different type of antigen. The 'switching on' of a particular gene involves the duplication of that gene, and the subsequent transposition (movement and insertion) of that duplicate gene into another region of the genome called the expression site. Once incorporated into the **expression site**, the duplicate gene is transcribed and translated into antigen. When the time comes for the next antigen to be produced, the corresponding gene is duplicated and the duplicate copy is inserted into the expression site, in place of the previous duplicated gene, which by this time has been removed and lost.

There are three other aspects of antigenic variation that should be mentioned. The first is that it occurs even in the absence of antibody, which indicates that trypanosomes are somehow 'pre-programmed' to produce a sequence of antigens even in the absence of external stimuli. The second point is that if trypanosomes are removed from a host and are recycled through a tsetse fly, they revert to producing one of the basic antigens when they enter a new host, irrespective of which antigen was last produced in the previous host. This also indicates a degree of 'pre-programming'. Finally, it is obvious that the practical implication of antigenic variation is that it is very difficult to produce a vaccine that will be effective against the large number of different antigens that each host is likely to encounter.

The phenomenon of antigenic variation is an important example of host–pathogen interaction. And it is all the more important because it occurs not only in trypanosomes but in other protozoa including members of the genus *Plasmodium*, which causes malaria, and the genus *Babesia*, which causes babesiosus or tick fever, an important disease of cattle that was mentioned in Chapter 8.

## Resistance in hosts

There is no shortage of examples of genetic variation in hosts for resistance to pathogens or parasites. Indeed, this type of variation is present in most, if not all, populations of hosts, in relation to most, if not all, parasites and pathogens that have been investigated. The genetic variation exists between and within breeds, and is usually multifactorial. Among the many documented examples are genetic variation for resistance to various bacteria, viruses, and protozoa in chickens; for resistance to bacteria in turkeys; for resistance to bacteria, viruses, and protozoa in fish; for resistance to insects (fly strike), bacteria (fleece rot, footrot), nematodes, and various viruses in sheep; for resistance to bacteria (atrophic rhinitis and scours) in pigs; and for resistance to arthropods (cattle tick, horn fly, stable fly), nematodes, trypanosomes, and bacteria (mastitis) in cattle. We shall consider just two examples below, in which genes for resistance have been identified.

### Resistance to neonatal scours in pigs

As we saw in Chapter 5, a major cause of neonatal scours in pigs are the strains of *E. coli* having a cell-surface antigen called K88. But not all piglets are susceptible to K88 *E. coli*. In particular, only those piglets with a K88 receptor on the walls of their intestines are susceptible; those that lack the receptor are resistant. As reported in Chapter 5, the presence or absence of the K88 receptor is determined by two alleles at an autosomal locus, with the allele for presence of the receptor being completely dominant to that for lack of the receptor. Thus resistance to neonatal *E. coli* scours in pigs is under the control of two alleles at a single locus, with resistance being recessive to susceptibility.

### Resistance to Marek's disease in chickens

Marek's disease in chickens is a neoplastic disease in which the growth of tumour cells is caused by a DNA virus. When a population of the Cornell random-bred control strain of chickens was selected for resistance to Marek's disease, mortality from the disease decreased dramatically from around 50 per cent to less than 10 per cent in only four generations. In another line taken from the same control population, selection for susceptibility increased the mortality to over 90 per cent in the same period. In terms of the concepts discussed in Chapter 6, selection had produced large changes in liability to Marek's disease. The fact that selection was able to alter liability so quickly indicates that there was substantial genetic variation for liability in the base population. In other words, there was substantial genetic variation for resistance to the pathogen.

As briefly mentioned in Chapter 8, it has since been shown that there is a strong association between the MHC histoglobulin $B^{21}$ and resistance to Marek's disease. In fact, much of the change in liability in the selection lines described above was due to changes in the frequency of the $B^{21}$ allele. This is one of the first cases where a gene that contributes to multifactorial variation in host resistance has been identified. As described at the end of this chapter, many more such discoveries will be made in the future.

## Resistance in parasites and pathogens

We shall now turn to parasites and pathogens, firstly to review the extent of genetic variation in resistance in them, and then to examine the extent to which selection has exploited this variation. We shall consider just one example each from insects, helminths, and microorganisms. Similar examples exist for most, if not all, parasites and pathogens.

### Resistance to insecticides in sheep blowflies

The Australian sheep blowfly, *Lucilia cuprina*, is a major cause of loss of income in the Australian wool industry, through damage done by larvae to live sheep, and the consequent loss of wool production and death of sheep. Attempts by humans to control the blowfly have until recently concentrated mainly on spraying (jetting) with insecticides.

The use of insecticides soon gave rise to a predictable pattern of response in the blowfly. In 1955, for example, an organo-chlorine called dieldrin was released for use, and it was extremely effective at first, giving protection for around 8 weeks or longer after jetting. Within 3 years, however, its effectiveness had dramatically fallen, and sheep were being struck by blowflies only a week or two after jetting. It was said that the blowfly had become resistant to the chemical. In 1958, a new insecticide was released, this time an organo-phosphate called diazinon. It, too, was very effective at first, but, as with dieldrin, it soon lost its effectiveness. Other chemicals were released in an attempt to keep one step ahead of the blowfly. But in each case, it was only a matter of time before the blowfly became resistant.

It is now known that the blowflies became resistant to each chemical in turn because of very strong natural selection favouring alleles for resistance at one or more loci in the blowfly. These resistance alleles usually operate by coding for an enzyme that is able to detoxify the insecticide, or by coding for a variant of the enzyme against which the insecticide acts, such that the variant is still able to function in the presence of the insecticide. Not surprisingly, some of these resistance alleles are located at loci encoding cytochrome-P450 enzymes, which, as we saw in Chapter 9, play a key role in detoxifying drugs. Prior to the introduction of a particular chemical, the relevant resistance alleles are usually maintained at a low frequency in the overall population of flies by a balance between mutation and selection, which arises because resistance alleles, in the absence of the chemical, are usually disadvantageous. The introduction of a new insecticide produces an immediate change in the relative fitnesses of the three genotypes $RR$, $RS$, and $SS$ (where $R$ is the resistance allele and $S$ is the susceptibility allele), with the result that $RR$ now has the highest relative fitness and $SS$ the lowest. The inevitable consequence of this change in relative fitness is an increase in the frequency of the $R$ allele: the population of flies becomes more resistant.

Switching from one insecticide to another within the same class of chemical compound produces very little change if the mode of action of the chemical, and hence the nature of resistance, is the same in each case. On the other hand, replacing one type of compound with another may cause equally strong selection in favour of a resistance allele at a different locus, in which case the above story is repeated. If the first resistance allele also still exerts some effect on the new insecticide (if there is **cross-resistance**), it remains at a high frequency even after the original insecticide is withdrawn from use. This is what sometimes happens in practice. If there is no cross-resistance, the withdrawal of the original insecticide causes the relative fitnesses of the three genotypes to revert to their original values, and the resistance allele decreases in frequency to its original very low value (provided, of course, that it had not already become fixed in the population).

By using standard gene-mapping techniques, researchers have determined the location of resistance loci in the blowfly genome. There are, for example, two different loci with alleles that confer resistance to organo-phosphates; one on chromosome 4 and another on chromosome 6. The resistance alleles are incompletely dominant to the susceptibility alleles, and have been recorded at a very high frequency (0.98–1.00) in several natural populations of blowflies. Dieldrin resistance is determined by an allele at a third locus, located on chromosome 5. When dieldrin was withdrawn in 1958, the frequency of the resistance allele was around 0.4. Ten years later, its frequency had fallen to around 0.01, where it has remained ever since. The fact that resistance to organo-phosphates was developing during the period in which dieldrin resistance was declining indicates that there is no cross-resistance between dieldrin and organo-phosphates.

The above account indicates that the reason for blowflies becoming resistant to insecticides is basically very simple; it represents an excellent illustration of the principles of population genetics.

Not surprisingly, the real situation is a little more complicated than outlined above. There are, for example, modifying genes of relatively small effect that play a role in insecticide resistance. In other words, there is multifactorial resistance in addition to single-gene resistance. The longer a particular insecticide is used, the more are those modifying genes subjected to selection, with the result that the major resistance gene becomes less and less likely to decrease in frequency when the insecticide is eventually withdrawn. Despite complications such as this, the above picture highlights the important general principles involved in the development of insecticide resistance in many species of insect, and of resistance to chemicals in general.

We can conclude that the inevitable consequence of the widespread use of an insecticide is that insects become resistant to it.

## Resistance to anthelmintics

Once again, the same principles apply. For example, just three years after the release in the USA of drenches based on the compound thiabendazole (TBZ), resistant strains of *Haemonchus contortus* were detected. With the continual widespread use of this and other benzimidazoles (BZ) in several major sheep-producing regions of the world, resistance to various forms of BZ has now become a major problem. Worse still, worms that are resistant to BZ sometimes show resistance to other compounds used as drenches, including organo-phosphates, salicylanilides, and substituted nitrophenols.

Researchers have shown that in some cases, resistance is due to a particular allele with a relatively large effect at a single locus. For example, most of the variation in resistance to levamisole in *Trichostrongylus colubriformis* is due to a sex-linked recessive allele. In other cases, however, resistance appears to be multifactorial, being primarily determined by alleles of relatively small effect at an unknown number of loci.

## Resistance to antibiotics

In the years following the introduction and widespread use of penicillin, strain after strain of resistant bacteria was isolated. Other antibiotics were introduced, but resistant strains soon emerged. Worse still, many such strains were resistant to more than one antibiotic. The emergence of resistance was too rapid and widespread to be explained solely by the conventional process described for other species of pathogens and parasites in earlier sections, namely the increase in frequency of resistance genes, resulting from selection during the vertical transmission of those genes from generation to generation in the pathogen or parasite. In fact, the rapid and widespread emergence of antibiotic resistance in bacteria has been mainly due to the ability of bacteria to transfer genes horizontally (between contemporary individuals, within generations) as well as vertically (between generations).

There are three methods by which bacteria transfer genes horizontally. They are **transformation** (the release of naked DNA from one cell, and its uptake by another cell), **transduction** (the transfer of DNA from cell to cell by means of a bacteriophage), and **conjugation** (the transfer of DNA from one cell to another, following the joining together—mating—of the two cells). Antibiotic resistance genes can be transferred horizontally by all three methods, with conjugation probably being the most important. This process involves the transfer from one cell to another of a duplicate copy of a plasmid, which, as we saw in Chapter 2, is a circular segment of DNA that functions independently of the bacterial chromosome. The importance of conjugation lies in the fact that many important genes for antibiotic resistance are located on plasmids. Plasmids that carry one or more resistance genes are called **R factors**.

The importance of horizontal transfer of resistance arises because of the large number of bacteria present in the external and internal environment of animals and of humans. The use of antibiotics creates an environment favouring the survival of strains that possess R factors. These strains then act as a reservoir for the transfer of R factors to any other strains (including pathogenic strains) that happen to be present from time to time.

Many different types of R factors have been identified, including those that have a single gene for resistance to almost any of the antibiotics currently in use. But there are also plasmids known to have genes for resistance to more than one antibiotic. At first it was hard to see how such plasmids could arise, because the chance of more than one relevant mutation occurring in the same plasmid is very small. The answer to this puzzle came with the discovery in the mid-1970s of **transposons**, which are a type of transposable genetic element (TGE). As described in Chapter 1, TGEs are segments of DNA that can move from one site to another within and between chromosomes. In bacteria, transposons can move within and between plasmids and the main bacterial chromosome. They can also insert themselves into and remove themselves from bacteriophage DNA. The most important aspect of transposons is that they contain one or more genes in addition to those required for transposition. Unfortunately, these additional genes often confer resistance to antibiotics.

Although most transposons carry only one gene for antibiotic resistance, it is easy to see how plasmids with multiple resistance genes have arisen so rapidly; they simply accumulate the appropriate transposons. In fact, a plasmid carrying genes for resistance to several different antibiotics is really just a plasmid containing the appropriate transposons.

There is abundant evidence of the role played by transposition in the creation of plasmids with multiple resistance, and of the role played by conjugation in enabling the rapid spread of such plasmids, and hence of multiple resistance, both within and between species of bacteria. There is also abundant evidence to indicate that the extensive use of antibiotics throughout the world confers a strong selective advantage for bacteria carrying multiple resistance.

## Control of parasites and pathogens

Having illustrated the fact that parasites and pathogens show widespread genetic variation, we shall now consider some of the ways in which humans are attempting to control them, or at least to combat them.

### Screw-worm flies

There are two types of screw-worm fly: the Old World fly (*Chrysomya bezziana*) and the New World fly (*Cochliomyia hominivorax*). They are both parasites of warm-blooded animals. The damage they cause arises from the predilection of the larval stage for open wounds. The Old World larvae, for example, cause up to 30 per cent loss of calves in New Guinea due to navel strike, and, at the height of their activity (in the 1950s), the New World larvae resulted in an annual loss of around $100 million in cattle production in the southern states of the USA. Because of its economic importance, considerable effort has been directed at eradicating the screw-worm fly from the USA, with a large degree of success.

The biggest contribution to this success has been a method of biological control known as the **Sterile Insect Release Method**, SIRM. This method involves rearing large numbers of larvae of both sexes in the laboratory, and exposing the late-stage pupae to doses of radiation sufficiently high to render the resultant flies sterile. The sterile flies are then dropped from aeroplanes at rates of between 1600 and 4000 per square mile per week. The principle of the method is simply that if sufficient sterile flies can be released, most (and preferably all) wild-type flies mate with a sterile fly rather than with a wild-type (fertile) fly. Obviously this occurs only if very large numbers of sterile flies are released.

A judicious combination of SIRM and dipping of cattle resulted in the complete eradication of the screw-worm fly from south-eastern USA by 1959, only two years after the programme had begun. The south-western eradication programme, which was a much more ambitious task, was commenced in 1962. By 1971 a fly-free barrier 200 to 300 miles wide had been established along the USA–Mexico border, and all areas north of this barrier were free of the fly. Since then, the Mexican–American Commission for the Eradication of Screw-worm (MACES) has gradually moved the barrier southwards. By 1991, the fly had been eradicated from Mexico. Obviously, the narrower the stretch of land over which the barrier has to extend, the easier and cheaper it is to maintain. Because of this, the aim is to move the barrier down to Panama, which should be reached by 1996.

Despite the success of the eradication programme, the screw-worm fly was not yet prepared to admit complete defeat. In 1988, an outbreak was reported in Libya, most probably having arisen from the importation of infested meat from South America. The establishment of the screw-worm fly on the African continent caused very serious concern in many countries, since it seemed likely that it could spread throughout Africa, and thence to southern Europe, the Middle East, and Asia. In northern Africa alone, it was estimated that the annual cost of treatment and prevention would be $360 million. And the threat to wildlife and humans (which it also attacks), especially in central Africa, was extremely serious.

In the face of this potential catastrophe, the Food and Agriculture Organisation of the United Nations (FAO) set up a Screw-worm Task Force which established the Screw-worm Emergency Centre for North Africa (SECNA) in mid-1990. After intensive investigations of possible courses of action, it was decided that an SIRM programme would be most appropriate, and that MACES would be asked to supply the sterile pupae. Although this would mean chartering aircraft to fly the pupae across the Atlantic Ocean from Mexico to Libya, it would be cheaper and quicker than establishing a new facility in Libya.

Shipments commenced in December 1990 at the rate of 3.5 million flies per week, and were gradually increased until by May 1991, 40 million flies were being flown across the Atlantic Ocean each week. This programme continued until October 1991, by which time it was evident that the screw-worm fly had been eradicated from Libya. The total cost of this operation was around $75 million, of which $25 million was provided by Libya, with the remainder coming from other countries. Given the devastation that would have resulted if the fly had become established, it is not surprising to learn that an independent economic analysis of the programme indicated a benefit:cost ratio of 50:1.

The use of SIRM in helping to eradicate the screw-worm fly, both in North America and in Libya, is commonly regarded as one of the most successful of all human attempts at biological control.

Although it has come to be regarded as a form of genetic control, the SIRM itself involves no genetics. It does, however, have genetical implications in relation to problems caused by adaptation of laboratory-reared flies, and also in relation to issues such as the possibility of selection for mating preference. (The SIRM obviously imposes very strong natural selection for the ability of wild-type flies to identify and mate with wild-type flies rather than laboratory-reared flies.) In addition, the sterilization procedure can be regarded as giving rise to dominant lethal alleles.

## Other insects

The conventional SIRM involves the maintenance of laboratory-reared insects right up to the adult stage (including irradiation at the late pupal stage), and the release of adults from aeroplanes or other vehicles. If a genetic source of sterility could be used as an alternative to radiation, the provision of labour and facilities for irradiation would be unnecessary, and the insects could be released at the larval stage, which is much simpler and far cheaper. Another substantial advantage of larval release is that the resultant adults are likely to be much better acclimatized, having pupated naturally in the soil, and having then emerged naturally into the area where they are expected to perform.

What are potential sources of genetic sterility? A possible answer could be some of the chromosomal rearrangements which were described in Chapter 4. Of course, in that chapter, we were discussing the effect of chromosomal rearrangements on fecundity of animals. But exactly the same principles apply to insects. With this in mind, there has been considerable research into the creation (by once-only irradiation) of strains of laboratory-raised insects that carry one or more reciprocal translocations between autosomes and the Y chromosome. All males in such stocks are heterozygous for the translocation, and consequently show the reduced fecundity that is characteristic of such chromosomal rearrangements. If the autosome involved in the translocation contains normal (wild-type) alleles at all loci, and if the translocation is introduced into a laboratory population that is homozygous for a deleterious recessive allele (e.g. for eye colour or wing deformities) at a locus on the same autosome, males survive (because they have one wild-type allele on the translocated autosome, in addition to being homozygous for the deleterious allele on their normal autosomes) but females do not, because, not having a Y chromosome, they lack the translocated autosome and hence lack the wild-type allele.

The combination of reduced fecundity and deleterious recessives has the potential for powerful biological control of insects. This and other possibilities have not yet reached the stage where they have replaced conventional SIRM. But there is a good chance that some of them will prove to be successful in the future.

## Worms

In principle, the techniques described above for the biological control of insects are also applicable to worms. In practice, relatively little research has been conducted in this area.

In the foreseeable future, animal producers have to combat worms as best they can, by drenching. Fortunately, there is now a wealth of information

available on the extent of cross-resistance between different classes of anthelmintics, which forms the basis of recommendations for the timing and rota-
tion of drenches, with the aim of slowing the spread of resistance.

### Bacteria

The long-term outlook for the control of bacteria is not good. As described
earlier, bacteria have very effective means of transferring genes for antibiotic
resistance horizontally as well as vertically, and the continued wide-spread
use of antibiotics has led to an alarming increase in the occurrence of resistant
bacteria. One of the few steps that could be taken to ease the selection
pressure for resistant bacteria would be to limit the use of antibiotics, for
example, by banning the use of antibiotics as additives in animal food. But
this use of antibiotics is such a lucrative business that there is very strong
opposition to suggestions that it should be banned, with the result that antibiotics are still used far more widely than is necessary for purely therapeutic
needs. It seems that we will have to learn to live with ever-increasing resistance to antibiotics in bacteria.

## Increasing the level of resistance in hosts

In addition to the direct means of controlling pathogens and parasites described
above, it is possible to exert some indirect influence over them, by increasing
the level of resistance in hosts.

### Selecting for resistance in hosts

We have seen that there is genetic variation for resistance to most pathogens
and parasites in most domestic species. The most obvious way to exploit this
variation is to select for increased resistance. There are numerous examples
where this has been a successful strategy. However, there is a major limitation to this approach, namely that the whole population has to be deliberately
exposed to the pathogen or parasite. In some cases, e.g. internal parasites,
this often happens despite the best intentions of humans to prevent it, in
which case selection for resistance occurs naturally. But artificial selection for
resistance raises ethical problems. Even if these problems are surmounted,
the effectiveness of artificial selection for resistance may be severely limited
unless resistance can be measured on a continuous scale, or at least on a
scale with many different values (because if animals are classed simply as
resistant or susceptible, the effectiveness of selection varies with the pre-
valence of the disease, and the genetic variation that exists within each
class cannot be exploited). Because of these limitations, there is much interest
in finding other ways to exploit the widespread genetic variation that exists

for resistance in hosts. DNA markers offer the greatest hope for achieving this aim.

## DNA markers for resistance in hosts

The big challenge today is to find DNA markers for resistance, i.e. easily detectable DNA polymorphisms that are closely linked to, or are actually part of, genes that contribute to genetic variation in resistance. If such markers can be identified, selection can be conducted on the basis of a simple blood test (i.e. by genotyping animals at marker loci), without the need for exposing animals to the pathogen or parasite. Genes within the MHC are one obvious set of candidates for useful DNA markers, and these are being subjected to much current research. But there are many other genes involved in determining resistance to pathogens and parasites. The challenge is to identify these genes, and then to determine how best to utilize them. The development of genetic maps (described in Chapter 2) is an important step towards this goal, because these maps enable the whole genome of the host species to be searched systematically. Further details of the general approach to searching for genes contributing to multifactorial variation are given in Chapters 11 and 14.

## Transgenesis

In Chapter 2, we saw two different ways in which transgenesis may be able to create resistance in hosts—by developing animals that express part of the protein coat of pathogens or enzymes that are specifically targeted against parasites. No doubt other transgenic approaches to resistance will be developed. It is too early yet to know how successful any of these approaches will be. But the hopes (and money) of many people are riding on their potential to provide a major means of combating pathogens and parasites.

## Practical implications of host–pathogen interactions

In using any of the above approaches to alter resistance in the host, we must never forget the practical implications of the dynamic equilibria discussed at the beginning of this chapter. If you change one side of the ledger (e.g. the level of resistance in the host), the other side (pathogen or parasite) is automatically exposed to natural selection for overcoming whatever change has occurred. Ideally, the change in the host should be sufficient to provide an insurmountable hurdle to the pathogen or parasite. The challenge is in determining which change in the host is most likely to create such a hurdle. Whichever path is taken, we should not be complacent about the powers of natural selection to respond to the challenges that will be provided by the development of increased resistance in hosts.

## Further reading

Darwin, C. (1859). *The origin of species by means of natural selection*, (1st edn). John Murray, London.

### *Myxomatosis and rabbits*

Thompson, H. V. and King, C. M. (ed.) (1994). *The European rabbit*. Oxford University Press, Oxford.

Fenner, F. and Kerr, P. J. (1994). Evolution of the poxviruses, including the coevolution of virus and host in myxomatosis. In *Evolutionary biology of viruses*, (ed. S. S. Morse), pp. 273–92. Raven Press, New York.

### *Spongiform encephalopathies*

Allen, I. V. (ed.) (1993). Spongiform encephalopathies. *British Medical Bulletin*, **49**, (4), 725–1016.

Bradley, R., Wilesmith, J. W., Matthews, D., Meldrum, K. C., Will, R. G., Chillaud, T., *et al.* (1993). Bovine spongiform encephalopathy in the United Kingdom—memorandum from a WHO meeting. *Bulletin of the World Health Organization*, **71**, 691–4.

Bradley, R. (ed.) (1994). Bovine spongiform encephalopathy. *Livestock Production Science*, **38**, 1–59.

Collinge, J. (ed.) (1994). Molecular biology of prion diseases. *Philosophical Transactions of the Royal Society of London Series B*, **343**, 353–463.

Goldmann, W., Hunter, N., Smith, G., Foster, J., and Hope, J. (1994). PrP genotype and agent effects in scrapie—change in allelic interaction with different isolates of agent in sheep, a natural host of scrapie. *Journal of General Virology*, **75**, 989–95.

Marsh, R. F. (1994). Symposium on risk assessment of the possible occurrence of bovine spongiform encephalopathy in the United States—Madison, Wisconsin September 8, 1993—Preface. *Journal of the American Veterinary Medical Association*, **204**, 70–3.

Prusiner, S. B. (1993). Genetic and infectious prion diseases. *Archives of Neurology*, **50**, 1129–53.

Prusiner, S. B. and Dearmond, S. J. (1994). Prion diseases and neurodegeneration. *Annual Review of Neuroscience*, **17**, 311–39.

Savey, M., Belli, P., and Coudert, M. (1993). Bovine spongiform encephalopathy in Europe—present and future. *Veterinary Research*, **24**, 213–25.

Straub, O. C. (1994). Report on a symposium—transmissible spongiform encephalopathies. *Tierarztliche Umschau*, **49**, 50–2.

Weaver, A. D. (1992). Bovine spongiform encephalopathy—its clinical features and epidemiology in the United-Kingdom and significance for the United-States. *Compendium on Continuing Education for the Practicing Veterinarian*, **14**, 1647–56.

Westaway, D., Zuliani, V., Cooper, C. M., Dacosta, M., Neuman, S., Jenny, A. L., *et al.* (1994). Homozygosity for prion protein alleles encoding glutamine-171 renders sheep susceptible to natural scrapie. *Genes & Development*, **8**, 959–69.

Wyatt, J. M., Pearson, G. R., and Gruffydd-Jones, T. J. (1993). Feline spongiform encephalopathy. *Feline Practice*, **21**, 7–9.

## Trypanosomes

Myler, P. J. (1993). Molecular variation in trypanosomes. *Acta Tropica*, **53**, 205–25.
Vanderploeg, L. H. T., Gottesdiener, K., and Lee, M. G. S. (1992). Antigenic variation in African trypanosomes. *Trends in Genetics*, **8**, 452–7.

## Variation in pathogens/parasites

Robertson, B. D. and Meyer, T. F. (1992). Genetic variation in pathogenic bacteria. *Trends in Genetics*, **8**, 422–7.
Schmidhempel, P. and Koella, J. C. (1994). Variability and its implications for host–parasite interactions. *Parasitology Today*, **10**, 98–102.

## Resistance in hosts

Decastro, J. J. and Newson, R. M. (1993). Host resistance in cattle tick control. *Parasitology Today*, **9**, 13–17.
Fivaz, B. H., Dewaal, D. T., and Lander, K. (1992). Indigenous and crossbred cattle—a comparison of resistance to ticks and implications for their strategic control in Zimbabwe. *Tropical Animal Health and Production*, **24**, 81–9.
Gray, G. D. and Gill, H. S. (1993). Host genes, parasites and parasitic infections. *International Journal for Parasitology*, **23**, 485–94.
Michaels, R. D., Whipp, S. C., and Rothschild, M. F. (1994). Resistance of Chinese Meishan, Fengjing, and Minzhu pigs to the K88Ac(+) strain of *Escherichia coli*. *American Journal of Veterinary Research*, **55**, 333–8.
Stamm, M. and Sorg, I. (1993). [Intestinal receptors for adhesive fimbriae of *Escherichia coli* in pigs—a review.]. *Schweizer Archiv für Tierheilkunde*, **135**, 89–95.
Wakelin, D. (1992). Genetic variation in resistance to parasitic infection: experimental approaches and practical applications. *Research in Veterinary Science*, **53**, 139–47.
Wakelin, D. (1992). Immunogenetic and evolutionary influences on the host–parasite relationship: review. *Developmental and Comparative Immunology*, **16**, 345–53.
Wakelin, D. and Blackwell, J. M. (ed.) (1988). *Genetics of resistance to bacterial and parasitic infection*. Taylor and Francis, London.

## Resistance to drugs, general

Bacchi, C. J. (1993). Resistance to clinical drugs in African trypanosomes. *Parasitology Today*, **9**, 190–3.
Chapman, H. D. (1993). Resistance to anticoccidial drugs in fowl. *Parasitology Today*, **9**, 159–62.
Denholm, I. and Rowland, M. W. (1992). Tactics for managing pesticide resistance in arthropods—theory and practice. *Annual Review of Entomology*, **37**, 91–112.
Hennessy, D. R. (1994). The disposition of antiparasitic drugs in relation to the development of resistance by parasites of livestock. *Acta Tropica*, **56**, 125–41.
Herd, R. P. (1993). Control strategies for ruminant and equine parasites to counter resistance, encystment, and ecotoxicity in the USA. *Veterinary Parasitology*, **48**, 327–36.

## Resistance to insecticides

Ffrenchconstant, R. H. (1994). The molecular and population genetics of cyclodiene insecticide resistance. *Insect Biochemistry and Molecular Biology*, 24, 335–45.

Hodgson, E., Rose, R. L., Goh, D. K. S., Rock, G. C., and Roe, R. M. (1993). Insect cytochrome-P-450—metabolism and resistance to insecticides. *Biochemical Society Transactions*, 21, 1060–5.

McKenzie, J. A. and Batterham, P. (1994). The genetic, molecular and phenotypic consequences of selection for insecticide resistance. *Trends in Ecology & Evolution*, 9, 166–9.

Roush, R. T. (1993). Occurrence, genetics and management of insecticide resistance. *Parasitology Today*, 9, 174–9.

Whyard, S., Russell, R. J., and Walker, V. K. (1994). Insecticide resistance and malathion carboxylesterase in the sheep blowfly, *Lucilia cuprina*. *Biochemical Genetics*, 32, 9–24.

## Resistance to anthelmintics

Barger, I. A. (1993). Control of gastrointestinal nematodes in Australia in the 21st century. *Veterinary Parasitology*, 46, 23–32.

Coles, G. C., Borgsteede, F. H. M., and Geerts, S. (1994). Recommendations for the control of anthelmintic resistant nematodes of farm animals in the EU. *Veterinary Record*, 134, 205–6.

Craig, T. M. (1993). Anthelmintic resistance. *Veterinary Parasitology*, 46, 121–31.

Jackson, F. (1993). Anthelmintic resistance—the state of play. *British Veterinary Journal*, 149, 123–38.

Lacey, E. and Gill, J. H. (1994). Biochemistry of benzimidazole resistance. *Acta Tropica*, 56, 245–62.

Lanusse, C. E. and Prichard, R. K. (1993). Relationship between pharmacological properties and clinical efficacy of ruminant anthelmintics—invited review paper. *Veterinary Parasitology*, 49, 123–58.

Le Jambre, L. F. (1993). Molecular variation in Trichostrongylid nematodes from sheep and cattle. *Acta Tropica*, 53, 331–43.

Schillinger, D. and Hasslinger, M. A. (1994). Benzimidazole resistance in small strongyles of horses—occurrence in Germany and strategies for avoiding resistance. *Revue de Médecine Vétérinaire*, 145, 119–24.

Shoop, W. L. (1993). Ivermectin resistance. *Parasitology Today*, 9, 154–9.

Waller, P. J. (1993). Towards sustainable nematode parasite control of livestock. *Veterinary Parasitology*, 48, 295–309.

Waller, P. J. (1994). The development of anthelmintic resistance in ruminant livestock. *Acta Tropica*, 56, 233–43.

## Resistance to antibiotics

Chin, G. J. and Marx, J. (ed.) (1994). Resistance to antibiotics. *Science*, 264, 359–93.

Espinasse, J. (1993). Responsible use of antimicrobials in veterinary medicine—perspectives in France. *Veterinary Microbiology*, 35, 289–301.

Haesebrouck, F. and Devriese, L. (1994). Antimicrobial drug resistance and oral antibiotic medication in farm animals. *Vlaams Diergeneeskundig Tijdschrift*, **63**, 3–6.

Jergens, A. E. (1994). Rational use of antimicrobials for gastrointestinal disease in small animals. *Journal of the American Animal Hospital Association*, **30**, 123–31.

Kidd, A. R. M. (1993). European perspectives on the regulation of antimicrobial drugs. *Veterinary and Human Toxicology*, **35**, (Suppl. 1), 6–9.

Lens, S. (1993). The role of the pharmaceutical animal health industry in post–marketing surveillance of resistance. *Veterinary Microbiology*, **35**, 339–47.

Martel, J. L. and Coudert, M. (1993). Bacterial resistance monitoring in animals—the French national experiences of surveillance schemes. *Veterinary Microbiology*, **35**, 321–38.

Mitsuhashi, S. (1993). Drug resistance in bacteria—history, genetics and biochemistry. *Journal of International Medical Research*, **21**, 1–14.

Smith, J. T. and Lewin, C. S. (1993). Mechanisms of antimicrobial resistance and implications for epidemiology. *Veterinary Microbiology*, **35**, 233–42.

Smith, W. J. (1993). Antibiotics in feed, with special reference to pigs—a veterinary viewpoint. *Animal Feed Science and Technology*, **45**, 57–64.

Wray, C., McLaren, I.M., and Beedell, Y.E. (1993). Bacterial resistance monitoring of Salmonellas isolated from animals: national experience of surveillance schemes in the United Kingdom. *Veterinary Microbiology*, **35**, 313–9.

## Screw-worm fly eradication

Lindquist, D. A., Abusowa, M., and Hall, M. J. R. (1992). The New World screw-worm fly in Libya—a review of its introduction and eradication. *Medical and Veterinary Entomology*, **6**, 2–8.

Vargasteran, M., Hursey, B. S., and Cunningham, E. P. (1994). Eradication of the screwworm from Libya using the sterile insect technique. *Parasitology Today*, **10**, 119–22.

## Breeding for resistance in hosts

Albers, G. A. A. (1993). Breeding for disease resistance—fact and fiction. *Archiv für Geflugelkunde*, **57**, 56–8.

Anon. (ed.) (1994). Workshop on genetic improvement of resistance to mastitis based on SCC. *Journal of Dairy Science*, **77**, 616–58.

Kloosterman, A., Parmentier, H. K., and Ploeger, H. W. (1992). Breeding cattle and sheep for resistance to gastrointestinal nematodes. *Parasitology Today*, **8**, 330–5.

Fjalestad, K. T., Gjedrem, T., and Gjerde, B. (1993). Genetic improvement of disease resistance in fish—an overview. *Aquaculture*, **111**, 65–74.

Flock, D. K. (1993). Improvement of disease resistance in poultry by conventional breeding techniques. *Archiv für Geflugelkunde*, **57**, 49–55.

Ollivier, L. and Renjifo, X. (1991). Use of genetic resistance to K88 colibacillosis in pig breeding schemes. *Génétique, Sélection, Evolution*, **23**, 235–48.

Owen, J. B. and Axford, R. F. E. (ed.) (1991). *Breeding for resistance in farm animals*. CAB International, Wallingford, England.

Shook, G. E. and Schutz, M. M. (1994). Selection on somatic cell score to improve resistance to mastitis in the United States. *Journal of Dairy Science*, **77**, 648–58.

# 11 Genetic and environmental control of inherited disorders

In Chapter 10 we saw that there is genetic variation in hosts for resistance to parasites and pathogens, and we saw how this can be utilized to breed animals with enhanced resistance. It remains for us now to turn our attention to diseases that are not caused by parasites or pathogens, i.e. to inherited disorders. As we saw in Chapter 6, the heritability for liability to any disorder is usually greater than zero; there is usually some genetic variation in liability to any disorder. This raises the possibility of artificial selection for decreased liability as a means of decreasing the incidence of the disorder.

However, the existence of genetic variation in liability is associated with a popular misconception; many people believe that if a disorder shows any sign of being inherited, there is nothing that can be done about it apart from selecting against it.

One purpose of this chapter is to show that this belief is wrong. By considering several examples, we will see that there are many potential non-genetic means of alleviating inherited disorders. Having proved this point, we shall go on to consider some examples of genetic control of inherited disorders.

## Environmental control of inherited disorders

### Hip dysplasia

The heritability of liability to hip dysplasia is certainly greater than zero, but it is certainly possible to decrease its incidence by non-genetic means.

For example, there is quite convincing evidence that restricted feeding during the growing phase can increase the average age of onset and reduce the incidence of hip dysplasia. In other words, restricted feeding during the growing phase can reduce the liability to hip dysplasia. There is also some evidence that dietary electrolyte balance affects liability to hip dysplasia.

This indicates that food intake and possibly dietary electrolyte balance are components (obviously non-genetic components) of liability to hip dysplasia. Another non-genetic factor that may alter liability to hip dysplasia is exercise during the growing phase. Although convincing data are lacking, many breeders believe that restricting exercise reduces the incidence and severity of hip dysplasia.

The main conclusion to draw from these observations is very straightforward. The fact that liability to hip dysplasia can be reduced by non-genetic means does not mean that hip dysplasia is a non-genetic disorder. It simply means that there are certain non-genetic factors, as well as many genetic factors, that contribute to the variation in liability to hip dysplasia.

## Muscular dystrophy in chickens

The heritability of liability to muscular dystrophy, MD, is quite high in all species studied. But research into MD in chickens has shown that administration of penicillamine delays the onset of clinical signs, and that exercise plus injections of diphenylhydantoin improves the ability of MD chickens to right themselves from a lying position.

Once again, this evidence is not at all in conflict with the existence of genetic variation in liability to MD. It does, however, point the way to possible non-genetic methods of alleviating the effects of MD, that may be very useful in practice.

## Phenylketonuria

The simplest and probably the best example of an environmental solution to a genetical problem involves phenylketonuria, PKU, which is a recessive disorder in humans caused by a deficiency of the enzyme phenylalanine hydroxylase. Affected individuals are unable to break down the amino acid phenylalanine, which builds up in the body, leading to severe mental retardation. As soon as the biochemical basis of this disorder was discovered, a simple non-genetic treatment became evident. It followed logically from the well-known fact that humans are unable to synthesize phenylalanine; our only source of this amino acid is the food we eat. Obviously, a simple solution to this inherited disorder is to remove phenylalanine from the diet of individuals homozygous for the defective allele. While this creates difficulties for both child and parents, it is far preferable to the alternative of the child suffering permanent mental retardation. And fortunately, the restricted diet can be relaxed towards the end of the teenage years, because by then, the lack of this enzyme ceases to be harmful.

## The paradox of inherited disorders

In all the examples discussed above, we have seen that it is possible to alleviate inherited disorders by non-genetic means, even if the heritability of liability is quite high. Indeed, in the case of PKU, broad-sense heritability (described in Chapter 6) is 100 per cent, because under normal circumstances, there are no non-genetic factors contributing to variation in liability to PKU. However, one particular non-genetic factor can be changed easily, with dramatic effects; the removal of phenylalanine from the diet of homozygote recessives reduces their liability to such an extent that they now have a liability on the other side of the threshold.

These cases described above illustrate a very important principle, which can be called the paradox of inherited disorders, and can be stated as follows: the more that is learnt about the genetic basis of an inherited disorder, the more it is likely that a non-genetic treatment will be developed.

## Transplantation and corrective surgery

While somewhat different from the non-genetic factors discussed above, transplantation and corrective surgery can both be regarded as non-genetic means of alleviating inherited disorders.

Transplantation of bone marrow, liver, or kidney, from normal animals to affected animals, has the potential to provide the necessary enzyme or blood-clotting factor in individuals suffering inherited deficiencies of these polypeptides. This type of treatment has produced positive results for disorders such as citrullinaemia, haemolytic anaemia due to pyruvate kinase deficiency, Gaucher's disease, and von Willebrand's disease.

Corrective surgery is also sometimes used to alleviate an inherited disorder. For example, some veterinarians have claimed that cutting the pectineus muscle alleviates hip dysplasia in dogs. The evidence for this is somewhat controversial, but the operation is quite popular in some countries. And there are numerous other examples where surgery has been used to 'hide' structural defects.

## Genetic effects of environmental control

Non-genetic control certainly alleviates inherited disorders. In the case of PKU, the simple change in diet has essentially eradicated the disorder. It has not, of course, removed the mutant alleles that cause PKU, and this raises an important question about non-genetic control of inherited disorders. If individuals carrying defective alleles are enabled to survive and reproduce, and hence pass on harmful or even lethal alleles, will there be an increase in the frequency of these alleles in the future, giving rise to an ever-increasing number of individuals requiring treatment?

The basic principles of population genetics tell us that if we remove selection pressure from a previously harmful allele so that all genotypes have equal fitness, on average the frequency of each allele will remain constant, except for the effect of mutation, which will tend to increase the frequency of the previously undesirable allele, but at an imperceptibly low rate.

Thus, in principle, there will be no extra problems created in the future by the use of non-genetic control of inherited disorders, provided that all genotypes have an equal chance of contributing alleles to the next generation. In practice, however, this proviso is often not met. For example, if an animal commands a large stud fee but has an inherited disorder, it is tempting to correct or treat the disorder and then to use that animal as extensively as possible. In effect, this increases the relative fitness of the undesirable genotype and consequently increases the frequency of the undesirable allele or alleles. In practice, therefore, non-genetic control of genetic disorders should be used with caution, and animals so treated should not be allowed to make large contributions to the next generation. They can, however, be used repeatedly in crossbred matings to produce commercial (non-pedigreed) animals, such as those that will be slaughtered for meat. Or if they are companion animals, they can be neutered and sold as pets.

## Genetic control of single-gene disorders

Genetic control programmes involve preventing certain individuals from contributing their genes to subsequent generations. This is called **culling**. When used in this sense, culling does not mean that animals have to be killed. Indeed, as noted above, they can be neutered and sold as pets, or if they are farm animals, they can be mated to animals from another breed, with the aim of producing commercial animals that will not be used for breeding.

### Clinical screening

There are many single-gene disorders that are considered to be serious problems but which do not prevent affected individuals from reproducing. Well-known examples include the inherited eye disorders of dogs, such as progressive retinal atrophy, retinal dysplasia, and various forms of cataract. If the disorder can be detected by clinical examination prior to reproductive age, it should be possible to select against the disorder.

The simplest programme involves culling affected animals. If the disorder is recessive, this involves selection against homozygotes for the harmful recessive allele. If all pedigreed offspring in a breed are screened, and if all affected offspring are culled, this amounts to complete selection against recessive homozygotes, the results of which were discussed in Chapter 5. A more effective programme involves culling all parents of affected animals as well as affected animals themselves. If the disorder is recessive, this amounts to partial selection against heterozygotes in addition to selection against homozygote recessives.

In terms of genetic control programmes, the halothane test for malignant hyperthermia syndrome (MHS) in pigs is a form of clinical screening. Prior to the cloning of the halothane gene, the halothane test was used extensively throughout the world to reduce the frequency of PSS.

### The general principle of genetic control of single-gene disorders

Since autosomal recessive disorders are by far the most common type of single-gene disorders, the following discussion will be primarily in terms of that type of disorder. With only minor adjustments, most of the discussion applies equally to other types of single-gene disorders.

The major principle of genetic control of recessive disorders is very simple: irrespective of how high the frequency of an undesirable recessive allele becomes, the frequency of affected offspring can be reduced immediately to zero if all matings involve at least one parent that is homozygous for the normal allele.

From this principle, it follows that the aim of genetic control programmes is to distinguish homozygotes (non-carriers) from heterozygotes (carriers). There are several methods for achieving this aim.

## Pedigree analysis

Pedigree analysis involves studying available pedigrees, with the aim of estimating the probability that a normal prospective parent is homozygous. While straightforward in principle, the mathematics are quite complex. However, algorithms have been written to perform the necessary calculations, and software incorporating such algorithms is becoming increasingly available to individual breeders. Such software is very useful as a means of decreasing the frequency of undesirable alleles without involving breeders in any major expense or trouble: the computer programme tells them which animals are most likely to be homozygous, and it is these animals that should be used in future matings.

## Test matings

Test matings involve considerable extra effort, expense and time. But they can be very useful. The most common options involve mating the prospective parent with:

(1) homozygotes for the recessive allele, or
(2) known heterozygotes, or
(3) progeny of the prospective parent, or
(4) a random sample of the population.

There are two possible outcomes from a test mating. If an offspring from a test mating is affected and hence is homozygous for the undesirable allele (*aa*), that offspring must have received one of its a alleles from the prospective parent. Obviously, in this case the prospective parent must be a carrier. The other possible outcome is that the offspring is normal, in which case there are two alternative explanations: either the prospective parent is homozygous for the normal allele (*AA*), or it is really a carrier (*Aa*) but by chance remained undetected because it passed on its *A* allele rather than its *a* allele. The aim of a test-mating programme is to distinguish as efficiently as possible between these two alternatives.

Consider matings with homozygous recessives. If the prospective parent is a carrier, a test mating of this type can be written as $Aa \times aa$, with the expected results being one-half $Aa$ (normal) offspring and one-half $aa$ (affected) offspring. Recalling that the carrier parent remains undetected if an $Aa$ offspring is produced, the chance of a carrier parent remaining undetected after producing one offspring is 0.5. Since the genotype of each offspring is independent of the genotypes of all other offspring, the chance of a carrier parent remaining undetected after two offspring is $0.5 \times 0.5 = (0.5)^2 = 0.25$; after three offspring it is $(0.5)^3 = 0.125$; and after $n$ offspring it is $(0.5)^n$. Thus, for each additional offspring, the chance of a carrier parent remaining undetected decreases by one-half.

The important question that has to be asked in practice is: how many offspring do we need to observe in order for there to be only a very small chance of a carrier parent remaining undetected? Suppose, for example, that we would like the chance that a carrier remains undetected to be no greater than 5 per cent. In this case, we require sufficient offspring per prospective parent to ensure that $(0.5)^n$ is less than or equal to 5 per cent. By solving the equation $(0.5)^n \leq 0.05$, we conclude that $n = 5$ is the required number of offspring. If we want the chance to be 1 per cent, the required number is $n = 7$.

It should be obvious that we can never prove that a parent is homozygous normal in a test mating. All we can do is to reduce the chance of the parent being undetected as a carrier, to some acceptably low level. On the other hand, as soon as the first affected offspring is produced, we have proved that the parent of that offspring is a carrier.

The principle is the same for the other types of test matings listed above; the main difference is in the chance of a carrier remaining undetected. Full details of how this is derived for each type of test mating are provided in *Veterinary genetics* (pp. 319–22). The results are shown in Table 11.1. It can be seen that matings to homozygous recessives are most efficient. If such individuals are not available, the next best option is to use known carriers. Although the last two types of test matings appear to be much less efficient, they do have certain advantages. For example, they do not involve the expense of establishing and maintaining a special group of tester animals. More importantly, they provide a test for undesirable recessive alleles at all loci rather than just at one locus, as is the case for the first two types of matings. In comparing the last two types of matings, Table 11.1 suggests that it is more efficient to mate a prospective parent to its offspring than to a random sample of the population, unless the recessive allele is quite common in the population. Against this, however, is the fact that the use of offspring as testers greatly increases the time required to test a prospective parent. The final type of mating is the one that occurs naturally in progeny-testing schemes such as those occurring throughout the world in the dairy industry. Notice that the efficiency of the test increases as the frequency of the recessive gene increases. This means that the higher the frequency of the gene, the sooner will carriers be detected. When the practical implications of this type of test

**Table 11.1** The number of offspring required in test matings for a recessive gene. In the fourth type of test mating, $q$ is the frequency of the recessive gene in the general population

| Prospective parent mated to: | Chance that a carrier remains undetected with $n$ offspring | Number of offspring required to reduce the chance of non-detection to: | | |
|---|---|---|---|---|
| | | 0.05 | 0.01 | 0.001 |
| 1. Homozygote recessives | $(0.5)^n$ | 5 | 7 | 10 |
| 2. Known carriers | $(0.75)^n$ | 11 | 16 | 24 |
| 3. Offspring of prospective parent | $(0.875)^n$ | 23 | 35 | 52 |
| 4. Individuals chosen at random | $(1 - 0.5q)^n$, where $q$ equals | | | |
| | 0.2 | 29 | 44 | 66 |
| | 0.1 | 59 | 90 | 135 |
| | 0.01 | 598 | 919 | 1379 |

mating are investigated over several consecutive generations, it turns out that this is a very efficient means of ensuring that undesirable alleles are kept at low frequencies.

One final point should be mentioned. It concerns the use of multiple ovulation and embryo transfer (MOET) and/or early fetal recovery to increase the effectiveness of test-mating programmes. MOET can be used to increase the number of males tested with a given number of females, or to enable the test mating of females that would otherwise never produce sufficient offspring in a lifetime. Artificial termination of pregnancy at the earliest stage at which the disorder is detectable in the fetus also increases the number of test matings that can be achieved in a given time. Both of these techniques have been used commercially in testing males and females for bovine syndactyly.

## Biochemical screening

If the disorder is caused by the deficiency of a polypeptide, and if the identity of the polypeptide is known, and if it is possible to measure the quantity or activity of that polypeptide in a laboratory test on a sample of blood or other readily-available tissue, biochemical screening is a possibility for distinguishing carriers from non-carriers. This type of screening makes use of the phenomenon of gene dosage, which was discussed in Chapters 1 and 3. A good example of this in animals is provided by mannosidosis, which is a lysosomal storage disease due to a deficiency of alpha-mannosidase (Appendix 3.1). Because heterozygotes have one normal and one abnormal allele, they show approximately half the level of enzyme activity in blood plasma compared with homozygous normals. Biochemical screening for this enzyme was used in very successful control programmes conducted in Angus cattle and related breeds in New Zealand and Australia during the 1970s and 1980s.

While straightforward in principle, there are various practical difficulties that can be encountered with biochemical screening. For example, there is often substantial variation in enzyme level within a genotype, due to various non-genetic factors and genes at other loci. This can result in some animals having enzyme levels midway between the averages of the two genotypes. Such cases are difficult to resolve. In addition, there is always the potential complication caused by blood-cell chimerism (Chapter 4) in cattle, if the animal commenced its *in-utero* life as a twin. If the enzyme level is estimated from blood cells, such animals may show their twin's enzyme level, rather than their own.

## DNA markers

Since the development of the molecular techniques described in Chapter 2, there has been unprecedented activity in generating large numbers of poly-morphic DNA markers for domestic animals.

How can DNA markers be used in the control of single-gene disorders? The first step involves deciding which markers to use. The second step involves obtaining DNA from the members of at least two consecutive gener-ations of families in which the disorder is segregating, and genotyping each animal at the disorder locus and at one or more marker loci. A linkage analysis is then conducted (like the one described in Chapter 1), in order to estimate the recombination fraction between the disorder locus and each marker locus.

## Choice of markers

One way to search for a useful marker is the so-called **candidate-gene** approach. This involves investigating what is known about the biochemistry and/or the genetics of the disorder in all species in which it has been reported, with a view to identifying genes that could possibly correspond to the disorder locus. An example of this approach is provided by the search for a marker for the halothane locus. A wealth of basic physiological and biochemical research over many years led to the suggestion that the gene for the calcium-release channel (CRC, also known as the ryanodine receptor—see Chapter 9) might be the halothane gene. As soon as the CRC gene was cloned in one species of mammal, it was a relatively straightforward task to clone it in other species, and to test whether it was linked to the halothane gene in each species. In pig families, and in some (but not all) human families, the recombination fraction

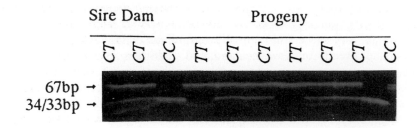

**Fig. 11.1** A PCR–RFLP test (using the enzyme *Hha*I) for MHS in pigs, which determines the genotype at the site of the causal mutation in the calcium-release-channel gene. CC = homozygous normal, CT = heterozygous, TT = homozygous for *hal*.

turned out to be zero, i.e. the CRC gene is completely linked to the halothane gene. As described in Chapter 9, further research has since shown that the CRC gene is actually the halothane gene, and a C→T substitution at position 1843 is the actual cause of the defective (*hal*) allele in populations of pigs throughout the world. Since this base substitution creates or destroys the recognition sequence for several restriction enzymes, it was a simple matter to develop a PCR-RFLP genotyping test for this mutation. Pigs can therefore be genotyped at the halothane locus on the basis of the polymorphism that actually causes the disorder (Fig. 11.1).

Not all candidate-gene searches turn out to be as successful as this one: many candidate genes turn out not to be linked to the disorder locus.

A set of mapped markers provides a powerful alternative to the candidate-gene approach. If the markers are equally spaced along all chromosomes, at least two of the markers must be linked to each locus in the genome (one on either side). As described in Chapter 2, more and more mapped markers are becoming available in all domestic species. The disadvantage of this approach is the expense and effort involved in genotyping all available members of several families at tens (if not hundreds) of marker loci, in order to obtain a complete coverage of all chromosomes. The advantage is that, after all the effort, you can be certain of identifying at least two markers that are linked to the disorder locus.

Once linked markers have been identified, more markers can be generated in the vicinity of the linked markers. By testing these new markers on the same families, the most likely location of the disorder locus becomes more and more tightly focused, until its location can be pinpointed to a region covered by just one YAC clone (see Chapter 2) from a set of contiguous overlapping clones that cover the entire genome. The clone can then be searched for coding sequences (open reading frames) or other tell-tale signs of structural genes, such as exon/intron boundaries or conserved promoters. At the same time, comparative mapping will be providing longer and longer lists of actual structural genes which are likely to be located in that region, and which could possibly be the disorder locus in question. Eventually, one of these approaches should result in the disorder locus being identified at the molecular level. This whole approach of moving from linked markers to the actual gene is called **positional cloning**.

## DNA markers in the control of single-gene disorders

The simplest situation is where the DNA-marker polymorphism actually corresponds to the causal mutation, as with MHS. In cases such as this, it is a straightforward matter to determine whether any animal is a homozygote or a heterozygote, simply by genotyping that animal for the causal mutation (Fig. 11.1).

What if we have a DNA marker polymorphism that is linked to the disorder locus, but is not the actual causal mutation? How can this be used to distinguish homozygotes from heterozygotes? Unfortunately such a marker cannot be used to determine with certainty the disorder-locus genotype of any animal; but it can provide an estimate of the probability of the animal having a particular genotype (homozygous or heterozygous) at the disorder locus. There are two ways in which this can be done.

### Using linked markers within families

In this approach, it is necessary to genotype the parents and grandparents of the animal at the marker locus, as well as the animal itself. It is also necessary to know which parents and grandparents are heterozygous at the disorder locus (on the basis of whether or not they have produced affected offspring from previous matings). Then, by deducing which marker allele is on the same chromosome (haplotype) as the defective allele in the parents, and taking account of the recombination fraction (i.e. the chance of crossing over) between the marker locus and the disorder locus, it is possible to estimate the probability of the animal being a carrier.

Any linked marker can be used within families in this manner. Obviously, the lower the recombination fraction between the marker and the disorder locus, the greater the accuracy of the estimate of genotype probability.

### Using linked markers in populations

An alternative way to use a linked marker is at the population level. By this we mean that members of a population are genotyped at the marker locus, and then this knowledge alone is used to estimate the probability of each member of that population being a carrier at the disorder locus. How useful are markers when used in this way?

In order to answer this question, we must introduce a concept called **gametic equilibrium** (also called **linkage equilibrium**). In order to understand this concept, we have to consider the possible gametes (which are equivalent to haplotypes) that can occur in a population, in relation to a marker locus and a disorder locus. Suppose that there are two alleles at each locus: $M_1$ and $M_2$ at the marker locus, and $D$ and $d$ at the disorder locus, with $d$ being the deleterious allele.

If the two loci are in gametic equilibrium, the frequency of each of the four possible haplotypes ($M_1 D$, $M_1 d$, $M_2 D$, and $M_2 d$) equals the product of the relevant gene frequencies. For example, the frequency of the $M_1 d$ haplotype equals the product of the frequencies of $M_1$ and $d$. Another way to look at this is to say that with gametic equilibrium, the $d$ allele occurs with the same frequency in haplotypes containing the $M_1$ marker as in haplotypes carrying the $M_2$ marker. At the population level, the practical consequence of gametic equilibrium is that the marker locus is no use as a predictor of genotype at the disorder locus, because the frequency of any genotype at the disorder locus is the same within each genotypic class at the marker locus.

On the other hand, if there is a non-random association between the two loci at the population level, we say there is **gametic disequilibrium**. For example, allele $M_1$ could be associated with allele $d$ more frequently than expected on the basis of their gene frequencies. In extreme cases of disequilibrium, each allele at the marker locus occurs only with one of the alleles at the disorder locus, and never with the other allele, e.g. $M_1$ occurs only with $d$. In such cases, the marker genotype is a perfect predictor of genotype at the disorder locus. In general, the greater the disequilibrium between a disorder locus and a marker locus, and the more similar the frequencies of the disorder and marker alleles, the more useful is the marker locus.

Disequilibrium can arise if selection favours particular combinations of alleles at different loci, or it can be generated by mutation, migration or genetic drift. Once it has arisen from whatever cause, disequilibrium decreases by a proportion $(1 - c)$ every generation, where $c$ is the recombination fraction between the two loci. Readers will recall from Chapter 1 that the maximum value of $c$ is 0.5, even for loci located on separate chromosomes. This means that if two loci are completely unlinked, the disequilibrium between them decreases by one-half per generation. If they are linked, then the closer the linkage, the slower is the decrease of the disequilibrium.

It should now be evident that there is a range of possible circumstances in which a DNA marker and a deleterious allele might be associated in a population. At one extreme, the marker might be completely unlinked to the disorder locus, e.g. it could be on a different chromosome, but a recent importation (even of just one animal) could have generated substantial disequilibrium. In this case, the marker is of only very limited use, because its non-random association with the defective allele (the very thing that makes it useful) decreases by one-half every generation. At the other extreme, the marker might be located very close to the disorder locus (it could even be located within the locus, but still be many kb away from the causal mutation), in which case the disequilibrium could have existed for many generations, and will be decaying at an imperceptibly slow rate. In this case, the marker will be a very useful predictor of disorder-locus genotype at the population level for many, many years.

Unfortunately, there is no way of knowing the extent of disequilibrium between any pair of loci, without actually going to the trouble of measuring it, which involves genotyping large numbers of unrelated animals at both loci in the population in which the marker is to be used. When this has been done, some very closely linked loci show substantial disequilibrium, while others just as closely linked show none at all. Also, two loci can show strong disequilibrium in one population, but equilibrium in another population.

All we can say is that if there is a strong association at the population level between a marker and a deleterious allele, there must be strong disequilibrium between the two loci in that population. The further apart the two loci are, the less useful is the association, because the faster it disappears with each passing generation. Conversely, the tighter the linkage between the marker and the disorder locus, the longer the disequilibrium remains, and hence the more useful is the marker as a predictor of disorder-locus genotype, simply on the basis of genotyping individual animals for the marker locus. However, a linked marker, even if only a few kilobases away from the causal mutation, is rarely as useful as being able to genotype individuals for the causal mutation itself.

## Some potential limitations

New mutations are occurring all the time, albeit at a slow rate. This means that even if a stage is reached where the actual causal mutation of a particular inherited disorder has been identified and is used as the basis of a genotyping test, it is always possible that a new mutation will occur at a different site in the same gene, or even in another gene, giving rise to the same clinical signs. We must always be prepared, therefore, for a well-established DNA genotyping test to 'miss' some carriers of defective alleles. In haemophilia A and other X-linked disorders in humans, for example, about one-third of affected individuals have novel mutations.

This means that we can never hope to keep up with the occurrence of harmful alleles, and we should therefore be prepared for any DNA test to fail sooner or later. Depending on the size of the gene, it may be possible without too much trouble to identify the new mutation, by sequencing or by DGGE or SSCP or similar techniques mentioned in Chapter 2. While the new mutation is being tracked down, it may be possible to find a DNA polymorphism (e.g. a microsatellite) within the gene, or near the gene, which can be used as a new marker. Within families, this new marker will be very useful as a guide to genotype at the site of the new mutation, because it will be very tightly linked to the new mutation. Its usefulness at the population level depends on the extent of disequilibrium between the polymorphic site identified in the test, and the site of the new mutation. It also depends on the extent to which the alleles that are in disequilibrium have the same frequencies; the greater the difference in frequencies, the less useful is the marker.

Another potential limitation of DNA markers is that they may not be polymorphic in all families. If a family is homozygous at a marker locus, the marker is useless in that family. In general, the greater the number of alleles at a marker locus, the greater is the proportion of families in which the marker is informative. Because of this, there is currently much research effort to locate highly polymorphic DNA markers (such as microsatellites) throughout the genome.

### DNA markers—in summary

The most desirable situation is where animals can be genotyped at the site of the mutation that causes the disorder. However, even this situation is less than perfect if new mutations causing the same disorder occur elsewhere in the gene. If this happens, the options are to identify the new mutation and/or find a polymorphism in or near the gene which can be used as a linked marker. If the actual gene is not known, the best that can be achieved is a linked marker.

Within families, the usefulness of a linked marker depends on the recombination fraction between the marker and the causal mutation.

Within populations, the usefulness of a linked marker depends on the disequilibrium, the recombination fraction between the marker and the causal mutation, and the similarity of allele frequencies at the two loci. The greater the disequilibrium, and the greater the similarity of allele frequencies, the greater is the initial usefulness of the marker. The smaller the recombination fraction, the slower is the erosion of the usefulness of the marker.

## Gene therapy

Gene therapy is a logical extension of transplantation. One of the major problems of transplantation, namely the problem of rejection, can be overcome if the patient's own cells are removed, 'repaired' by the addition of normal genes, and then replaced. Alternatively, normal genes can be inserted into the appropriate tissue *in vivo* by indirect means, such as via a harmless virus or a liposome carrying the normal host gene. Considerable research effort is being devoted to gene therapy, and substantial progress has been made. There are still, however, major practical problems to be solved.

Even if it can be made to work regularly and effectively, gene therapy is applicable only to those disorders in which the relevant gene is expressed in a tissue that is accessible, either directly or indirectly. In any case, it is doubtful whether such therapy will be of much practical use in domestic animals. The reason for this is that the molecular technology for heterozygote detection is likely to progress at least as fast as that of gene therapy, so that by the time gene therapy becomes a practical reality, heterozygote detection will most likely be available for the majority of single-gene disorders. Once this stage is reached, it will be far easier to prevent the birth of affected animals by genotyping prospective parents, and arranging appropriate matings. Only in species like humans, where this type of control is unacceptable, is the addition of normal genes to previously defective cells likely to have much impact. However, most of the development work for human gene therapy uses animal models of human disorders, in which veterinarians have a major interest.

## Genetic control of multifactorial disorders

The genetic control of multifactorial disorders is best illustrated by hip dysplasia in dogs.

Hip dysplasia is probably the best known of all animal disorders that are familial but not due to a single gene; it has been the subject of more research, and more controversy, than any other similar disorder. One of the causes of controversy is that hip dysplasia is traditionally diagnosed not on clinical signs but by subjective evaluation of a radiograph, as illustrated in Chapter 6. The problem with this approach is that in most populations, the incidence of abnormal hips as diagnosed by radiography is much higher than the incidence of clinical hip dysplasia (CHD). This immediately creates a credibility gap between veterinarians and breeders, because all too often a dog that can jump a fence six feet high is diagnosed as being dysplastic according to its radiograph. The solution to this problem is for breeders and veterinarians to distinguish between the trait that we wish to improve (called the breeding objective) and the trait that is actually measured (called the selection criterion): see Chapter 16. In the present context, the breeding objective is clearly CHD. Since CHD is very difficult to measure, and may not be expressed at a young age, the selection criterion in most hip dysplasia control programmes is 'radiographic' hip dysplasia (RHD), which is readily assessable at an early age. The fact that RHD is assessed subjectively does not detract from its usefulness as a selection criterion. All that is required is that RHD be measured on an arbitrary scale, and that this measurement has a positive genetic correlation (see Chapter 14) with CHD. Although no estimates of this correlation have been made, the available evidence indicates that it is positive and sufficiently high to justify the use of RHD as the selection criterion in control programmes.

The heritability of RHD has been estimated on many occasions, with estimates usually falling in the range 0.25–0.40. This is sufficiently high to justify a selection programme based on simple mass selection, which is selection of individuals according to their own phenotype. As mentioned above, phenotype for RHD is usually measured on an arbitrary scale. For example, in the control programme run jointly by the British Veterinary Association (BVA) and the German Shepherd League (GSL) (which is now the standard scheme for almost all breeds in the UK, New Zealand, and Australia), nine different radiographic features of each hip are each assessed on a scale from 0 (ideal) to 6 (worst), giving a total potential range of subjective scores from 0 to 108. With such a large range of possible scores, selection on RHD is essentially the same as selection on a continuously varying trait such as body weight; in effect, the BVA/GSL scoring system has changed RHD from a threshold trait to a conventional multifactorial (quantitative) trait. This provides a substantial advantage to breeders wishing to decrease the incidence and severity of hip dysplasia.

For any multifactorial disorder that can be classified into many categories, selection against the disorder is exactly the same in principle as selection for a production trait such as growth rate or fleece weight. Details of how such selection can be practiced are given in Chapter 16.

There are many disorders which at present can still only be categorized into a small number of classes, as exemplified by the congenital heart defects discussed in Chapter 6, or even just into two classes—affected or normal. While it is more difficult to decrease the incidence of such threshold traits, it is still possible to make substantial progress from selection. The basis of success lies in the conclusions that were reached about familial disorders in Chapter 6, namely that:

(1) the more severely an individual is affected, the more frequent and severe is the disorder in the offspring of that affected individual, and
(2) among normal individuals, the lower their genetic relationship with affected individuals and the larger the proportion of their relatives that are normal, the less frequent and severe is the disorder in their offspring.

In the early stages of a control programme, when the incidence is still quite high, the first of these conclusions is particularly relevant; all potential parents should be ranked according to severity, and as many as possible should be culled according to severity. As the incidence decreases over time, a stage is reached when the least affected category of potential parents contains more animals than are needed as actual parents. This is the stage at which the second conclusion becomes relevant; the aim then is to select those animals having the lowest genetic relationship with affected animals, and the largest proportion of normal relatives. As the programme progresses, affected animals gradually disappear from the pedigrees of selected animals.

## Use of DNA markers

As mentioned in Chapters 6 and 7, as sets of mapped DNA markers become increasingly available in each domestic species, linkage analyses between the markers and multifactorial disorders will lead to the identification of markers that are linked to genes that contribute to variation in the disorder, and eventually will lead to identification of the genes themselves. Identification of linked markers will be of immediate assistance in selecting against the disorder, although the inevitable decay of disequilibrium between the marker and the gene, as discussed above, will limit the usefulness of this approach at the population level. In the longer term, the identification of the genes themselves will enable more effective selection (along the lines discussed above for single-gene disorders), and will lead to a far better understanding about the underlying causes of the disorder, which in turn may well lead to various non-genetic means of controlling the disorder.

## Genetic control—some final points

### The bare essentials

Breeders are being confronted continually by inherited disorders. While one or other of the above approaches can certainly help in many circumstances, there remains a need for simple advice that can be put into practice immediately by individual breeders. What should this advice be? By far the simplest and most effective way to minimize the occurrence of inherited disorders is to minimize the mating of relatives. The reasons for this, and the means of achieving it, are described in Chapter 13.

### Insurance schemes

Irrespective of whether or not a control programme is available for a single-gene disorder, there is always the option of insuring against an animal being shown to be a carrier of a defective allele, either as a result of a test, or by throwing a defective offspring. Furthermore, this option can be extended to multifactorial disorders, providing agreement can be reached in relation to the definition of disorders. If a policy is taken out on each animal sold for breeding purposes, everyone benefits: buyers are secure in the knowledge that if the animal does produce affected offspring, they will at least get their money back; vendors are saved the trauma of defending themselves against dissatisfied customers; and the breed as a whole benefits because of the positive incentive for inherited disorders to be brought out into the open.

### The art of the possible

Amid growing concern about the obvious problems associated with the occurrence of inherited disorders, well-meaning veterinary authorities sometimes devise sets of guidelines for the control of inherited disorders. These guidelines often include a list of 'prohibited' alleles, i.e. animals must be shown to be *not* carrying each of the harmful alleles on the list before they can be registered in a breed society or imported or used in artificial insemination. The aim of such guidelines is to reach a stage where all populations are free of all deleterious alleles. Whilst this aim is certainly laudable in theory, it is, unfortunately, completely unrealistic in practice. The reason for this is that mutations can occur at any time at any locus. And, given that there are probably between 50 000 and 100 000 genes in each species of domestic animal, there are potentially tens of thousands of defective alleles. Even though the rate of mutation is very low, the inevitable consequence of the above biological facts is that almost all animals, including the purest of purebreds (plus the readers of this book, and its author!), are carrying several severely deleterious alleles. Given this biological reality, it is obviously point-less to try to achieve a situation where a population is free of all harmful alleles. In fact, the only way to achieve this state would be to cull almost all animals!

As soon as these biological realities are grasped, it is obvious that we have to learn to live with harmful alleles. For autosomal recessive disorders, which are by far the most common, it has already been stressed that so long as at least one parent is not carrying the harmful allele, *no* affected offspring will be produced. In other words, the incidence of the disorder can be reduced to zero, simply by ensuring that each mating involves at least one non-carrier. Obviously the harmful allele is still present in the population, but the disorder itself will have disappeared, which is all we can realistically hope for.

In order to achieve this, it is necessary to have a simple means of geno-typing individuals for known harmful alleles. Wherever such tests exist, breed societies and artificial-breeding organizations should be encouraged to geno-type breeding animals for known harmful alleles, and to widely publicize the results of the tests. An atmosphere needs to be developed in which breeders are rewarded for telling others about which harmful alleles their animals carry, rather than, as in most cases at present, being persecuted or, at the very least, being financially penalized through lost sales of breeding stock. Breeders must realize that having harmful alleles is a biological inevitability rather than something to be ashamed of. Moreover, if they are willing to go public about the occurrence of harmful alleles, the incidence of inherited disorders can be dramatically reduced, because this information enables breeders to avoid those matings that are likely to produce animals with inherited disorders.

## The problems created by some breed standards

Most breeds have an official standard to which all breeders aspire, and which forms the basis for the decisions of judges at shows. Unfortunately, the official standards of some breeds actually encourage breeders to select for inherited disorders. The most obvious examples are those in which the breed standard (or a favoured phenotype) is based on heterozygosity for a defective gene, e.g. Scottish Fold cats, Manx cats, Merle dogs, and Overo horses (see Chapter 12). However, there are many other, more subtle, cases (especially in companion animals) where the breed standard encourages breeders to select for undesirable features. Overcoming these problems involves changing the culture of breed societies, which is obviously not a simple task. All that can be done in the short term is to be aware of the problems created by some of the current breed standards, and to try to encourage a gradual change in philosophy, with the eventual aim of having breed standards that are a reflection of healthy animals, and which are not conditional upon the presence of defective alleles.

## Further reading

### General

Collins, F. S. (1992). Positional cloning: let's not call it reverse any more. *Nature Genetics*, **1**, 3–6.

Owen, J. B. and Axford, R. F. E. (ed.) (1991). *Breeding for resistance in farm animals*. CAB International, Wallingford, England.

Patterson, D. F. (1993). Understanding and controlling inherited diseases in dogs and cats. *Tijdschrift Voor Diergeneeskunde*, **118**, (Suppl.), S23–7.

Smith, C. A. (1994). New hope for overcoming canine inherited disease. *Journal of the American Veterinary Medical Association*, **204**, 41–6.

Wilcock, B. (1990). The genetic disease crisis in purebred dogs. *Canadian Veterinary Journal*, **31**, 265–6.

### Pedigree analysis

Elsen, J. M., Leroy, P., and Goffinet, B. (1991). Comparison of 4 statistical tests for genotype determination at a major locus of progeny tested sires. *Journal of Animal Breeding and Genetics*, **108**, 167–73.

Fernando, R. L., Stricker, C., and Elston, R. C. (1993). An efficient algorithm to compute the posterior genotypic distribution for every member of a pedigree without loops. *Theoretical and Applied Genetics*, **87**, 89–93.

Goffinet, B., Elsen, J. M., and Leroy, P. (1990). Statistical tests for identification of the genotype at a major locus of progeny-tested sires. *Biometrics*, **46**, 583–94.

van Arendonk, J. A. M., Smith, C., and Kennedy, B. W. (1989). Method to estimate genotype probabilities at individual loci in farm livestock. *Theoretical and Applied Genetics*, **78**, 735–40.

### Control schemes

Anon. (1993). BVA/KC/ISDS eye scheme: notes on procedure. *Veterinary Record*, **128**, 137–41.

Bedford, P. G. C. (1994). WSAVA Kennel Clubs meeting—control of hereditary elbow disease in pedigree dogs. *Journal of Small Animal Practice*, **35**, 119–22.

Bell, D. R. and Brown, C. J. (1992). BVA/Kennel Club hip dysplasia scheme. *Veterinary Record*, **130**, 148.

Fuschini, E., Fries, R., and Stocker, H. (1992). Malformations and genetic disorders in cattle—registration, frequencies and control of hereditary diseases in the AI-derived Braunvieh population. *Wiener Tierarztliche Monatsschrift*, **79**, 161–5.

Laikre, L., Ryman, N., and Thompson, E. A. (1993). Hereditary blindness in a captive wolf (*Canis lupus*) population—frequency reduction of a deleterious allele in relation to gene conservation. *Conservation Biology*, **7**, 592–601.

Lingaas, F. and Klemetsdal, G. (1990). Breeding values and genetic trend for hip dysplasia in the Norwegian Golden Retriever population. *Journal of Animal Breeding and Genetics*, **107**, 437–43.

O'Brien, P. J., Shen, H., Cory, C. R., and Zhang, X. (1993). Use of a DNA-based test for the mutation associated with porcine stress syndrome (malignant hyperthermia) in 10,000 breeding swine. *Journal of the American Veterinary Medical Association*, **203**, 842–51.

Walde, I. and Neumann, W. (1991). International eye examination certificate for inherited eye diseases in dogs. *Wiener Tierarztliche Monatsschrift*, **78**, 284.

## *Gene therapy/transplantation*

Kay, M. A., Landen, C. N., Rothenberg, S. R., Taylor, L. A., Leland, F., Wiehle, S., *et al.* (1994). *In vivo* hepatic gene therapy—complete albeit transient correction of factor IX deficiency in hemophilia B dogs. *Proceedings of the National Academy of Sciences*, **91**, 2353–7.

Lozier, J. N., Thompson, A. R., Hu, P. C., Read, M., Brinkhous, K. M., High, K. A., and Curiel, D. T. (1994). Efficient transfection of primary cells in a canine hemophilia-B model using adenovirus polylysine DNA complexes. *Human Gene Therapy*, **5**, 313–22.

Mulligan, R. C. (1993). The basic science of gene therapy. *Science*, **260**, 926–32.

Taylor, R. M., Farrow, B. R. H., and Stewart, G. J. (1992). Amelioration of clinical disease following bone marrow transplantation in fucosidase-deficient dogs. *American Journal of Medical Genetics*, **42**, 628–32.

# Single genes in animal breeding

**12**

In previous chapters, we discussed many traits that are determined by a single gene, including blood-cell antigens and a large variety of disorders. There are many other single-gene traits, some of which are of particular importance to animal breeding. The aim of this chapter is to discuss such traits, and to consider some of the practical uses to which they can be put.

## Coat colour

Coat colour in mammals is due to the presence in hair and wool of pigment granules consisting of melanins in a protein framework. The melanins are formed by a series of metabolic pathways that convert the amino acid tyrosine into either **eumelanins** (dark colour) or **phaeomelanins** (light colour). Eumelanins are often described as black, but they include brown and derivatives of black and brown. Phaeomelanins contain sulphur. They are often described as yellow, but they can range from a rather bright yellow through to red. Melanin production occurs in organelles called **melanosomes** within cells called **melanocytes**. Once a melanosome has become filled with pigment, it is called a pigment granule, and is secreted from the cell.

Although much remains to be discovered about the genetic control of pigment formation, it is now generally accepted that at least six autosomal loci, each with multiple alleles, influence the production and distribution of pigment. The most interesting aspect of these six loci is that they appear to exist in all mammals. Although not all species of mammals have all known alleles at any locus, there are sufficient examples of similar coat colours and/ or patterns inherited in a similar way in several different species to present a convincing picture of homology of coat-colour and coat-pattern alleles among species. A summary of the six main loci is given in Table 12.1.

Other loci are known to be important in determining coat colour and pattern in certain species. In cats, for example, the autosomal Tabby locus has three alleles, giving rise to Abyssinian tabbies ($T^a$), striped tabbies ($T$), and blotched tabbies ($t^b$). Another easily recognizable locus in cats is the X-linked orange locus, which gives rise to the well-known tortoiseshell coat colour discussed in Chapter 1. The orange allele, $O$, prevents expression of eumelanins in much the same way as the yellow allele, $A^y$, does at the autosomal agouti locus. The non-orange allele, $o$, allows normal expression of eumelanins.

**Table 12.1** Characteristics of the six main loci determining coat colour in mammals. Each locus is autosomal

| Locus | Symbol | Main alleles | Effects and mode of action |
|---|---|---|---|
| Agouti | A | $A^y, A^w, A, a^t, a, a^e$ | Controls regional distribution of eumelanin and phaeomelanin over the body and in individual hairs. |
| Brown | B | $B^{lt}, B, b, b^l$ | Affects concentration of eumelanins. This locus encodes a tyrosinase-related protein. |
| Albino | C | $C, c^{ch}, c^b, c^s, c^a, c$ | Reduces intensity of pigmentation, first phaeomelanin and then eumelanin, until none is left in $cc$ (albino). This locus encodes the enzyme tyrosinase. |
| Dilute | D | $D, d, d^l$ | Dilutes both eumelanin and phaeomelanin by clumping pigment granules. This locus encodes a myosin heavy chain. |
| Extension | E | $E^d, E, e^{br}, e$ | Extends eumelanin or phaeomelanin pigment in body as a whole, with $e^{br}$ giving a eumelanin/phaeomelanin variegation. This locus encodes a membrane-transporter protein. |
| Pink-eyed dilution | P | $P, p, p^s$ | Main effect on eumelanosomes, with dark colours much more diluted than light ones. This locus encodes the melanocyte-stimulating hormone receptor. |

Another coat-colour locus of particular interest is dominant white spotting, which was illustrated in the photograph of the tortoiseshell cat in Chapter 1 (Fig. 1.13). There are two interesting effects of this gene. First, in animals with some white fur, the white is usually on the belly and other ventral surfaces rather than on the back or dorsal surfaces. Second, the larger the total area of white, the larger are the individual patches of orange and non-orange in tortoiseshell cats. The explanation for these two observations comes from research in mice, where the white-spotting gene is known to be one of a number of genes that regulate normal growth and proliferation of cells. In fact, it encodes a protein that protrudes through the cell membrane, relaying 'messages' from outside to inside the cell. The transmembrane domain of the protein is a receptor for a **growth factor** (a protein produced by one type of cell, that acts on another type of cell). The domain inside the cell has tyrosine kinase activity. When a growth factor binds to the receptor on the outside of the cell, this stimulates tyrosine kinase activity inside the cell, which sets off a cascade of phosphorylations, resulting in activation of transcription factors

(Chapter 1), which in turn activate genes, resulting in multiplication of stem cells, including melanocyte precursor cells, in the developing embryo. This whole process is known as a **signal transduction pathway**. During embryonic development, the precursor cells migrate from the neural crest down either side of the body, eventually meeting at the centre of the belly. The cells then proliferate sideways until they meet neighbouring cells, thereby filling up all available areas, resulting in a solid mass of melanocytes over the entire body.

The white-spotting allele produces a defective transmembrane protein which is less efficient at relaying messages. This results in fewer melanocyte precursor cells, possibly with poorer mobility. The migration consequently stops part-way down the sides, and, since there are fewer cells, each cell proliferates to a greater extent before meeting a neighbouring cell, giving rise to larger pigmented areas derived from each precursor cell. This provides an explanation for the two observed effects of the white-spotting allele; the white areas are those that were never reached by the melanocyte precursor cells; and the larger the area not reached by these cells, the larger is each patch of cells derived from a single cell.

Another interesting aspect of the white-spotting gene is that if it is activated at the wrong time, the result can be excess and uncontrolled proliferation of stem cells; in other words, cancer. In fact, at some time in the past, a retrovirus 'picked up' a copy of the white-spotting gene and incorporated it into its own genome. When this retrovirus infects mice, it activates its own copy of this gene at inappropriate times, causing sarcoma. Retroviral genes that cause cancer are called **oncogenes**. The original host version of an oncogene is called a **proto-oncogene**. Thus, the white-spotting gene is actually a proto-oncogene. In this particular case, the proto-oncogene was discovered and named as *c-kit* (where 'c' indicates that it is a cellular gene) long before its identity with the white-spotting gene was established. The corresponding oncogene is called *v-kit*, where 'v' indicates the viral form of the gene. Mutations at the *c-kit* gene in humans cause piebaldism, which is the human equivalent of white spotting.

There is one more interesting point. In mice, there is another coat-colour gene called steel, which is on a different chromosome to white spotting, and whose mutants give rise to the same phenotype as white spotting. The protein encoded by steel is in fact the growth factor that binds to the receptor portion of the white-spotting gene product—it is the so-called **ligand** for the white-spotting receptor. Thus, the white-spotting phenotype can result either from a faulty white-spotting gene or a faulty steel gene. If either gene is faulty, the appropriate message does not get through, and cell proliferation is incomplete. Similarly, piebaldism in humans can result from mutations at *c-kit* or at the human steel gene. This is another good example of genetic heterogeneity, which was first encountered in Chapter 3. Incidentally, there is now much interest in using molecular techniques to mass-produce the protein encoded by the steel gene (which is called stem cell factor) from various species (including dog), because of its considerable potential as a drug for treatment of anaemia and other conditions in which stem-cell proliferation needs additional stimulation.

A gene that may be similar to the white-spotting gene gives rise to the Overo coat-colour pattern in horses. As with white spotting, the Overo pattern is characterized by pigment spreading down both sides from the dorsal midline, giving way to lack of pigment (i.e. white) primarily on the ventral surfaces. Homozygosity for the Overo allele results in white or nearly white foals which die within a few days of birth: the so-called lethal white foal syndrome (LWFS). The cause of death is intestinal obstruction caused by a lack of nerve cells in the distal portion of the large intestine (aganglionic megacolon), which is thought to be due to a fault in the proliferation and/or migration of nerve stem cells from the neural crest of the developing embryo. This is an another example of pleiotropy (see Chapter 5), i.e. a single gene affects two or more apparently unconnected traits; in this case, coat colour and agangliosis. This pleiotropy is a reflection of the effect of the Overo allele on proliferation and/or migration of various types of stem cells from the neural crest. Interestingly, the homologous disorder in humans (Hirschprung disease) is due to mutations in a proto-oncogene. A similar lethal defect occurs in grey and white Karakul lambs.

Another locus which may be similar to the white-spotting gene is the autosomal merle locus in dogs, with alleles *m* (normal) and *M* (merle). The *M allele is co-dominant with respect to coat colour, but is recessive with respect to a number of defects:* MM dogs have serious eye defects (including reduction in size, i.e. microphthalmia, and sometimes absence, i.e. anophthalmia), are partially or completely deaf, and are often sterile.

## Complications

Although the inheritance of coat colours is straightforward in principle, there are several complications that arise in practice.

One of these is **epistasis**, or interaction between loci. An example of epistasis is the complete masking of the various tabby alleles at the tabby locus by the non-agouti allele; it is usually impossible to tell which tabby allele or alleles are present in cats that are homozygous for non-agouti, because such cats are uniformly black.

Another complication is that alleles at different loci can sometimes be used with more-or-less equal validity to explain a certain coat colour. Nowhere is this more evident than in horse coat colour, which unfortunately has been a source of much confusion to scientists and breeders alike.

Despite this problem, there are two rules for coat-colour inheritance in horses that are valid. The Chestnut Rule states that the mating of chestnut with chestnut will not produce a black, brown, bay, or grey; and the Grey Rule states that a grey horse must have at least one grey parent. Both of these rules have now been sufficiently tested for them to be of considerable value in checking the validity of pedigrees. If, for example, the result of a certain mating appears to break one of these rules, the progeny of that mating should not be registered until a thorough check of the pedigree has been made, because it is most likely that an error has been made in recording the pedigree.

## Trademark genes

With segregation of so many coat-colour loci in various domestic species, it has been possible for enthusiasts to develop a large number of different genotypes, many of which are recognized as distinct varieties or even as distinct breeds. While there may now be other genetic differences between varieties and between breeds, it is important to realize that, in many cases, what are now called different breeds originally differed by alleles at only one or a few coat-colour loci. These differences in coat colour have in many cases become the trademark of the breed. In some cases, such as palomino horses, the coat-colour trademark happens to be due to heterozygosity at a coat-colour locus (in this case, the E locus), which means that it is impossible to obtain a population that will breed true for the trademark.

## Carpet wool

The Romney breed has been the predominant sheep breed in New Zealand since the 1920s. A typical New Zealand Romney fleece consists of a majority of unpigmented wool fibres, which are solid, and a minority of hair fibres, which have a hollow core (called a medulla) running down the centre of the fibre. Traditionally, there has been strong selection against medullated (hairy) fibres in the New Zealand Romney.

In 1931, a purebred Romney ram lamb with an exceptionally hairy fleece was born on a property belonging to a Mr Nielson. It was given to Professor Dry at what is now Massey University, where it was eventually shown that the extreme hairiness was due to an autosomal, incompletely dominant allele which is now designated $N^d$ ($N$ for Nielson, and $d$ for Dry), which must have resulted from a mutation of the normal, non-hairy allele, $n$. Fleeces from sheep that are homozygous for $N^d$ have approximately 65 per cent by weight of medullated fibres, which is ideal for carpet manufacture. Heterozygotes ($N^d n$) have a level of medullation that is intermediate between the two homozygotes. Being virtually free of pigmentation, and having good spinning qualities, wool resulting from the $N^d$ allele soon became popular with carpet-wool manufacturers, and the allele became known as the carpet-wool gene. The numbers of $N^d N^d$ and $N^d n$ sheep were increased as rapidly as possible, giving rise to a new breed called the Drysdale, which is now the basis of a firmly established carpet wool industry.

Other carpet-wool genes have appeared from time to time. For example, the $N^t$ gene, which is completely dominant to $n$, has given rise to another carpet-wool breed, the Tukidale. And a mutation at a different locus in Tasmanian Romneys has given rise to the Elliottdale breed of carpet-wool sheep.

## Prolificacy in sheep

Another sheep gene that has created considerable interest is the Booroola fecundity gene, $Fec(B)$, which is the major cause of the prolificacy seen in the Booroola strain of Australian Merino. This gene received considerable publicity in 1993, when, after linkage analyses involving more than 100 microsatellite markers, two markers were identified as being linked to it. Subsequent analyses, making good use of the strong chromosomal homologies that exist between sheep, cattle and humans (Chapter 2), showed that the gene is located on chromosome 6. Another prolificacy gene has been discovered in sheep in New Zealand. Whereas the Booroola gene is autosomal, this gene (called the Inverdale fecundity gene, $FecX(I)$) is X-linked. Unfortunately, homozygotes for $FecX(I)$ have non-functional 'streak' ovaries.

## Polledness

In general terms, the presence or absence of horns can be attributed to the action of two alleles at an autosomal locus, with polled ($P$) being dominant to horned ($p$). Many breeds of domestic animals are horned and are therefore homozygous for $p$. With increasing concern over the practical problems of carcase damage and difficult handling that are often associated with horned animals, many practical breeders now prefer their animals to be polled. The main difficulty inherent in creating a polled version of any breed is the usual difficulty of attempting to select in favour of a dominant allele, as discussed in Chapter 5: it is very difficult to achieve complete homozygosity, because the recessive (horned) allele remains 'hidden' in heterozygotes. A major step towards resolving this problem was achieved in 1993, when two linked, mapped microsatellite markers were identified in cattle, locating the gene on chromosome 1.

A rather unusual problem arises with the occurrence of the polled gene in goats. In normal circumstances in other species of mammals, individuals that have two X chromosomes develop into normal females. And even in goats, XX individuals that are horned ($pp$) or heterozygous for polled ($Pp$) are normal females. But all XX goats that are homozygous for the polled allele are intersexes. In addition, a proportion of XY goats that are homozygous for the polled allele are sterile. This is another example of pleiotropy.

## Muscular hypertrophy in cattle and sheep

'Double muscling' is the popular but somewhat misleading term for this trait. Its advantages include a substantially higher percentage of muscle and lower percentage of fat, and increased efficiency of food conversion. In cattle, its association with substantially increased dystocia has been sufficient to limit its popularity. However, the allele for muscular hypertrophy has reached a high frequency in the Belgian Blue, in which the additional financial rewards are sufficient to justify the veterinary assistance required to avoid the dystocia problem. In contrast to cattle, the trait was only recently observed in sheep. Linkage analyses have already identified two linked markers on sheep chromosome 18.

## Dwarf poultry

There are alleles at several different loci in the domestic chicken that give rise to birds with a markedly lower mature body size. Most of these so-called dwarfing genes seriously affect viability or hatchability and are therefore of no commercial interest. There is, however, a Z-linked dwarfing gene that appears to have some commercial value. It encodes the chicken growth hormone receptor (GHR), and the *dw* allele at this locus produces a defective transcript that is only three-quarters the length of the normal transcript. In at least one strain of broilers, this is due to a deletion in the GHR gene (Appendix 3.1).

For practical purposes, the *dw* allele can be regarded as recessive. Thus dwarf males are $Z^{dw}Z^{dw}$ and dwarf females are $Z^{dw}W$. Several broiler-breeder lines homozygous for *dw* have been developed. These *dw* lines are used as a source of female parents which are mated to males from a normal broiler strain. Mainly because of reduced feed consumption and a smaller space requirement, *dw* broiler-breeder lines are more economical than normal broiler lines.

## Genes for sexing chickens

Poultry breeders are continually faced with the need to separate day-old chicks into males and females. The conventional method by which sexes are distinguished is vent sexing, which requires skilled operators and which is therefore relatively expensive.

A much cheaper alternative, now widely used commercially, is to exploit genetically-determined differences between the sexes which can be distinguished easily in day-old chicks by unskilled workers. The most commonly used differences arise from segregation of alleles at two Z-linked loci: the

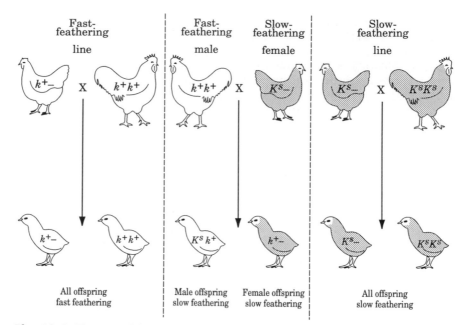

**Fig. 12.1** The use of fast-feathering/slow-feathering Z-linked sexing in chickens.

feathering locus, with the slow-feathering allele ($K^s$) being dominant to rapid-feathering ($k^+$); and a feather-colour locus, with silver ($S$) being dominant to gold ($s$). Since all four alleles exert discernible effects in day-old chicks, either pair of alleles can be used to enable sexing to be carried out by unskilled workers, as shown in Fig. 12.1.

Interestingly, the slow feathering ($K^s$) allele appears to be an insertion mutation, resulting from the insertion of a DNA copy of the RNA genome of the avian leucosis virus, which is a retrovirus. The DNA copy is called $ev21$ (endogenous viral gene number 21), and is inherited like any host gene. This gene is a mixed blessing. While it is obviously advantageous in terms of the slow-feathering phenotype it has created, it is disadvantageous because it produces infectious viral particles (called endogenous viruses). These viruses are transmitted congenitally from hens with $K^s$ to all of their offspring. This does not seem to harm those offspring that also inherit $K^s$, i.e. the slow-feathering offspring. But in the offspring that have not inherited $K^s$ (i.e. the fast-feathering offspring), the presence of endogenous viral particles induces immunological tolerance to the virus, which renders them unable to mount an effective immune response against exogenous viral particles, resulting in poorer performance and increased mortality due to tumours induced by the exogenous virus. By referring to Fig. 12.1, readers should be able to deduce that all the females in the offspring generation will therefore be at risk in the presence of exogenous avian leukosis virus. Fortunately, there are various ways to overcome at least some of this disadvantage, such as vaccination of the slow-feathering dams, who then provide protection to their offspring via the transfer of maternal antibodies.

Because of these complications, some effort is being devoted to identifying Z-linked loci with suitable alleles that are not insertion mutations, that could be used for auto-sexing. One which has been showing some promise is sex-linked imperfect albinism.

## Pedigree checking

Many breeding animals are bought on the strength of a pedigree. In some situations such as thoroughbred yearling sales, the pedigree is the major source of information available. Obviously, it is very important for the buyer to be certain that the available pedigree information is correct.

In view of the risk of incorrect pedigrees occurring from time to time (because of honest or not-so-honest mistakes), breed societies are often keen to conduct random checks on pedigrees, and to verify the pedigree of each animal sold at official sales. This is done by checking that the pedigrees are compatible with Mendelian inheritance at one or more identifiable loci. Traditionally, this has involved examination of inheritance patterns at coat-colour and blood-group loci, but these loci do not usually provide a very powerful test.

The most powerful test is provided by minisatellites (DNA fingerprinting) or by microsatellites, both of which were described in Chapter 2. In fact, there is now a rapid move to the use of molecular techniques (either Southern analysis or PCR) based on minisatellite or microsatellite sequences. An example of a paternity test using DNA fingerprinting is given in Fig. 12.2. Band 6 is absent from the dam, but is present in four pups. It must therefore have come from the sire. But sire A lacks this band; he is therefore excluded as a potential sire. In contrast, sire B has this band, which means that he could have been the sire of the litter. Notice that it is not possible to prove that sire B was in fact the actual sire; the evidence merely fails to exclude him.

When testing parentage, it is important to remember that, because of blood-cell chimerism (Chapter 4), an animal may show more than just its own DNA fingerprint (or in extreme cases, may show its twin's DNA fingerprint rather than its own). Before dogmatically excluding an animal on the basis of a blood test, therefore, it would be wise to obtain a DNA sample from some other tissue, such as skin or hair follicle.

Besides being very useful in paternity testing in domestic animals, mini-satellites and microsatellites are also very useful for testing paternity in wild populations (e.g. birds and lions), identifying the source of biological material (such as tusks 'poached' from elephants), assessing the level of inbreeding and relationship within populations of free-ranging animals, assessing the evolutionary relationship (genetic distance) between populations (Chapter 5), and increasing the efficiency of introgression programmes (see Chapter 18).

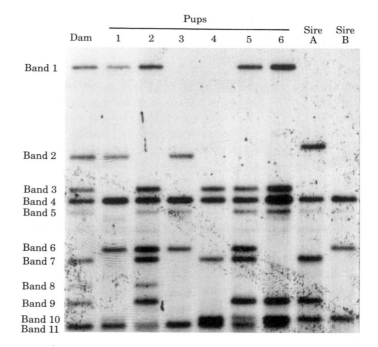

**Fig. 12.2** A paternity test in dogs using Southern analysis with the enzyme *Hae*III and a multi-locus human minisatellite probe consisting of 29 tandem repeats of a 16 bp core sequence.

# Further reading

## General

Crittenden, L. B. (1991). Retroviral elements in the genome of the chicken: implications for poultry genetics and breeding. *Critical Reviews in Poultry Biology*, **3**, 73–109.

## Coat colour

Bultman, S. J., Klebig, M. L., Michaud, E. J., Sweet, H. O., Davisson, M. T., and Woychik, R.P. (1994). Molecular analysis of reverse mutations from nonagouti (*a*) to black-and-tan (*aᵗ*) and white-bellied agouti (*Aᵂ*) reveals alternative forms of agouti transcripts. *Genes and Development*, **8**, 481–90.

Fleischman, R. A. (1993). From white spots to stem cells—the role of the kit receptor in mammalian development. *Trends in Genetics*, **9**, 285–90.

Hudon, J. (1994). Biotechnological applications of research on animal pigmentation. *Biotechnology Advances*, **12**, 49–69.

Lauvergne, J. J., Silvestrelli, M., Langlois, B., Renieri, C., Poirel, D., Antaldi, G. G. V. (1991). A new scheme for describing horse coat colour. *Livestock Production Science*, **27**, 219–29.

McCabe, L., Griffin, L. D., Kinzer, A., Chandler, M., Beckwith, J. B., and McCabe, R. B. (1990). Overo lethal white foal syndrome: equine model of aganglionic megacolon (Hirschsprung disease). *American Journal of Medical Genetics*, **36**, 336–40.

Morrison-Graham, K. and Takahashi, Y. (1993). Steel factor and c-kit receptor—from mutants to a growth factor system. *Bioessays*, **15**, 77–83.

Searle, A. G. (1968). *Comparative genetics of coat colour in mammals*. Logos Press, London.

## DNA fingerprinting

Baker, C. S., Gilbert, D. A., Weinrich, M. T., Lambertsen, R., Calambokidis, J., McArdle, B., Chambers, G. K., and O'Brien, S. J. (1993). Population character-istics of DNA fingerprints in humpback whales (*Megaptera novaeangliae*). *Journal of Heredity*, **84**, 281–90.

Binns, M. (1993). DNA fingerprinting as an epidemiological tool. *British Veterinary Journal*, **149**, 121–2.

Decker, M. D., Parker, P. G., Minchella, D. J., and Rabenold, K. N. (1993). Monogamy in black vultures—genetic evidence from DNA fingerprinting. *Behavioral Ecology*, **4**, 29–35.

Ewen, K. R., Templesmith, P. D., Bowden, D. K., Marinopoulos, J., Renfree, M. B., and Yan, H. (1993). DNA fingerprinting in relation to male dominance and paternity in a captive colony of Tammar wallabies (*Macropus eugenii*). *Journal of Reproduction and Fertility*, **99**, 33–7.

Fondrk, M. K., Page, R. E., and Hunt, G. J. (1993). Paternity analysis of worker honeybees using random amplified polymorphic DNA. *Naturwissenschaften*, **80**, 226–31.

Galbraith, D. A. (1994). *A practical introduction to DNA fingerprinting*. Chapman and Hall, London.

Grobet, L. and Hanset, R. (1993). Identification and parentage testing by the use of DNA fingerprints in domestic species. *Annales de Medecine Veterinaire*, **137**, 123–32.

Groen, A. F. (1993). A note on the use of DNA fingerprints to assess the coefficient of inbreeding in populations with unknown pedigree. *Journal of Animal Breeding and Genetics*, **110**, 156–60.

Hermans, I. F., Morris, C. A., Chambers, G. K., Towers, N. R., and Jordan, T. W. (1993). Assessment of DNA fingerprinting for determining genetic diversity in sheep populations. *Animal Genetics*, **24**, 385–8.

Trommelen, G. J. M., Dendaas, J. H. G., Vijg, J., and Uitterlinden, A. G. (1993). DNA profiling of cattle using microsatellite and minisatellite core probes. *Animal Genetics*, **24**, 235–41.

## Linked markers

Cockett, N. E., Jackson, S. P., Shay, T. L., Nielsen, D., Moore, S. S., Steele, M. R., *et al.* (1994). Chromosomal localization of the callipyge gene in sheep (*Ovis aries*) using bovine DNA markers. *Proceedings of the National Academy of Sciences, USA*, **91**, 3019–23.

Georges, M., Drinkwater, R., King, T., Mishra, A., Moore, S. S., Nielsen, D., *et al.* (1993). Microsatellite mapping of a gene affecting horn development in *Bos taurus*. *Nature Genetics*, **4**, 206–10.

Lanneluc, I., Drinkwater, R. D., Elsen, J. M., Hetzel, D. J. S., Nguyen, T. C., Piper, L. R., *et al.* (1994). Genetic markers for the Booroola Fecundity (Fec) gene in sheep. *Mammalian Genome*, **5**, 26–33.

Montgomery, G. W., Crawford, A. M., Penty, J. M., Dodds, K. G., Ede, A. J., Henry, H. M., *et al.* (1993). The ovine Booroola fecundity gene (FecB) is linked to markers from a region of human chromosome 4q. *Nature Genetics*, **4**, 410–4.

# Relationship and inbreeding 13

The aim of this chapter is to provide an understanding of the concepts of relationship and inbreeding, which have important practical applications in the breeding of companion animals, the control of inherited diseases, the management of zoo populations and endangered species, the estimation of heritability, and in artificial selection programmes.

## The inbreeding coefficient

The simplest case involves considering a single locus in two offspring, B and C, that have one parent, A, in common. Using arrows to indicate the direction of inheritance, this situation can be represented as follows:

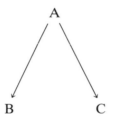

A is called the **common ancestor** of B and C. At any locus, there is a chance that B and C each received a copy of the same gene (the same segment of DNA) that existed in A. When this happens, we say that B and C have genes that are **identical by descent** from A. Genes are identical by descent if they are copies of a segment of DNA that occurs in a common ancestor.

Suppose that B and C mate and produce an offspring, O:

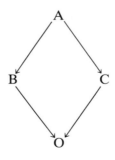

At any locus, if B and C have genes that are identical by descent, there is a chance that O inherits two genes that are identical by descent, one from A through B, and the other from A through C. We are now ready for a definition: the **inbreeding coefficient** of an individual is the probability that the two genes present at a locus in that individual are identical by descent. The inbreeding coefficient is usually given the symbol $F$.

If an individual has two genes that are identical by descent at a certain locus, the individual must be homozygous at that locus. Thus the inbreeding coefficient is a reflection of homozygosity. However, it does not measure homozygosity in an absolute sense. The reason for this will be explained later in this chapter.

We shall now consider relationship in some detail, before returning to inbreeding.


## Relationship

The most common situation, and the one most easily understood, is where neither of the related individuals is inbred. In this section, therefore, unless otherwise stated we shall assume that relatives are not inbred, i.e. we shall assume that $F = 0$ for each relative.


### *Direct relationship*

The most basic relationship is that between a parent (P) and its offspring (O). At any locus an offspring has two genes, one of which (the paternal gene) is a copy of one of its father's genes, and the other of which (the maternal gene) is a copy of one of its mother's genes. Since the same is true for all loci, we can say that an offspring has exactly ½ of its genes in common with each of its parents. We can now state a simple definition: the **relationship** between two non-inbred individuals is the expected proportion of genes that the two have in common. The relationship between offspring and parent, therefore, is ½.

What is the relationship between offspring (O) and grandparent (GP)? In order to answer this question, we need to follow the transmission of genes from a particular grandparent ($GP_1$) to a parent (P) to an offspring (O). It is obvious that $GP_1$ transmits exactly ½ of its genes to P who in turn transmits exactly ½ of its genes to O. On average therefore, O receives $½ \times ½ = ¼$ of its genes from $GP_1$. Thus, the relationship between an offspring and any one of its grandparents is ¼.

By an argument similar to that used above, the relationship between an offspring and any one of its great-grandparents is $½ \times ½ \times ½ = ⅛$. It should now be evident that the relationship between an individual and an ancestor decreases by ½ for each generation that separates the individual from that ancestor. Thus, the relationship between an individual and an ancestor is

$(\frac{1}{2})^n$, where $n$ is the number of generations between the individual and the ancestor in the pathway of direct descent from the ancestor to the individual.

It follows that irrespective of how superior a particular ancestor may have been, if it occurs only once in an individual's pedigree and several generations back in the pedigree, there is only a small chance that the individual in question inherited any of that ancestor's genes. It is therefore pointless to select an individual solely because its pedigree contains a distant ancestor that happened to be very famous.

The situation is a little different if a particular ancestor occurs more than once in a pedigree. In this case, each occurrence of the ancestor in the pedigree provides an independent opportunity for the individual to have inherited the ancestor's genes. The total relationship is the sum of the independent contributions from each pathway of direct descent. Thus, if an ancestor occurs several times in a pedigree, and not too far back in the pedigree, the relationship between the individual and the ancestor could be quite high. This is what happens with **line breeding**.

The relationships considered above are called **direct relationships** because they refer to relationships that can be traced in a direct line or pathway of descent from an ancestor to a descendent. The other type of relationship is where two individuals have an ancestor in common, and may therefore each have inherited the same gene from that ancestor. This is called **collateral relationship**.

## Collateral relationship

We shall return to the simplest situation described earlier, which involves two offspring, B and C, and their parent, A. Having one parent in common, B and C are called **half-sibs**. As we saw earlier, if B and C each receive a copy of the same gene at any locus in A, we can say that B and C have genes that are identical by descent from A. We can now consider a more general definition of relationship: the **relationship** between any two individuals is the expected number of genes at a locus in one individual that are identical by descent with a randomly chosen gene at the same locus in the other individual. This definition is correct in all situations, whether the related individuals are inbred or not. If the related individuals are not inbred, this definition is equivalent to the simpler one given earlier.

As with direct relatives, the relationship between two collateral relatives decreases by $\frac{1}{2}$ for each generation that separates the two relatives along a certain pathway. The only difference is that in the case of collateral relatives, the pathway between them consists of two lines of descent; from the common ancestor to one relative and from the common ancestor to the other relative. To emphasize this, the total number of generations separating two collateral relatives is written as $n + n'$, where $n$ is the number of generations between the common ancestor and the first relative, and $n'$ is the number of generations between the common ancestor and the second relative. Thus for any pathway, the relationship between two collateral relatives is $(\frac{1}{2})^{n+n'}$.

Sometimes there may be more than one pathway through a certain common ancestor, and sometimes there may be more than one common ancestor. In all these cases, the overall relationship is the sum of the relationships contributed by each pathway.

## The inbreeding coefficient revisited

We are now in a position to derive an equation for calculating the inbreeding coefficient, by giving further consideration to the case where individual A has two offspring B and C, who mate to produce offspring O.

Consider a randomly chosen gene that B passes on to O. In order to calculate the inbreeding coefficient of O, we need to calculate the probability that the other gene at the same locus in O (the gene from C) is identical by descent with the gene from B. We can do this by noting that the relationship between B and C is the expected number of genes in C that are identical by descent with a randomly chosen gene at the same locus in B. However, the randomly chosen gene in B is the gene that was passed from B to O. Since there is a chance of $\frac{1}{2}$ that any gene in C is passed on to O, it follows that the probability that O receives a gene from C that is identical by descent with the gene that O received from B, is equal to the relationship between B and C, multiplied by $\frac{1}{2}$.

In general, the **inbreeding coefficient** of any individual is $\frac{1}{2}$ the relationship between the parents of that individual. To calculate the inbreeding coefficient of any individual, therefore, all we have to do is to calculate the relationship between its parents, and then multiply by $\frac{1}{2}$. If the relationship of the parents is not known, the inbreeding coefficient of their offspring is assumed to be zero. The justification for this will be given later in this chapter.

## A general expression for relationship and inbreeding

We can now derive a general expression for calculating the relationship between any two individuals, and hence determining the inbreeding coefficient of their offspring.

First we need to consider the effect on relationship if the common ancestor in a certain pathway is itself inbred, i.e. if the common ancestor has an inbreeding coefficient greater than zero.

If the common ancestor is inbred, there is a greater chance that it transmits the same gene to each of the collateral relatives descended from it, which increases the chance that the two relatives each have genes that are identical by descent. We can cater for this by multiplying the contribution of each pathway by $(1 + F_A)$, where $F_A$ is the inbreeding coefficient of the common ancestor in that pathway. As before, if we know nothing of the parents of a certain common ancestor, the inbreeding coefficient of that ancestor is assumed to be zero.

Combining all of the above discussions, we end up with the relationship between any two individuals being given by

$$a = \sum_{i=1}^{p} (\tfrac{1}{2})^{n_i + n_i'} (1 + F_{A_i})$$

where $a$ is the symbol for relationship, $\Sigma$ indicates summation, $p$ is the number of pathways, $n_i$ is the number of generations between the common ancestor and the first relative (along the $i$th pathway), $n_i'$ is the number of generations between the common ancestor and the second relative (along the $i$th pathway), and $F_{A_i}$ is the inbreeding coefficient of the common ancestor in the $i$th pathway. In the case of direct relationships, there is only one line of descent for each pathway, and so $n_i' = 0$ for each pathway.

The relationship calculated by the above formula is called the **additive relationship**, which is why it is given the symbol $a$. It is also sometimes called the **numerator relationship**. It corresponds to the exact definition of relationship, namely the expected number of genes at a locus in one individual that are identical by descent with a randomly chosen gene at the same locus in the other individual. If neither of the relatives is inbred, it also equals the proportion of genes in common between the two relatives.

Once the additive relationship has been calculated for any pair of individuals, it is a simple matter to calculate the inbreeding coefficient, $F$, of the offspring of these two individuals as

$$F = \tfrac{1}{2}a.$$

Examples of the use of these two formulae are given in Appendix 13.1 of *Veterinary Genetics*.

In principle, the use of these two equations for calculating relationships and inbreeding coefficients is relatively straightforward. In practice, however, it can be very complex and tedious, especially for large pedigrees. Fortunately, these are exactly the type of calculations that can readily be performed by computers, and there are now several public-domain algorithms that calculate relationships and inbreeding coefficients from three-column lists of individual, sire and dam. Anyone requiring such an algorithm for their personal computer should contact their local geneticist, who should either be able to provide one, or know where to obtain one.

## The base population

It was stated earlier that the inbreeding coefficient does not measure homozygosity in an absolute sense. In fact, it measures the decrease in heterozygosity relative to a base population in which all individuals are assumed to be unrelated and to have zero inbreeding. In other words, it measures the extent to which an individual is less heterozygous than individuals that are assumed to have zero inbreeding.

How can measures of relationship and inbreeding be of any use when their actual magnitudes are dependent on the arbitrary choice of a base population, the members of which are conveniently assumed to have no ancestors in common? At first sight, it is difficult to reconcile this with the fact that if we go back a sufficient number of generations, any two individuals must have ancestors in common and hence must be related. In practice, this does not present a problem, so long as we remember that coefficients of relationship and inbreeding are relative, rather than absolute, quantities. Thus, if an individual has a zero inbreeding coefficient relative to a particular base population, we know that this individual has the same level of heterozygosity as members of that base population. If the actual level of heterozygosity in that base population is quite low, due, say, to substantial mating of close relatives amongst the ancestors of that base population, the individual with an inbreeding coefficient of zero actually has quite a low level of heterozygosity. The important point is, however, that if a second individual has an inbreeding coefficient of 0.3 relative to the same base population, we immediately know that this second individual is 30 per cent less heterozygous than the individual whose inbreeding coefficient is zero. This highlights the fact that inbreeding coefficients enable the relative levels of heterozygosity to be compared among individuals whose pedigrees can be traced back to the same base population.

## Inbreeding in populations

**Inbreeding** is the mating of related individuals. In previous sections, we have seen that the greater the relationship between two individuals, the greater is the inbreeding coefficient of their offspring. We have also seen that the greater the inbreeding coefficient of an individual, the lower is the chance of that individual being heterozygous. It follows that the greater the extent of inbreeding within a population, the lower the frequency of heterozygotes within that population. In the extreme case where all members of a population are completely inbred ($F = 1$), all individuals are homozygous at all loci, and the frequency of heterozygotes is zero.

From this, it is apparent that inbreeding changes genotype frequencies: it decreases the frequency of heterozygotes, and increases the frequency of homozygotes. However, it is important to realize that inbreeding does not, on average, change gene frequencies: the effect of the decrease in heterozygosity is simply to relocate genes from heterozygotes to homozygotes.

## Inbreeding depression

In Chapter 5, we saw that harmful recessive genes are maintained in populations by a balance between selection and mutation, and that the majority of these genes are hidden in heterozygotes. Since inbreeding decreases the frequency of heterozygotes, it tends to bring these harmful recessive genes out into the open, in the form of homozygotes. Consider, for example, a recessive gene with a frequency of 0.05. In a non-inbred, random-mating population, the frequency of homozygotes for this gene, and hence the frequency of the recessive phenotype, is $(0.05)^2 = 2.5$ per thousand. The frequency of heterozygotes is $2 \times 0.05 \times 0.95 = 0.095 = 95$ per thousand. An individual that has an inbreeding coefficient of $F = 0.4$ relative to this base population is 40 per cent less heterozygous; its actual level of heterozygosity is $(1 - 0.4)(0.095) = 0.058$. The loss in heterozygosity is $0.4 \times 0.095 = 0.038 = 38$ per thousand. Since this loss in heterozygosity is apportioned equally between the two types of homozygotes (19 per thousand to each homozygote), the frequency of homozygote recessives has risen from 2.5 per thousand to $(2.5 + 19.0) = 21.5$ per thousand, which is a very large increase.

Since many harmful recessive genes are lethal, inbreeding increases the frequency of embryonic death (spontaneous abortion) and stillbirths. Those harmful recessive genes with less severe effects contribute to a decrease in productive and/or reproductive performance of animals. The decrease in performance resulting from inbreeding is called **inbreeding depression**. The role of harmful recessive genes in leading to inbreeding depression, as discussed above, is just one example taken from the overall set of causes of inbreeding depression. In general, inbreeding depression occurs at any locus at which the performance (phenotype) of the heterozygote is greater than the midpoint between the two homozygotes. In other words, inbreeding depression occurs whenever genes that increase performance (or improve phenotype) show any degree of dominance at a locus. The greater the departure of the performance or phenotype of heterozygotes from a level intermediate between the homozygotes, the greater the inbreeding depression. Also, the closer the gene frequencies are to intermediate values, the greater the inbreeding depression.

Inbreeding depression is generally greatest for traits associated with natural fitness such as viability and reproductive ability, because there is more dominance at the loci affecting these traits than at loci affecting other traits.

Inbreeding depression has been very well documented in domestic animals. In general, performance in reproductive traits and viability traits decreases at the rate of around 1 per cent of the mean, for every 1 per cent increase in the inbreeding coefficient. Traits that are not directly associated with reproduction or viability usually decrease at less than 1 per cent of the mean. If we take

1 per cent inbreeding depression per one per cent increase in $F$ as a general guide, this means that if, for example, a sire is mated with his half-sister, the performance of the resultant offspring (which has $F = 12.5$ per cent) in a trait such as net reproductive rate is expected to be 12.5 per cent less than that of a non-inbred contemporary. There is, of course, substantial variation around this prediction; in some cases, the offspring of such a mating show very little inbreeding depression at all; and in other cases, the decrease in performance is much greater than 12.5 per cent. But it is very important to realize that, on average, inbreeding does result in substantial decreases in performance, especially for fitness traits.

The rates of inbreeding depression that occur in fitness traits, combined with the increased frequency of genetic defects and abnormalities (including spontaneous abortion and stillbirths) caused by inbreeding, have meant that most attempts to create highly inbred lines of domestic animals have failed. However, there are some lines of chickens that have inbreeding coefficients approaching $F = 1$, simply because with chickens, inbreeding can be conducted on a scale sufficiently large to allow for the huge wastage. For example, one inbreeding programme in chickens commenced with 279 different lines. After 15 generations of full-sib mating (i.e. matings between individuals with both parents in common, which is the most intense form of inbreeding possible in animals), only eight lines survived! With inbreeding having such drastic effects, it is obviously not a particularly progressive practice. And, since linebreeding is merely a type of inbreeding, the same conclusion applies to linebreeding.

## Control of inherited disorders

Bearing in mind that inbreeding affects all loci in the same way, it is evident that inbreeding within a stud or a breed increases the frequency of all disorders for which there are defective recessive alleles in that stud or breed. It does this by increasing the frequency of homozygotes; it does not, on average, increase the frequency of the recessive genes. As soon as this effect of inbreeding is appreciated, it is obvious that one of the major ways of controlling inherited diseases is to arrange matings so as to minimize the level of inbreeding in offspring. In other words, breeders should aim for matings between individuals that are as unrelated as possible. Of course, in practice there are limitations on the extent to which this can be done. But it remains the single most effective way in which individual breeders can control inherited disorders. To help them achieve this aim, there are several software packages (using the algorithms mentioned earlier) that calculate the relationship between all potential mating pairs among available animals, thereby enabling breeders to choose the matings that minimize the level of inbreeding. As before, your local geneticist should be able to provide assistance in obtaining such software.

## Endangered species and zoo animals

The plight of endangered species is causing increasing concern throughout the world. There are many well documented cases of species whose total numbers in the wild have dropped to alarmingly low levels. When this happens, it is inevitable that many alleles are lost, because the smaller the number of survivors, the greater the genetic bottleneck (see Chapter 5). In the extreme case, if only one male and one female remain, the maximum number of alleles at any locus is four (if both are heterozygous for different alleles). But in many cases, the remaining individuals are related, which means that our imaginary couple could easily each be homozygous for the same allele.

When a species is threatened with extinction in the wild, one possibility is to capture the survivors, and to attempt to breed them in captivity, with the ultimate aim of increasing the population size sufficiently so that descendants can be released back into the wild. These so-called **captive breeding programmes** are becoming increasingly popular, especially in zoos, and some have already achieved their aim. However, it is important to realize the limitations of such programmes. First, even if the population size were eventually to grow to hundreds of thousands, the level of heterozygosity is the same as in the few original survivors, because increasing the population size does not in itself create new alleles. In fact, of course, the only source of new alleles is mutation, and unfortunately, mutation is a painfully slow means of regenerating lost alleles.

In addition, since inbreeding depression of fitness traits is a universal phenomenon, it poses a very serious threat to captive breeding programmes. Suppose, for example, that among the survivors of a particular species, only one pair produces offspring. When these parents die, and the only surviving offspring are ready to reproduce, there is no alternative but to mate full-sibs, which results in offspring with 25 per cent inbreeding, which in turn could drastically reduce the chance of this next generation of offspring surviving. It is possible, therefore, that a captive breeding programme could actually end in the extinction of the species, despite the best intentions of the people involved. However, if the survivors were all closely related in the first place, there may be relatively little inbreeding depression in subsequent generations, because the survivors already share many genes. The important conclusion to be drawn is that captive breeding programmes are not without their risks, and that people should not be too optimistic about the results of any particular programme. In many cases, however, there is no other option.

At a less extreme level, it is becoming increasingly common for zoos to keep pedigree records, and to calculate the relationship between all possible mating pairs that could occur in a particular species. Often these calculations are done jointly for several different zoos, with a view to exchanging animals (or semen) if this would lead to a substantially lower increase in the level of inbreeding. This is a very useful practical application of the ideas presented in this chapter.

## Further reading

### Calculating relationship and inbreeding

Meuwissen, T. H. E. and Luo, Z. (1992). Computing inbreeding coefficients in large populations. *Génétique Sélection Evolution*, **24**, 305–13.

Tier, B. (1990). Computing inbreeding coefficients quickly. *Génétique Sélection Evolution*, **22**, 419–30.

### Inbreeding and inbreeding depression

Burrow, H. M. (1993). *The effects of inbreeding in beef cattle. Animal Breeding Abstracts*, **61**, 737–51.

Cook, W. R. and Kirk, N. W. (1991). Hereditary diseases of the horse and their prevention. *Irish Veterinary Journal*, **44**, 59–66.

Ercanbrack, S. K. and Knight, A. D. (1993). 10-year linear trends in reproduction and wool production among inbred and noninbred lines of Rambouillet, Targhee, and Columbia sheep. *Journal of Animal Science*, **71**, 341–54.

Hintz, R. L. and Foose, T. J. (1982). Inbreeding, mortality and sex ratio in gaur (*Bos gaurus*) under captivity. *Journal of Heredity*, **73**, 297–8.

Lacy, R. C. (1993). Impacts of inbreeding in natural and captive populations of vertebrates—implications for conservation. *Perspectives in Biology and Medicine*, **36**, 480–96.

Miglior, F., Szkotnicki, B., and Burnside, E. B. (1992). Analysis of levels of inbreeding and inbreeding depression in Jersey cattle. *Journal of Dairy Science*, **75**, 1112–18.

Prodhomme, P. and Lauvergne, J. J. (1993). The Merino Rambouillet flock in the national sheep fold in France. *Small Ruminant Research*, **10**, 303–15.

Ubbink, G. J., Knol, B. W., and Bouw, J. (1992). The relationship between homozygosity and the occurrence of specific diseases in Bouvier-Belge-Des-Flandres dogs in the Netherlands—inbreeding and disease in the Bouvier dog. *Veterinary Quarterly*, **14**, 137–40.

Wiener, G., Lee, G. J., and Woolliams, J. A. (1992). Effects of rapid inbreeding and of crossing of inbred lines . . . of sheep. *Animal Production*, **55**, 89–99, 101–14, 15–21.

Vanwyk, J. B., Erasmus, G. J., and Konstantinov, K. V. (1993). Inbreeding in the Elsenburg Dormer sheep stud. *South African Journal of Animal Science*, **23**, 77–80.

### Conservation programmes

Ellegren, H., Hartman, G., Johansson, M., and Andersson, L. (1993). Major histocompatibility complex monomorphism and low levels of DNA fingerprinting variability in a reintroduced and rapidly expanding population of beavers. *Proceedings of the National Academy of Sciences*, **90**, 8150–3.

Glosser, J. W. (1993). Conservation and wildlife preservation challenges for veterinarians. *Journal of the American Veterinary Medical Association*, **202**, 1078–81.

Hedrick, P. W. and Miller, P. S. (1992). Conservation genetics—techniques and fundamentals. *Ecological Applications*, **2**, 30–46.

Loeschcke, V., Tomiuk, J., and Jain, S. K. (ed.) (1994). *Conservation genetics*. Birkhauser Verlag, Basel.

Mace, G., Olney, P. J., and Feistner, A. (ed.) (1993). *Creative conservation: interactive management of wild and captive animals*. Chapman and Hall, London.

Markerkraus, L. and Grisham, J. (1993). Captive breeding of cheetahs in North American zoos—1987–1991. *Zoo Biology*, **12**, 5–18.

Moore, H. D. M., Holt, W. V., and Mace, G. M. (ed.) (1992). *Biotechnology and the conservation of genetic diversity*. Clarendon Press, Oxford.

Rahbek, C. (1993). Captive breeding—a useful tool in the preservation of biodiversity. *Biodiversity and Conservation*, **2**, 426–37.

Robinson, T. J. and Elder, F. F. B. (1993). Cytogenetics—its role in wildlife management and the genetic conservation of mammals. *Biological Conservation*, **63**, 47–51.

Ryder, O. A. (1993). Przewalski's horse—prospects for reintroduction into the wild. *Conservation Biology*, **7**, 13–5.

Short, J., Bradshaw, S. D., Giles, J., Prince, R. I. T., and Wilson, G. R. (1992). Reintroduction of macropods (Marsupialia, Macropodoidea) in Australia—a review. *Biological Conservation*, **62**, 189–204.

Spencer, L. (1993). Zoo and wildlife veterinarians examine their role in conservation. *Journal of the American Veterinary Medical Association*, **202**, 714–7.

Stüwe, M. and Nievergelt, B. (1991). Recovery of Alpine Ibex from near extinction—the result of effective protection, captive breeding, and reintroductions. *Applied Animal Behaviour Science*, **29**, 379-87.

Tear, T. H., Scott, J. M., Hayward, P. H., and Griffith, B. (1993). Status and prospects for success of the Endangered Species Act—a look at recovery plans. *Science*, **262**, 976–7.

Willis, K. (1993). Use of animals with unknown ancestries in scientifically managed breeding programs. *Zoo Biology*, **12**, 161–72.

# 14  Quantitative variation

The majority of traits of interest in animal breeding are continuously varying in the sense that animals cannot be readily classified into distinct classes. Milk production, fleece weight, body weight, and speed over a certain distance are just a few examples of continuously varying traits. Even a trait like egg production, which is not strictly continuous, can be considered as continuously varying because there are a large number of classes into which hens can be fitted according to the number of eggs laid in a certain period. Continuously varying traits are called **quantitative traits** or **metric traits**, and variation in them is called **quantitative variation** or **continuous variation**. Because they are measured on a continuous scale, it is not immediately obvious how variation in quantitative traits can result from the action of genes, which of course are discrete entities. The aim of this chapter is to describe the basis of quantitative variation, and to show how it can be partitioned into genetic and non-genetic components.

## Quantitative traits

Since quantitative variation is a statistical concept, we have to use statistical methods to investigate it.

We shall start with a frequency distribution of first-lactation milk yields in Friesians, as illustrated in Fig. 14.1. The two main statistical concepts (**mean** and **variance**) are explained in the caption to this figure. Even though milk yield is measured on a continuous scale, heifers have to be divided into an arbitrary number of small classes in order to construct the distribution. Once this is done, it becomes apparent that the distribution is more-or-less symmetrical and that it corresponds quite closely to a Normal distribution. To illustrate this, the mean and the variance of the actual distribution in Fig. 14.1 have been calculated, and a Normal distribution with the same mean and the same variance has been superimposed on the actual distribution. It can be seen that the Normal distribution provides quite a good description of the data, and the same conclusion applies to most quantitative traits. This is fortunate, because many of the applications of quantitative genetics involve the assumption that the data follow a Normal distribution. For traits that are not Normally distributed, e.g. faecal worm-egg counts, it is usually possible to find a simple transformation, such as square-root or logarithmic, that enables the useful properties of the Normal distribution to be exploited.

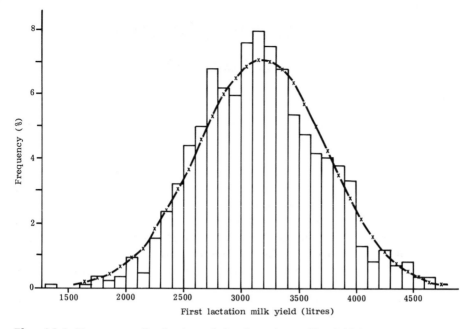

**Fig. 14.1** Frequency distribution of first-lactation milk yield in a population of Friesian cows. If $P_i$ is the performance (milk yield) of the $i$th heifer, if $n$ is the total number of heifers, and if $\Sigma$ indicates summation from $i = 1$ to $i = n$, the mean is estimated as $\Sigma P_i/n$, and the variance is estimated as $\{\Sigma P_i^2 - (\Sigma P_i)^2/n\}/(n - 1)$. In this population, the mean is 3180 litres and the variance is 315352 (litres)$^2$. A Normal distribution with this mean and variance has been superimposed on the frequency distribution.

How does continuous variation arise from the action of discrete genes? In order to answer this question, we shall start by considering just one locus. Imagine that there are two alleles at this locus, with allele $A$ increasing milk yield by one litre and allele $a$ giving no increase in milk yield. Imagine further that there is no dominance at this locus, so that the three genotypes $aa$, $Aa$, and $AA$ contribute 0, 1, and 2 litres to milk yield. If the frequency of each allele in a herd of cows is 0.5, the frequency distribution of milk yield resulting from variation at this one locus is symmetrical and consists of the three classes, as shown in Fig. 14.2a. Suppose now that exactly the same situation exists at a second locus, with the three genotypes $bb$, $Bb$, and $BB$ also contributing 0, 1, and 2 litres to milk yield. Considering these two loci together, the resultant frequency distribution now has five classes and is shown in Fig. 14.2b. As we increase the number of loci contributing to the quantitative trait, we increase the number of classes. Not all alleles have the same effect on milk yield. If there are several loci with a very small effect, the difference between some of the classes is as small as the error of measurement of milk yield, and it is no longer possible always to place heifers in their

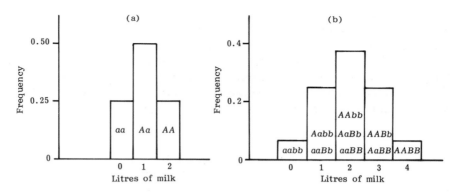

**Fig. 14.2** Frequency distribution of milk yield resulting from variation at (a) a single locus, and (b) two loci.

correct class: the edges of the different classes are blurred. Besides the effect of alleles at a number of loci, there are many non-genetic (environmental) factors that affect milk yield, and these also tend to blur the edges of the discontinuous classes. If the effect of a particular allele is very large relative to the total variation, discrete classes are still evident even in the presence of environmental factors. However, the majority of alleles affecting quantitative traits have an effect that is sufficiently small so as to be not readily detectable.

We can conclude that quantitative traits are determined by the combined action of alleles at many loci, most of which have a relatively small effect on the trait; plus non-genetic (environmental) factors.

## The performance of an individual animal

The performance of an animal for a particular trait is called its **phenotypic value**, P, for that trait. The two factors that together determine phenotypic value are **genotypic value**, G, and environmental deviation, E. The genotypic value of an animal refers to the combined effect of all the animal's genes at all loci that affect the trait, taking account of the way in which the genes are paired together into a genotype. The environmental deviation represents the combined effect of all non-genetic factors that have influenced the phenotypic value. For any trait in any animal, G is determined at conception, while E represents the combined effect of all factors that have influenced the trait in that animal between conception and the time when P is measured.

The above paragraph can be summarized by writing the phenotypic value of an animal for a particular trait as

$$P = G + E \qquad (14.1)$$

where E can be either positive or negative, depending on the combined effect of all non-genetic factors that have influenced the trait in that animal.

From a practical point of view, one of the most important attributes of an animal is its value as a breeder, as judged by the average performance of its offspring for any trait, when compared with the average performance of all offspring. The difference in performance between a particular offspring and the population mean is called the **deviation** of that offspring from the population mean. Using this concept, we can now define two terms that are of vital practical importance in animal improvement programmes throughout the world.

If an animal is mated with a random sample of animals from a population, that animal's **progeny difference** for a certain trait is the average deviation of its offspring from the population mean for that trait. An animal's **breeding value** for a trait is twice the progeny difference for that trait.

The average performance of offspring is doubled in the definition of breeding value because only half of the genes of any offspring come from the animal in question; the other half come from the random sample of animals to which it was mated. In other words, progeny difference reflects the average merit of gametes, each of which is a sample half of an animal's genes, while breeding value reflects the merit of all of the animal's genes. Since breeding value is simply twice the progeny difference, there is no need to discuss each term separately. In the remainder of this book, we shall use only one of them, namely breeding value. But obviously the reader can replace progeny difference for breeding value at any time, simply by remembering that progeny difference = ½ (breeding value).

The genotypic value for any trait is obviously a reflection of the effect of an animal's genotype at all loci that affect the trait. In contrast, breeding value is a reflection of the genes that are passed on to offspring. In fact, an animal's breeding value is directly proportional to the number of favourable genes that it has, while its genotypic value reflects the way in which those genes are combined into its particular genotype. In other words, an animal's breeding value is determined by adding together the effect of each gene considered on its own, whereas its genotypic value is determined by the combined effect of pairs of genes at each locus that contributes to the trait. In order to emphasize this additive nature of breeding value, it is given the symbol $A$. If there is no dominance at any locus that affects the trait, by definition the heterozygote is exactly intermediate between the two homozygotes at each locus. In this case gene action is entirely additive, and genotypic value ($G$) equals breeding value ($A$). Conversely, if there is dominance at any locus, genotypic value is determined by breeding value and by the type and extent of dominance.

This can be expressed symbolically as

$$G = A + D,  \tag{14.2}$$

where $D$ is the deviation due to dominance, which can be positive or negative.

Next, we need to take account of interaction between loci, which is called epistasis (see Chapter 12). If there is no epistasis, the genotypic value is entirely determined by breeding value and dominance deviation. If there is epistasis between any of the loci that affect the trait, this is an independent source of deviation from the additive gene action that determines the breeding value. We can cater for epistatic interactions by adding another term to our expression for genotypic value, to give

$$G = A + D + I, \tag{14.3}$$

where $I$ is the overall deviation due to interactions between loci. The combined deviations due to dominance and epistasis are sometimes called **non-additive** deviations, because they both arise from non-additive gene action. If gene action is entirely additive within and between loci, $D = I = 0$, and $G = A$.

Combining equations (14.1) and (14.3), we can now write

$$\begin{aligned} P &= G + E \\ &= A + D + I + E \end{aligned} \tag{14.4}$$

as an adequate description of the components of an animal's phenotypic value.


## The differences between animals

The most popular parameter used for measuring the extent to which animals differ from each other is the variance, which we have already encountered in this chapter. The extent to which animals differ in their phenotypic values is measured by the **phenotypic variance**, $V_P$. This is the quantity that can be estimated easily (as shown in the caption to Fig. 14.1) for any trait on which a reasonable number of observations (values of $P$) are available. Given an estimate of $V_P$ so calculated, we can make use of our knowledge about the components of $P$ (as shown in equation (14.4)) to learn something about the components of $V_P$. In fact, for every component of $P$ there is a corresponding component of $V_P$. Thus, we can write

$$V_P = V_A + V_D + V_I + V_E \tag{14.5}$$

where $V_A$ is variance in breeding values, $V_D$ is variance in dominance deviations, $V_I$ is variance in deviations due to epistatic interactions, and $V_E$ is variance in non-genetic (environmental) deviations.

Equation (14.5) represents the partitioning of $V_P$ into a set of components. Because breeding values represent the additive effect of genes, $V_A$ is often called the **additive genetic variance**. In contrast, $V_D$ and $V_I$ are components of **non-additive genetic variance**. The sum of the first three components is the **total genetic variance**, or the **genotypic variance**, $V_G$, which measures the extent to which different animals have different genotypes. Since genotypes are determined at conception, $V_G$ measures the extent to which animals differ in factors that are fixed at the moment of conception. The other component, $V_E$, measures the extent to which animals differ in all non-genetic factors that have influenced the trait from the moment of conception to the time when phenotypic value was measured.

There is one important difference to note between equations (14.1)–(14.4), and equation (14.5). In the first four equations, each component can have a positive or negative sign. This means that we cannot think in terms of a phenotypic value being divided into proportions attributable to $A$ or $D$ or $I$ or $E$. On the other hand, the components of $V_P$ are always positive and so they do represent proportions of $V_P$. We can see this most easily by dividing through equation (14.5) by $V_P$ to give

$$1 = \frac{V_A}{V_P} + \frac{V_D}{V_P} + \frac{V_I}{V_P} + \frac{V_E}{V_P}. \qquad (14.6)$$

The relative contribution of any component to $V_P$ is simply the proportion of $V_P$ attributable to that component.

## Heritability

Breeding values are of prime importance in selection programmes, because the main aim when deciding which animals to use as breeders is to choose those that are going to have the best offspring. We are likely, therefore, to be interested in the proportion of phenotypic variance attributable to variance in breeding values. This is represented by the fraction $V_A / V_P$, which is called **heritability** and which is given the symbol $h^2$. Strictly speaking, it is called heritability in the **narrow sense**, in contrast to the ratio $V_G/V_P$, which is heritability in the **broad sense**, and which describes the relative contribution of genotypic variance to $V_P$. Since $V_A$ is never greater than $V_G$, it is evident that narrow-sense heritability is never greater than broad-sense heritability. Because the concept of heritability is most commonly used with animals in relation to selection programmes, and because it is breeding values that are of prime importance in selection programmes, the term heritability is normally used in the narrow sense unless otherwise stated.

### Response to selection

The aim of selection programmes is to select those animals with the highest breeding values. We have also seen that heritability indicates the relative contribution of variation in breeding values to phenotypic variance. We can link these two observations together and explain why heritability is such an important concept, by considering two extreme situations in relation to response to selection.

Consider a population of animals at breeding age. We shall call these animals **candidates** for selection. Suppose that a measurement of phenotypic value for each candidate has been made, so that candidates can be ranked and $V_P$ can be calculated. The top 20 per cent of candidates are to be selected as parents of the next generation, and the remaining 80 per cent are to be culled.

We shall start by supposing that heritability is zero, which means that $V_A$ is zero. If there is no variation in breeding values, all candidates have exactly the same breeding value. Thus, any of the top 20 per cent of candidates must have exactly the same breeding value as any other candidate in the population. Consequently, when the top 20 per cent of candidates are selected and mated, the average performance of their offspring is exactly the same as the average performance of the offspring of any other candidate. The end result is that the offspring distribution has the same mean as the unselected parental distribution, as shown in Fig. 14.3. When $h^2 = 0$, none of the superiority of the selected candidates is passed on to their offspring.

At the other extreme, we can assume that heritability is one, which means that the whole of $V_P$ is due to variation in breeding values. Since the only differences between candidates are now differences in breeding values, the top 20 per cent of candidates have the top 20 per cent of breeding values; ranking the candidates in order of phenotypic value is equivalent to ranking them on breeding value. In this case, the superiority of selected candidates is due solely to superiority in breeding value and hence we expect the offspring mean to equal the mean of selected candidates, as also shown in Fig. 14.3. When $h^2 = 1$, all of the superiority of selected candidates is passed on to their offspring.

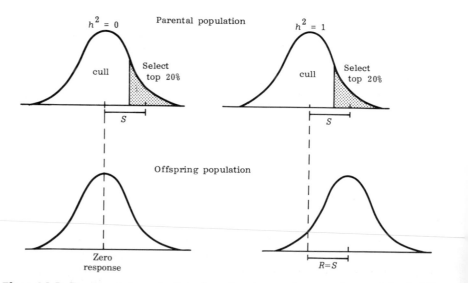

**Fig. 14.3** Response to selection for the two extreme values of heritability, namely zero and one.

In order to summarize the conclusions to be drawn from Fig. 14.3, we need to introduce two new terms. The first is **selection differential**, $S$, which is the average phenotypic superiority of the candidates selected as parents. It is equal to the mean phenotypic value of the candidates selected as parents minus the mean phenotypic value of the whole population from which they were selected. The other term is **response to selection**, $R$. Providing there has been no change in the environment between generations, response to selection equals the mean phenotypic value of the offspring population minus the mean phenotypic value of the whole population from which the parents were selected.

In the previous paragraphs, we have seen that if $h^2 = 0$ then $R = 0$, and if $h^2 = 1$ then $R = S$. In fact, these two extreme situations are just special cases of the general prediction

$$R = h^2 S, \tag{14.7}$$

which is true for all values of heritability. From this statement we can obtain a very practical definition of heritability which indicates its importance in determining response to selection: heritability is the proportion of phenotypic superiority of parents that is seen in their offspring.

It is now obvious that we need to know the heritability of a trait if we are to predict how rapidly it will respond to selection. How do we determine the heritability of a trait?

## Estimation of heritability

The basis of methods for estimating heritability is resemblance between relatives. In fact, the usual way to estimate heritability for any trait is to estimate the extent of resemblance between relatives for that particular trait, and then to divide by the additive relationship between the relatives.

The most common classes of relatives are full-sibs, half-sibs, or parents and their offspring. With the increasing success of embryo splitting, sets of identical twins are also becoming more readily available. Statistical methodologies have been developed for estimating resemblance, and hence heritability, from measurements made on any class of relatives.

In practice, of course, populations usually contain varying numbers of several different classes of relatives, including distant relatives. Not surprisingly, the most efficient way to estimate heritability is to perform a single analysis that simultaneously estimates the resemblance and calculates the relationship between all members of a particular population. The statistical technique that achieves this is called REML, which stands for *restricted maximum likelihood*. Although REML is computationally demanding, a development known as derivative-free REML has greatly expanded its practical utility. New methods of estimating heritability are continually being developed. The MCMC approach (Chapter 7), for example, shows considerable promise.

**Table 14.1** Representative values of heritability

|  | Per cent |
| --- | --- |
| **Horses** | |
| Log of earnings—jumping | 20 |
| Best time | 25 |
| Pulling ability | 25 |
| **Dairy cattle** | |
| Protein yield | 25 |
| Milk yield | 25 |
| Butterfat yield | 25 |
| **Beef cattle** | |
| Survival to weaning | 5 |
| Weaning weight | 25 |
| Postweaning gain | 35 |
| Efficiency of gain | 35 |
| Final weight | 40 |
| Marbling | 40 |
| Percentage retail product | 65 |
| **Sheep** | |
| Probability of conceiving (fertility) | 5 |
| Number of lambs per pregnancy (fecundity) | 15 |
| Clean fleece weight | 40 |
| Fibre diameter | 45 |
| Staple length | 50 |
| Greasy fleece weight | 60 |
| **Pigs** | |
| Litter size | 10 |
| Killing-out percentage | 20 |
| Daily gain | 25 |
| Food conversion ratio | 35 |
| Eye muscle area | 50 |
| Carcase lean proportion | 50 |
| **Fish (Salmon/Trout)** | |
| Survival | 5 |
| Body length | 10 |
| Body weight | 20 |
| **Chickens** | |
| Fertility | 5 |
| Hatchability | 5 |
| Liveability | 5 |
| Hen-housed egg production | 10 |
| Body weight | 50 |
| Egg weight | 55 |

There is another way to estimate heritability—from the results of selection. From equation (14.7), it can be seen that if we know how much selection was applied ($S$) and if we measure the response ($R$), we can estimate $h^2$. An estimate obtained in this way is called **realized heritability**.

Since $V_A$ and $V_P$ can vary from population to population, and from time to time within a population, and since estimates are subject to sampling variation, it is not surprising that heritability estimates for the same trait vary from one estimate to the next. However, for any particular trait there is a certain degree of similarity between estimates. Table 14.1 lists representative heritability values for various traits in domestic animals. In general, those traits most closely associated with viability and reproductive ability have lower heritability than other traits. This has important practical implications, as we shall see in Chapter 19.

## Correlations between traits

As we saw in Chapter 12, it is common for a single gene to affect more than one trait. When the traits are quantitative (i.e. determined by many genes and many non-genetic factors), the extent to which two traits are determined by the same set of genes is called the **genetic correlation**, $r_G$. Another measure of association between two traits is the **phenotypic correlation**, $r_P$, which is the correlation between the performance in each trait; it reflects the extent to which performance in one trait is associated with performance in the other trait.

Correlations between traits are estimated using statistical analyses very similar to those used for estimating heritabilities. Increasingly, multi-trait derivative-free REML analyses are being used to obtain estimates of the heritability of each of a number of traits, together with estimates of correlations between all pair-wise combinations of the traits. Values for genetic and phenotypic correlations amongst some traits commonly measured in domestic animals are given in Table 14.2. These correlations have important practical implications in breeding programmes, as we shall see in Chapter 16.

## Quantitative trait loci (QTL)

We have seen that genetic variation in quantitative traits is due to segregation at many loci. These loci used to be called **polygenes**, but are now called **quantitative trait loci** (QTL). There are good grounds for believing that there is a range in the size of effects of the QTL for any trait, from a few with relatively large effects, down to a large number having very small effects. The developments in molecular biology (described in Chapter 2) now make it feasible to identify QTL.

If a large number of animals are genotyped for a set of mapped markers on

**Table 14.2** Examples of genetic ($r_G$) and phenotypic ($r_P$) correlations

|  | $r_G$ | $r_P$ |
|---|---|---|
| Dairy |  |  |
|    Milk yield: fat yield | +0.80 | +0.90 |
|    Milk yield: protein yield | +0.90 | +0.95 |
|    Fat yield: protein yield | +0.90 | +0.95 |
| Pigs |  |  |
|    Growth rate: food conversion ratio | −0.80 | −0.75 |
|    Growth rate: food intake | +0.40 | +0.45 |
|    Growth rate: backfat thickness | −0.25 | −0.10 |
| Sheep |  |  |
|    Clean fleece weight: yield | +0.50 | +0.40 |
|    Clean fleece weight: staple length | +0.40 | +0.30 |
|    Clean fleece weight: greasy fleece weight | +0.60 | +0.80 |
| Chickens |  |  |
|    Egg number: age at first egg | −0.35 | −0.25 |
|    Egg number: body weight | −0.20 | 0.00 |
|    Egg number: egg weight | −0.30 | −0.05 |

all chromosomes, and are also measured for a quantitative trait, then, by considering the interval between each pair-wise combination of adjacent markers, it is possible to conduct analyses which identify the most likely map locations for QTL, and their effect on the trait. This is called **interval mapping**. Unfortunately, even if the data set is quite extensive, interval mapping is a somewhat inexact science, giving rise to imprecise estimates of QTL location and size of QTL effect. However, as more and more markers are identified in the intervals containing QTL, each region can be broken down into an ever-increasing number of smaller and smaller regions, which, when analysed with more powerful methods for interval mapping, will give rise to increasingly accurate and precise estimates of QTL location and effect.

As soon as markers linked to QTL have been identified, they can be used in selection programmes. This use of markers (called **marker-assisted selection, MAS**) is described in Chapter 16.

In the fullness of time, as the regions become smaller and smaller, as the power of interval mapping increases, and as comparative mapping provides longer and longer lists of actual structural genes that could possibly be the QTL in question, those structural genes that seem likely to have something to do with the trait (candidate genes) can be investigated, to see if they actually do contribute to the genetic variation in the trait. Alternatively, a set of contiguous YAC clones which span an interval containing a QTL can be searched for coding sequences, as described in Chapter 11. Sooner or later, the QTL will be identified at the molecular level. As mentioned in Chapter 11, this approach is called positional cloning.

Once QTL have been identified, their biochemical and physiological roles can be studied. The results of these studies may suggest non-genetic ways in which the action of a QTL can be enhanced. Or it may be possible to create new, more favourable, alleles at these loci. At the very least, knowledge about the role of QTL will greatly increase our understanding of the nature of genetic variation in economically important traits, which in turn will provide the knowledge necessary to maintain that variation, and to utilize it in the most efficient, effective and sustainable manner.

## Further reading

### Estimation of genetic parameters

Becker, W. A. (1984). *Manual of quantitative genetics*, (4th edn). Academic Enterprises, PO Box 666, Pullman, Washington, USA.

Foulley, J. L. (1993). A simple argument showing how to derive restricted maximum likelihood. *Journal of Dairy Science*, **76**, 2320–4.

Searle, S. R. (1991). Henderson, C. R., the statistician—and his contributions to variance components estimation. *Journal of Dairy Science*, **74**, 4035–44.

Thompson, R. and Atkins, K. D. (1994). Sources of information for estimating heritability from selection experiments. *Genetical Research*, **63**, 49–55.

### Genetic parameters

Davis, G. P. (1993). Genetic parameters for tropical beef cattle in northern Australia—a review. *Australian Journal of Agricultural Research*, **44**, 179–98.

Koots, K. R., Gibson, J. P., Smith, C., and Wilton, J. W. (1994). Analyses of published genetic parameter estimates for beef production traits. *Animal Breeding Abstracts*, **62**, 309–38, 825–53.

Miller, R. H. (1991). A compilation of heritability estimates for farm animals. In *Handbook of animal science* (ed. P. A. Putnam), pp. 151–60. Academic Press, San Diego.

Sumner, R. M. W. and Bigham, M. L. (1993). Biology of fibre growth and possible genetic and non-genetic means of influencing fibre growth in sheep and goats—a review. *Livestock Production Science*, **33**, 1–29.

### Quantitative trait loci

Andersson, L., Haley, C. S., Ellegren, H., Knott, S. A., Johansson, M., Andersson, K., *et al.* (1994). Genetic mapping of quantitative trait loci for growth and fatness in pigs. *Science*, **263**, 1771–4.

Tanksley, S. D. (1993). Mapping polygenes. *Annual Review of Genetics*, **27**, 205–33.

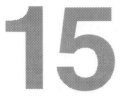

# **Selection between populations**

Artificial selection occurs whenever humans choose to breed from certain animals and not from others. The choice can be made between populations and/or within populations. In the former, it involves a decision as to the most appropriate source of breeding stock or commercial progeny. In the latter, it involves continual efforts to alter a population by breeding from only those animals which by some criteria are the most desirable within that population. In both cases, selection is exploiting genetic variation.

The aim of this chapter is to discuss the main points involved in selection between populations. It is followed, in Chapter 16, by a discussion of selection within populations.

## **Comparison between populations**

Most breeders have their favourite breed or strain, and most have their own reasons for their particular preference. It is obvious that individual preferences differ a great deal among breeders, even among breeders engaged in very similar enterprises in the same area; it is not difficult to think of many situations in which completely different breeds or strains are used by different breeders for the same purpose.

In deciding which breeds or strains to use, breeders are carrying out selection between populations. For many years, this type of selection was in most cases a very subjective process, because breeders had no useful information on the relative merits of different populations. The only way to obtain such information is to conduct large and well-designed comparisons of different populations, a job that no single breeder can ever hope to carry out, because of the relatively long time required, and because of the large numbers of animals needed in order to produce useful results. However, governments, universities, breed societies, and some other large institutions sometimes have the resources necessary for comparisons, and organizations such as these have become actively involved in this type of work, both within countries and between countries.

### *Design of comparisons*

Deciding on the best design for comparisons is quite a complicated business, and should be undertaken only after consultation with people experienced in this area. The factors that must be taken into account include randomization, equality of treatment, the type of comparison, the number of sires, and the number of repeat measurements.

The question of randomization arises at several levels. In many situations it is best if each population is represented by a random sample of animals. If this is not possible, great care should be taken to see that the method and extent of selection of animals is as similar as possible for each population. Also, if the animals are to be evaluated according to the performance of their progeny when mated to a so-called **tester** population, the mates must be chosen at random from the tester population. Furthermore, if the comparison is to be conducted at more than one site, there must be a random allocation of stock from each population to each site.

The requirement that all stock be treated equally is so obvious that it should not need to be mentioned. However, because there are sometimes quite large profits or losses to be made depending on the outcome of a comparison, all possible precautions should be taken to ensure that the comparison is conducted in a manner that minimizes the chances of any population receiving favoured treatment.

Another factor that affects the efficiency of distinguishing between populations is the type of comparison that is conducted. For example, a **direct comparison** (all populations under test being compared at the same location) is more efficient than an **indirect comparison** (each population being measured in a different location, with comparisons being made indirectly through a tester population measured in all locations). Also, a comparison between straightbred offspring (where each offspring in the comparison is the progeny of a male and a female belonging to one of the populations under test) is more efficient than a comparison between crossbred offspring (where the offspring being compared are obtained from mating just one sex, usually male, from the populations under test, to a random sample of members of a tester population).

Another factor that plays a major role in determining the efficiency of a comparison is the number of measurements made on each population under test. There are two important generalizations that can be made in relation to this factor. Firstly, the efficiency of a comparison is determined primarily by the number of sires represented in each population under test, rather than by the number of offspring per sire. Indeed, comparisons involving only, say, two or three sires per population are virtually worthless, even if hundreds of offspring from each sire have been measured, because the average performance of the offspring will be much more a reflection of the average breeding value of those particular sires than of the population from which the sires came. Thus, when planning a comparison, it is vitally important to ensure that each population under test is represented by as many sires as possible. Another point to note is that unless the traits being measured have a very low repeatability (see Chapter 16), it is usually better to measure a different set of offspring each season or year than to take repeated measurements on the same set of offspring.

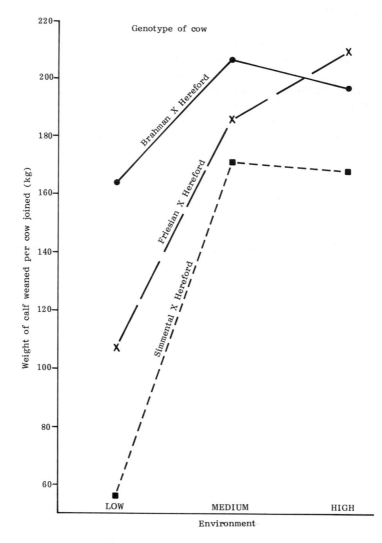

**Fig. 15.1** Examples of genotype–environment interaction (G × E) in beef production.

## Genotype–environment interaction

Comparisons generally involve testing the performance of groups of animals under one or a limited number of environments. The Food and Agricultural Organisation (FAO), for example, conducted a large-scale comparison of various Friesian strains from around the world, by using appropriate semen on a large number of cows on collective farms in Poland. Do the results obtained in Poland apply to other countries as well? In other words, would the bulls within countries of origin, and the countries of origin themselves, rank in the same order if the trial had been conducted in, say, Canada or New Zealand?

If the results of comparisons vary depending on the environments in which they are conducted, we say there is **genotype–environment interaction**, G × E. In the examples of G × E illustrated in Fig. 15.1, three different cow genotypes were evaluated under low, medium, and high levels of nutrition on a research station at Grafton, NSW, Australia. All cows were mated to Hereford bulls. The results of this comparison illustrate the two types of G × E that occur. The first involves just a change in relative performance (low versus medium environments), while the second involves a change in ranking (medium versus high environments).

The problem with G × E is that in many cases it is difficult to predict in advance whether or not such an interaction is likely to be important. All that can be done in practice is to conduct the comparison in all relevant environments, which is usually not possible, or to interpret the results from a different environment cautiously, in the light of what is known in general about G × E in relation to the traits concerned.

## Further reading

### Comparisons

Amer, P. R., Kemp, R. A., and Smith, C. (1992). Genetic differences among the predominant beef cattle breeds in Canada—an analysis of published results. *Canadian Journal of Animal Science*, **72**, 759–71.

Amer, P. R., Kemp, R. A., Fox, G. C., and Smith, C. (1994). An economic comparison of beef cattle genotypes for feedlot traits at their optimal slaughter end point. *Canadian Journal of Animal Science*, **74**, 7–14.

Heil, G. and Hartmann, W. (1992). Combined summary of European random sample egg production tests completed in 1990. *World's Poultry Science Journal*, **48**, 269–70.

Hetzel, D. J. S. (1988). Comparative productivity of the Brahman and some indigenous Sanga and *Bos indicus* breeds of East and Southern Africa. *Animal Breeding Abstracts*, **56**, 143–55.

Sutherland, R. A., Webb, A. J., and King, J. W. B. (1985). A survey of world pig breeds and comparisons. *Animal Breeding Abstracts*, **53**, 1–22.

Zarnecki, A., Jamrozik, J., and Norman, H. D. (1991). Comparison of 10 Friesian strains in Poland for yield traits from 1st 3 parities. *Journal of Dairy Science*, **74**, 2303–8.

### Genotype–environment interaction

Cameron, N. D. (1993). Methodologies for estimation of genotype with environment interaction. *Livestock Production Science*, **35**, 237–49.

Hartmann, W. (1990). Implications of genotype environment interactions in animal breeding—genotype location interactions in poultry. *World's Poultry Science Journal*, **46**, 197–210.

Kinghorn, B. P. and Swan, A. A. (1991). A multitrait approach for data involving genotype × environment interaction. *Journal of Animal Breeding and Genetics*, **108**, 111–5.

Leenstra, F. and Cahaner, A. (1991). Genotype by environment interactions using fast-growing, lean or fat broiler chickens, originating from the Netherlands and Israel, raised at normal or low temperature. *Poultry Science*, **70**, 2028–39.

Stanton, T. L., Blake, R. W., Quaas, R. L., Van Vleck, L. D., and Carabano, M. J. (1991). Genotype by environment interaction for Holstein milk yield in Colombia, Mexico, and Puerto Rico. *Journal of Dairy Science*, **74**, 1700–14.

Sylven, S., Rye, M., and Simianer, H. (1991). Interaction of genotype with production system for slaughter weight in rainbow trout (*Oncorhynchus mykiss*). *Livestock Production Science*, **28**, 253–63.

Syrstad, O. (1990). Dairy cattle crossbreeding in the tropics—the importance of genotype × environment interaction. *Livestock Production Science*, **24**, 109–18.

Webb, A. J. and Curran, M. K. (1986). Selection regime by production system interaction in pig improvement: a review of possible causes and solutions. *Livestock Production Science*, **14**, 41–54.

# Selection within populations

16

Ever since animals were first domesticated, humans have been attempting to alter animal populations by means of artificial selection. The vast array of different breeds and strains of domestic animals in existence today is testimony to the effectiveness of such selection. Despite the many changes that have already occurred as a result of artificial selection, there are still many improvements needed, especially in terms of the economic efficiency of production of milk, eggs, wool, meat, and other animal products. And there is also a continual demand for faster horses, better showjumpers and more intelligent guidedogs. In most situations, the traits to be improved are quantitative traits.

The aim of this chapter is to describe how artificial selection is conducted in animal populations.

## Estimated breeding values and accuracy of selection

When selection is carried out for any trait, the usual aim is to select as parents those animals that have the highest breeding values for that trait, out of all the candidates available for selection, so as to achieve the highest possible average performance for that trait in the offspring of selected parents. If we knew exactly the actual breeding value (called the **true breeding value**) of each candidate, we could achieve this aim with maximum efficiency by ranking candidates according to their true breeding value, and selecting those at the top of the list.

In practice, however, we do not know an animal's true breeding value for any trait. Instead, all we have is one or more clues to the animal's true breeding value for various traits. These clues, which are called **selection criteria**, consist of one or more measurements of performance (phenotypic values) taken on the animal itself and/or one or more of its relatives. By means that are described below, we can use these clues to estimate the true breeding value of each animal for any trait, and the animals can then be ranked according to **estimated breeding value** (EBV) for the trait of interest. By ranking animals according to their EBV for a particular trait, we tend to rank them according to their true breeding value for that trait. The more accurate our estimate, the more accurate is the ranking.

It is convenient to think of accuracy on a scale from 0 per cent, where the clue provides no information on breeding value, to 100 per cent, where the clue is the true breeding value itself. If accuracy is 0 per cent, animals are, in effect, ranked at random; selecting those animals at the top of the list produces no response to selection, on average. At the other extreme, if accuracy is 100 per cent, animals are ranked according to their true breeding value, and response to selection is maximized.

Strictly speaking, **accuracy of selection** for any trait is the correlation between the available clues and the true breeding value for that trait. The symbol for accuracy is $r_{AC}$, where $r$ is the usual symbol for correlation, $A$ represents true breeding value, and $C$ stands for clues or criteria.

## Clues to a candidate's breeding value for a trait

At regular intervals during a selection programme, groups of candidates become available for selection and therefore have to be ranked in terms of estimated breeding value, EBV.

There are many potential clues to a candidate's true breeding value.

The simplest and most commonly available clue is a single measurement of its own performance. Measurement of the performance of candidates is called **performance testing**, and selection on the results of performance testing is called **individual selection** or **mass selection**. Other potential clues to a candidate's true breeding value include single measurements on a relative of a candidate (e.g. parent, sib, or offspring), or on groups of relatives, such as full-sibs (called a **dam family**) or half-sibs (called a **sire family**). Selection on ancestor performance is called **pedigree selection**, and on sib performance is called **sib selection**. Evaluating candidates on the performance of their offspring is called **progeny testing**. For some traits, it is possible to measure performance more than once on the same animal. Fleece weight, for example, can be measured each year on each sheep, and maternal ability of beef cows, as judged by the weaning weight of their calves, can be measured on the same cow each time she weans a calf. Such traits are said to be repeatable, and the correlation between repeated measurements on the same animal is called **repeatability**, which ranges from 0 per cent to 100 per cent.

For each of these sources of clues, it is possible to derive an expression for accuracy of selection, as shown in Appendix 16.2 of *Veterinary Genetics*. In all cases, accuracy is a function of heritability; the higher the heritability of a trait, the greater the accuracy of selection.

## Combining clues from more than one source

In practical selection programmes, clues to a candidate's true breeding value are often available from more than one source. In selecting hens for egg production, for example, data are usually available on the hen's own performance, on the average performance of the full-sib family of which she is a member (her dam-family average) and on the average performance of the half-sib family of which she is a member (her sire-family average). Corresponding male candidates can be ranked according to the same sire-family and dam-family averages, but obviously without any measurement of their own performance being included. With pigs, both male and female candidates are often ranked in terms of their own performance and that of their sibs.

The accuracy of selection increases as more clues are used. How can the clues be combined together into one overall estimate of a candidate's breeding value, and how can the resultant accuracy be determined?

Imagine that we have $k$ different clues,

$$C_1, C_2, \ldots, C_k,$$

where a clue may be:

(1) a single measurement or the average of repeated measurements on a candidate or on any relative, or
(2) the average performance of a group of the candidate's relatives, where the record available on each relative is either a single measurement or the average of repeated measurements.

The single overall estimate of a candidate's true breeding value that is obtained from these different clues is called a **selection index**. It is the sum of all the clues, with each clue being weighted in such a way as to maximize the accuracy of the index as an estimate of the candidate's true breeding value. The index is written as

$$I = \text{EBV} = b_1 C_1 + \ldots + b_k C_k, \tag{16.6}$$

where $I$ is the estimated breeding value, EBV, and where the $b$ values are weighting factors calculated so as to maximize the correlation between the index, $I$, and the candidate's true breeding value, $A$, i.e. to maximize accuracy of selection.

The general principles for calculating appropriate weighting factors so as to maximize accuracy are very straightforward—they involve a simple application of the standard method of maximizing a function, as taught in high-school calculus courses:

(1) write down an expression for the parameter to be maximized (in this case, accuracy);
(2) differentiate the expression with respect to each $b$ value;
(3) set the differentials equal to zero, thereby creating a set of so-called **normal equations**; and
(4) solve these equations simultaneously for the $b$ values.

The actual information required in order to calculate the $b$ values is the heritability of the trait, the additive relationships (Chapter 13) among all relatives who are providing clues, and the additive relationship between the candidate and these relatives. If groups of relatives (e.g. half-sibs) contribute a single clue (e.g. a sire-family average), the number of relatives in each group is also required. If a clue includes multiple measurements, the repeatability of the trait is required, as well as the number of repeat measurements. For those readers who would like more information on this procedure, full details are provided in Appendix 16.2.4 of *Veterinary Genetics*.

To take just one example from *Veterinary Genetics*, suppose there are two clues: the candidate's own performance, and the performance of one of its parents. If the heritability of the trait is 0.25, the $b$ values turn out to be $b_1 = 0.238$ and $b_2 = 0.095$. Notice that the candidate's own performance is more important than its parent's performance (the reason for this was explained in Chapter 13).

## Best linear unbiased prediction (BLUP)

In many practical situations, each candidate has a different set of clues, which means that a different set of $b$ values has to be calculated for each candidate before EBVs can be calculated.

Fortunately, it is now possible to calculate as many different sets of $b$ values as are required, and then to calculate EBVs, all in a single process, using the BLUP method of estimation. BLUP stands for *best linear unbiased prediction*, which describes the statistical properties of the estimates obtained using the method. In practical terms, EBVs obtained using the BLUP method have all the desirable properties of EBVs obtained from a conventional selection index. Indeed, the conventional selection index is a special case of BLUP. However, the real merit of the BLUP method is that it is more powerful than the conventional selection index approach. For example, BLUP can account for complications such as non-random mating, sires coming from more than one distinct group or population, environmental trends over time, herd differences in the average breeding value of dams, and bias due to selection and culling. It can also take account of identifiable non-genetic (environmental) factors such as month of calving or parity. Finally, and very importantly, since BLUP automatically calculates the correct $b$ values for the particular set of relatives from which clues are available for each candidate, it enables us to take correct account of the available clues from all the known relatives of a candidate. Another important advantage of BLUP is that since it can provide EBVs for all animals in a population (using the so-called **animal model**), a good indication of response to selection (**genetic trend**) can be obtained simply by calculating the average EBV of each age group within the population, and then plotting average EBV against year of birth.

Because of these substantial advantages, BLUP has become a very popular method for calculating EBVs in most livestock species. Further discussion of the BLUP method, and a simple practical example, are given in Appendix 16.3 of *Veterinary genetics*.

## Correlated traits

Selection for one trait almost always produces changes in other traits. A change in an unselected trait resulting from selection of another trait is called a **correlated response**. The magnitude of the correlated response depends, among other things, on the correlations between the two traits, which were discussed in Chapter 14. These correlations have important practical implications for breeding programmes.

Firstly, the direction and magnitude of correlated response in an unselected trait depends on the sign and the magnitude, respectively, of the genetic correlation between the unselected trait and the selected trait. If, for example, the genetic correlation between two traits is negative, an increase in the trait being selected produces a decrease in the unselected trait.

Secondly, the existence of genetic correlations raises the possibility of improving a trait that is difficult or expensive or even impossible to measure in practical conditions, by selecting on a correlated trait that is easy and cheap to measure. The practice of improving one trait by selecting on another is called **indirect selection**. It is used, for example, in broiler chickens, where growth rate has a high positive genetic correlation with food conversion efficiency. This means that food conversion efficiency can be improved by selecting solely on growth rate, without going to the considerable extra expense of actually measuring food consumption.

Thirdly, the existence of genetic correlations provides an important new source of clues to a candidate's breeding value for any trait; the performance of a candidate and/or of any relative in any trait that is correlated with the trait to be improved, provides additional clues to the candidate's breeding value for the trait to be improved. Thus, even if the trait to be improved can be measured easily and cheaply on candidates themselves, it may be useful to measure the performance of the candidate and/or of relatives for correlated traits, and to make use of all these measurements when estimating the breeding value of candidates.

This can be achieved by using a selection index or BLUP, in exactly the same manner as described earlier, except that now the list of potential clues includes correlated traits as well as, or instead of, the trait to be improved. For example, a sheep selection programme might involve the measurement of fleece weight and fibre diameter on all candidates. Even if no pedigree records are available, it would still be possible to use several different selection indexes, each using the same two clues, namely fleece weight and fibre diameter. For example, a selection index could be used for calculating each candidate's EBV for fleece weight, and another index could be used for calculating each candidate's EBV for fibre diameter. Other indexes could be derived for calculating each candidate's EBV for any trait that is correlated with the two measured traits, but which is not actually measured in the flock, e.g. body weight.

In each case, the clues for each index are exactly the same, namely the candidate's own performance in the two traits; the only difference between the indexes are the *b* values. For the fleece-weight index, the *b* values are calculated so as to maximize the correlation between the index and true breeding value for fleece weight; for the fibre-diameter index, the *b* values maximize the correlation between the index and true breeding value for fibre diameter; and for the body weight index, the *b* values maximize the correlation between the index and true breeding value for body weight.

For all indexes, the *b* values are calculated using exactly the same approach as described for single-trait selection. However, because the clues now consist of more than one trait, estimates of genetic and phenotypic correlations among the traits are required in addition to the heritabilities needed to calculate *b* values when the clues consist of measurements on only one trait.

If pedigree records are kept, the performance of relatives (for each trait) can be used as additional clues in each index. Alternatively, EBVs for each trait can be calculated using so-called multi-trait BLUP, which combines all available clues from all traits measured on the candidate and on all known relatives, automatically providing the optimum weight (*b* value) for each clue.

Irrespective of which method is used, the result is a list of EBVs for each trait for each candidate, so that candidates can be ranked for each trait. While this is very useful information, it is not the end of the matter, because when replacements are being selected, we need to rank candidates according to overall merit, taking account of their EBV for each trait.

## Selection for more than one trait

There are five steps involved in selecting for more than one trait.

### Step 1: decide on the breeding objectives

This involves drawing up a list of the traits that you would like to improve, irrespective of whether they are cheap or expensive or even impossible to measure on the candidate (called **breeding objectives**).

For example, in a pig selection programme, you may wish to improve growth rate, G, food conversion ratio, F, and percentage lean in the carcase, L. The first trait is easy to measure on candidates; the second is expensive to measure, and hence may be recorded on only a limited number of candidates; while the third trait is impossible to measure on candidates, since it can be recorded only from carcases.

## Step 2: decide on the selection criteria

As we have already seen, selection criteria are the traits that are actually measured on candidates and/or their relatives. These may be the same as the breeding objectives, or they may be different; there are no limitations on which traits can be used as selection criteria, providing that they are measurable, and providing that estimates of the relevant genetic and phenotypic parameters are available.

For the pig example just mentioned, suppose that the only two traits that are actually measured are growth rate, G, and backfat thickness, B. The first of these traits is one of the objectives, and is correlated with the other objectives; the second measured trait is not an objective, but is correlated with the objectives (see Table 14.2).

## Step 3: calculate the EBV for each breeding objective for each candidate

This involves using one of the approaches described earlier.

Each candidate's EBV for growth rate could be calculated just from the candidate's own performance for that trait. But the EBV would be estimated more accurately if a selection index were used to combine information from both clues (growth rate and backfat thickness) from each candidate, and preferably from relatives as well. For the other two objectives (the ones that are not actually measured), a selection index has to be used to combine clues from the measured traits on the candidates and/or on relatives. Alternatively, maximum accuracy of selection can be achieved if multi-trait BLUP is used to calculate the EBVs for each objective for each candidate.

## Step 4: determine the net economic value of improvement in each breeding objective

For each objective, the **net economic value**, $v$, is the additional profit expected from a unit improvement in that objective alone. This step is often not as simple as it might at first appear. However, software packages for calculating net economic values are gradually becoming available to individual breeders, who, with the help of suitably-trained advisers, can calculate a set of values appropriate to their particular circumstances.

In the past, and commonly still today, breeders have guessed the net economic value for each of their objectives. In many cases, this has been done subconsciously. The important thing to realize is that whenever there is more than one objective in a breeding programme, net economic values must be determined in one way or another before selection can be conducted. Furthermore, this statement is as true for the prehistoric humans who domesticated animals, as it is for present-day breeders.

*Step 5: carry out selection*

Once the net economic value has been either guessed or calculated for each breeding objective, there are two main ways in which selection is conducted.

## (1) Independent culling levels

This method involves selecting animals which exceed a particular level (the culling level) for each objective. In other words, an animal is not selected, i.e. is culled, if its EBV is worse than the culling level for any one objective, irrespective of how much its EBV may be better than the culling level for each of the other objectives. The actual culling levels are chosen so as to give, overall, a certain proportion of candidates selected. The method of calculating the correct culling levels is rather complicated, but in many cases the necessary calculations can now be done on a computer. Once calculated, the culling levels can be used in any selection programme for which they are relevant, without further use of a computer.

## (2) Index selection

This method involves ranking and selecting candidates according to their EBV for overall merit, which is yet another form of selection index. If, as in our pig example, there were two breeding objectives, the index would be:

$$I = \text{EBV for overall merit}$$
$$= v_1\text{EBV}_1 + v_2\text{EBV}_2,$$

where $v_1$ is the net economic value and $\text{EBV}_1$ is the estimated breeding value for the first breeding objective; and similarly for the second objective.

In most circumstances, index selection is the best option.

## The importance of inbreeding and genetic drift

In Chapter 13 we saw that the mating of relatives (inbreeding) results in a decrease in performance (inbreeding depression), especially for traits associated with viability and/or reproductive ability; as the level of inbreeding increases, so too does the incidence of embryonic mortality (spontaneous abortion), stillbirths, and single-gene recessive disorders. In addition, since inbreeding increases homozygosity, it results in a decrease in genetic variance, which, in turn, reduces the potential for improving a population by selection.

In Chapter 5, we saw that the smaller the population, the more likely it is that gene frequencies change due to chance (genetic drift) rather than due to selection.

In addition to their relevance described in the earlier chapters, inbreeding and genetic drift are very relevant to improvement programmes, where there is a great temptation to concentrate on just a few animals with very high

EBVs. The fewer the parents in a selection programme, the greater is the rate of inbreeding, and the greater is the chance that genetic drift results in the loss of favourable alleles (which reduces the improvement that can be achieved). In addition, the greater is the chance that genetic drift results in the whole improvement programme making no progress, or even going backwards!

The importance of inbreeding and genetic drift can be quantified in terms of a parameter called **effective population size**, $N_e$, which (as shown in Appendix 16.1 of *Veterinary genetics*) can be calculated as $N_e = (4sdL)/(s + d)$, where $s$ is the number of sires entering the population per year, $d$ is the number of dams entering the population each year, and $L$ is the average age of the male and the female parents when their offspring are born (i.e. the average of male and female **generation intervals**), in years. The increase in inbreeding per year, $\Delta F$, is approximately $\Delta F = 1/(2N_eL)$.

How, then, do we try to ensure that $\Delta F$ is at an acceptably low level? In practice, we generally follow two rather arbitrary rules, which are:

(1) avoid mating very close relatives such as full-sibs, or parents and offspring, and
(2) ensure that effective population size is sufficient for $\Delta F$ to be less than an arbitrarily chosen value, such as 1 per cent per year.

From the above equation, this amounts to ensuring that $N_e$ is larger than $50/L$. In very general terms, this is also a satisfactory criterion for avoiding the worst excesses of genetic drift.

## Sire-reference schemes

In the dairy industry, the widespread use of artificial insemination (AI) means that most dairy herds are linked together by the use of common bulls. Consequently, when EBVs are calculated for dairy cows and dairy bulls, the data from all herds can be treated as if they came from just one herd, and the resultant EBVs are comparable across all herds. At present, such calculations are usually done within regions or within countries. However, given the substantial international trade in dairy semen, there are many links between dairy herds throughout the world. Consequently, an international centre called Interbull has been established (in Sweden) with the aim of developing methods for combining data from different countries, to enable calculation of dairy EBVs that will be comparable throughout the world.

In stark contrast to the dairy situation, other livestock industries make relatively little use of AI, with the result that there are very few links between herds or flocks. This means that EBV calculations have to be done separately for each herd or flock, and consequently, EBVs from one herd or flock are not comparable with EBVs from another herd or flock. This is a major limitation for animal improvement: it greatly restricts the range of candidates for selection, and it substantially increases the likelihood of breeders en-countering problems with inbreeding and genetic drift.

One solution to this problem is for individual breeders to co-operate with each other, by agreeing that each herd or flock will share the use of one or more sires, either by AI or by transporting males. When a sire is used in several herds or flocks, he provides a link between them, which enables the EBVs of all animals in all of the co-operating herds or flocks to be calculated together, and hence to be comparable with each other. Such sires are called **reference sires**. Sire-reference schemes are operating in the beef-cattle, sheep and pig industries. Sometimes they are combined with a **central test**, in which candidate reference sires (or their sibs or progeny) are evaluated at a single site.

## Marker-assisted selection (MAS)

We saw in Chapter 14 that one of the benefits of genetic maps is the identifica-tion of DNA markers linked to quantitative trait loci (QTL). If candidates are genotyped for each linked marker, these genotypes can be used as additional clues to the true breeding value of each candidate for a trait. As also men-tioned in Chapter 14, this use of markers in improvement programmes is called marker-assisted selection (MAS).

As the number of markers continually increases, and as the effectiveness of the statistical tools for interval mapping also increases, so too will the esti-mates of QTL locations and effects become more accurate. In the long term, as described in Chapter 14, QTL will be identified right down to the coding sequence. Once this stage has been reached, there will no longer be any need for the linked markers or for MAS. However, given that this stage will not be reached for many decades yet, MAS is likely to play a role in improvement programmes for a very long time.

## Further reading

*Books*

Chapman, A. B. (ed.) (1985). *General and quantitative genetics*, World Animal Science Series, Vol. 4A. Elsevier, Amsterdam.

Falconer, D. S. (1989). *Introduction to quantitative genetics*, (3rd edn). Longman, London.

Gianola, D. and Hammond, K. (ed.) (1990). *Advances in statistical methods for genetic improvement of livestock*. Springer-Verlag, Berlin.

Hammond, K., Graser, H.-U., and McDonald, C. A. (ed.) (1992). *Animal breeding: the modern approach*. Postgraduate Foundation in Veterinary Science, University of Sydney.

Van Vleck, L. D., Pollak, E. J., and Oltenacu, E. A. B. (1987). *Genetics for the animal sciences*. Freeman, New York.

Van Vleck, L. D. (1993). *Selection index and introduction to mixed model methods*. CRC Press, Boca Raton.
Weller, J. L. (1994). *Economic aspects of animal breeding*. Chapman and Hall, London.
Willis, M. B. (1991). *Dalton's introduction to practical animal breeding*, (3rd edn). Blackwell Scientific, Oxford.

## Theory

Dekkers, J. C. M. (1992). Asymptotic response to selection on best linear unbiased predictors of breeding values. *Animal Production*, **54**, 351–60.
Goddard, M. E. (1992). Optimal effective population size for the global population of black and white dairy cattle. *Journal of Dairy Science*, **75**, 2902–11.
Groeneveld, E., Kovac, M., Wang, T. L., and Fernando, R. L. (1992). Computing algorithms in a general purpose BLUP package for multivariate prediction and estimation. *Archiv für Tierzucht*, **35**, 399–412.
Muir, W. M. and Xu, S. Z. (1991). An approximate method for optimum independent culling level selection for *n* stages of selection with explicit solutions. *Theoretical and Applied Genetics*, **82**, 457–65.
Quinton, M., Smith, C., and Goddard, M. E. (1992). Comparison of selection methods at the same level of inbreeding. *Journal of Animal Science*, **70**, 1060–7.
Wray, N. R. and Hill, W. G. (1989). Asymptotic rates of response from index selection. *Animal Production*, **49**, 217–27.
Woolliams, J. A., Wray, N. R., and Thompson, R. (1993). Prediction of long-term contributions and inbreeding in populations undergoing mass selection. *Genetical Research*, **62**, 231–42.
Wray, N. R., Woolliams, J. A., and Thompson, R. (1994). Prediction of rates of inbreeding in populations undergoing index selection. *Theoretical and Applied Genetics*, **87**, 878–92.

## Selection experiments

Falconer, D. S. (1992). Early selection experiments. *Annual Review of Genetics*, **26**, 1–14.
Hill, W. G. and Caballero, A. (1992). Artificial selection experiments. *Annual Review of Ecology and Systematics*, **23**, 287–310.

## Selection in practice

American Society of Animal Science (1991). *Journal of Animal Science*, **69**, (9). [A series of reviews of US improvement programmes in dairy, beef, sheep, pigs, and quarter horses.]
Brandt, H. (1993). BLUP developments in pig breeding. *Archiv für Tierzucht*, **36**, 189–95.
Burnside, E. B., Jansen, G. B., Civati, G., and Dadati, E. (1992). Observed and theoretical genetic trends in a large dairy population under intensive selection. *Journal of Dairy Science*, **75**, 2242–53.
Ewart, J. (1993). Evolution of genetic selection techniques and their application in the next decade. *British Poultry Science*, **34**, 3–10.

Gall, G. A. E., Bakar, Y., and Famula, T. (1993). Estimating genetic change from selection. *Aquaculture*, **111**, 75–88.

Haley, C. S., Avalos, E., and Smith, C. (1988). Selection for litter size in the pig. *Animal Breeding Abstracts*, **56**, 317–32.

Klemetsdal, G. (1992). Estimation of genetic trend in racehorse breeding. *Acta Agriculturae Scandinavica Section A—Animal Science*, **42**, 226–31.

McMillan, I., Fairfull, R. W., Gowe, R. S., and Gavora, J. S. (1990). Evidence for genetic improvement of layer stocks of chickens during 1950–80. *World's Poultry Science Journal*, **46**, 235–45.

McManus, C. and Thompson, R. (1993). Breeding objectives for red deer. *Animal Production*, **57**, 161–7.

Meinert, T. R., Pearson, R. E., and Hoyt, R. S. (1992). Estimates of genetic trend in an artificial insemination progeny test program and their association with herd characteristics. *Journal of Dairy Science*, **75**, 2254–64.

Newman, S., Morris, C. A., Baker, R. L., and Nicoll, G. B. (1992). Genetic improvement of beef cattle in New-Zealand—breeding objectives. *Livestock Production Science*, **32**, 111–30.

Philipsson, J. and Banos, G. (1993). Interbull—the international bull evaluation service—report on activities. *Livestock Production Science*, **37**, 235–7.

## Economic weights

Amer, P. R., Fox, G. C., and Smith, C. (1994). Economic weights from profit equations—appraising their accuracy in the long run. *Animal Production*, **58**, 11–18.

Amer, P. R. and Fox, G. C. (1992). Estimation of economic weights in genetic improvement using neoclassical production theory—an alternative to rescaling. *Animal Production*, **54**, 341–50.

## Marker-assisted selection

Smith C. & Smith D. B. (1993). The need for close linkages in marker-assisted selection for economic merit in livestock. *Animal Breeding Abstracts*, **61**, 197–204.

Visscher, P. M. and Haley, C. S. (1995). Utilizing genetic markers in pig breeding programmes. *Animal Breeding Abstracts*, **63**, 1–8.

# Breed structure

## 17

Not all animals in a breed contribute to genetic improvement within that breed; in most cases, breeds are structured so that only a minority of animals are given that opportunity.

The aim of this chapter is to describe the structure of breeds and to discuss the ways in which the structure can be modified so as to increase the overall genetic merit of the breed.

## The traditional pyramid

The structure of most breeds consists of a series of subgroups called tiers. Typically there are three tiers, namely **nucleus**, **multiplier**, and **commercial**. Occasionally there are only two (nucleus and commercial), and sometimes there are more than three (more than one level of multiplier). Irrespective of the number of tiers, the basic structure is much the same, being commonly represented in the shape of a pyramid, as shown in Fig. 17.1.

In a traditional pyramid, the nucleus tier consists of herds or flocks that breed their own male and female replacements. In some cases, they may occasionally import a sire or dam from another nucleus herd or flock. Multipliers

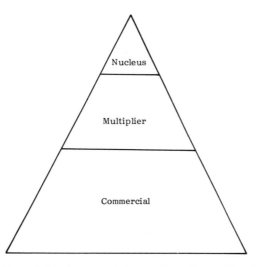

**Fig. 17.1** A typical breed structure consisting of three tiers in the shape of a pyramid.

take males and sometimes females from usually just one nucleus herd or flock, with the aim of producing sufficient breeding stock (males, and sometimes females) to satisfy the demands from herds or flocks in the commercial tier.

## Closed-nucleus breeding schemes

In the traditional pyramid, there is a one-way flow of genes within the pyramid, downwards from top to bottom. This means that the only source of cumulative genetic progress in commercial populations is improvement that occurs at the top of the pyramid, in the nucleus population. If the nucleus tier makes no genetic improvement, neither does the rest of the breed. However, even if the nucleus tier does make progress, this improvement is not seen immediately at lower levels of the pyramid; it takes time for genetic progress in one tier to be transmitted to the next tier. The resultant difference in average performance between any two adjacent tiers is called the **improvement lag**, which is usually expressed in terms of the number of years of genetic improvement that are represented by the difference in performance between adjacent tiers.

There are two factors that affect the size of the improvement lag. They are the age structure in the lower tiers, and the source and merit of sires and dams used in the lower tiers.

For example, the lag can be reduced by keeping sires and dams in the lower tiers for shorter periods of time before replacing them with younger stock. It can also be reduced by transferring females as well as males downwards between tiers. Even greater reductions result if some nucleus parents can be transferred directly to the commercial tier.

The effect of altering some of these factors is illustrated for the case of pigs in Fig. 17.2. The lag in a traditional pig structure, in which only sires are passed down, and only between adjacent tiers, is around 4 years (Fig. 17.2a). In contrast, if all sires used in both the multiplier and commercial tiers come from the nucleus tier and if, in addition, dams are transferred downwards between adjacent tiers, the lag can be reduced to around 1½ years, which is a substantial reduction (Fig. 17.2b).

In the breeding schemes discussed above, there is a downward-only flow of genes from the nucleus to the lower tiers. Because no genes flow into the nucleus tier, these schemes are called closed-nucleus breeding schemes. This type of structure is the most commonly encountered in practice; most of the traditional breeds of livestock and most of the modern pig and poultry breeding programmes have a closed-nucleus structure.

## Open-nucleus breeding schemes

Even if there is substantial improvement lag between tiers, there is usually sufficient variation within the lower tiers for some animals that are born in

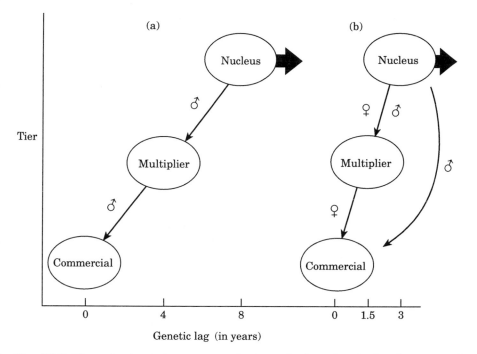

**Fig. 17.2** The reduction in improvement lag brought about by altering the source of sires and dams used in the lower tiers of a pig pyramid. Thick arrows indicate the direction of genetic improvement in the nucleus tier, and thin arrows show the direction of gene flow between tiers. In this example, the lag is that expected when unselected animals are passed down. If selected animals are passed down, the lag is smaller.

those tiers to have a higher performance than some animals in a higher tier. To the extent that higher performance is evidence of a superior breeding value, it would make good sense to transfer superior animals from a lower tier into a higher tier, and even (if they are sufficiently superior) into the nucleus tier. This amounts to opening the nucleus. Since traditionally the nucleus tier has consisted of studs of 'pedigree' animals registered with a breed society, the above proposal raises the possibility of introducing commercial (non-'pedigree') animals into 'pedigree' herds or flocks, which of course is not exactly in keeping with traditional stud-breeding philosophy. And yet there are definite advantages to be gained by opening the nucleus: the annual response to selection is increased, and the rate of inbreeding in the nucleus is substantially reduced.

For example, in a well-designed sheep or beef-cattle open-nucleus scheme, response to selection could be increased by 10 per cent to 15 per cent, and the rate of inbreeding could be halved, in comparison with a closed-nucleus scheme of the same overall size.

One popular form of an open-nucleus breeding scheme involves a group of breeders agreeing to co-operate in the formation and subsequent running of an open nucleus, in return for a regular supply of breeding stock (mostly males) from the nucleus, for use in their own herd or flock. There are several such schemes in practice now in sheep and to a lesser extent in cattle. They are often called group breeding schemes or co-operative breeding schemes.

One of the biggest practical difficulties with group breeding schemes is that very close and continuing co-operation is required between the co-operating breeders. The successful establishment of a group breeding scheme is therefore as much a matter of sociology as of genetics. However, a sufficient number of schemes have been running successfully for a sufficient time now to indicate that they can, given the right circumstances, be very beneficial to the co-operating breeders and to the industry as a whole.

If the advantages of open-nucleus schemes are as great as described, why do pig and poultry breeders still persist with closed-nucleus schemes? The main reason is that in pig and poultry breeding, nucleus herds and flocks are usually maintained under strict quarantine, with the aim of excluding as many diseases as possible. Opening these nucleus populations to regular importations from other herds or flocks involves an unacceptably high risk of introducing disease. This is an important point. It illustrates clearly that practical breeding programmes cannot be designed solely on the basis of genetic requirements. Quite often there are non-genetic constraints, such as requirements in relation to disease, that have a major influence on the final design of a breeding programme.

## Further reading

Anderson, S. and Curran, M. K. (1990). Selection and response within the nucleus of a sheep group-breeding scheme. *Animal Production*, **51**, 593–9.

Gearheart, W. W., Keller, D. S., and Smith, C. (1990). The use of elite nucleus units in beef cattle breeding. *Journal of Animal Science*, **68**, 1229–36.

Roden, J. A. (1994). Review of the theory of open nucleus breeding systems. *Animal Breeding Abstracts*, **62**, 151–7.

Shepherd, R. K. and Kinghorn, B. P. (1992). Optimising multitier open nucleus breeding schemes. *Theoretical and Applied Genetics*, **85**, 372–8.

Shepherd, R. K. and Kinghorn, B. P. (1993). A deterministic model of BLUP selection in 2 tier open nucleus breeding schemes. *Livestock Production Science*, **33**, 341–54.

Smith, C. (1988). Genetic improvement of livestock, using nucleus breeding units. *World Animal Review*, (65), 2–10.

# Crossing 18

Crossing is the mating of individuals from different populations (strains, breeds, or species). It is the second major method of exploiting genetic variation, selection being the first.

Animals that result from crossing are called **crossbreds**, as distinct from animals that result from matings within a population, which are called **straightbreds** or **purebreds**.

Many people think of crossing in terms of crosses between inbred lines, partly because of the considerable success achieved by this breeding method in plants, especially in maize. But as described in Chapter 13, the development of inbred lines in animals is very wasteful and costly, and hence is hardly ever used now, except possibly by one or two poultry-breeding organizations. Instead, crossing in animals is generally carried out between populations that have not been deliberately inbred but which have been isolated from each other for varying lengths of time.

The aim of this chapter is to describe the main methods of crossing that are used in practice, and to comment on the implications of each method.

## Regular crossing

Regular or systematic crossing occurs when the same cross is made on a regular basis, with the aim of producing a particular type of progeny. Regular crossing may be advantageous from two points of view.

Firstly, the crossbred progeny usually show **heterosis** or **hybrid vigour** for certain traits. Heterosis occurs when the average performance of crossbred progeny is superior to the average performance of the two parents. Various types of heterosis are recognized, including **parental heterosis** (either **maternal** or **paternal**), referring to the performance of animals as parents, and **individual heterosis**, referring to non-parental performance. The amount of heterosis for a particular trait can vary considerably, depending on the environment and on the populations being crossed. However, in general, (1) heterosis is greatest in traits most closely associated with reproduction and viability, and (2) the greater the genetic diversity between two populations of domesticated animals, the greater the heterosis in crosses between them.

The reasons for these conclusions can be briefly summarized as follows. Heterosis occurs only if there is non-additive gene action (dominance and/or epistasis) at loci affecting the trait; and the greater the difference in gene frequencies between the two populations being crossed, the greater the heterosis. Recalling from Chapter 13 that inbreeding depression occurs only if there is non-additive gene action, it is not surprising to find in general that the same traits that show heterosis also show inbreeding depression.

The second advantage of regular crossing is that **complementarity** may occur. This refers to the additional profitability obtained from crossing two populations, resulting not from heterosis but from the manner in which two or more traits complement each other.

For example, consider two populations of pigs, one (A) with a very high food conversion ratio but low litter size, and the other (B) with poor food conversion ratio but high litter size. Suppose that boars from A are regularly mated with sows from B to produce a crossbred pig that is raised solely for meat production. Even if there is no heterosis for food conversion ratio, i.e. even if the average performance of the crossbred pigs is exactly intermediate between that of the two parental populations, and if the litter size of B sows is the same when mated to either A or B boars, the overall profitability of this particular operation is likely to be much greater than the profitability of running either A or B alone, because the same total number of pigs is produced as from the most prolific population, B, but the food conversion ratio of each offspring is higher than that of offspring from B × B matings.

Certain crosses show more complementarity than others, depending on the extent to which the populations differ in reproductive performance and in production traits, and also depending on the 'direction' of the cross. The latter point can be illustrated by noting that there is far greater complementarity when the most prolific population is used as a source of dams rather than of sires.

There are two basic methods of regular crossing.

## Specific crossing

The simplest form of specific crossing is the **two-way cross**, in which animals from one population, A, are regularly mated to animals of a second population, B:

$$A \times B$$
$$\downarrow$$
$$(AB)$$

In this diagram A and B are straightbred parents, and (AB) represents the crossbred progeny, which are known as **first-cross** or F1 (first filial) progeny.

Sometimes the male parent in the cross always comes from one population and the female parent always comes from the other population, so as to obtain maximum benefit from complementarity. When this happens, the two parental populations are called the **sire line** and the **dam line** respectively. Obviously, in order to maintain the lines as separate entities, both males and females must be mated within a sire line and within a dam line; but only one of the sexes from each line (males in the sire line, and females in the dam line) makes a contribution to the cross.

The two-way specific cross produces offspring that are 100 per cent heterozygous, in the sense that they have one gene from each parental population at every locus. As such, they show 100 per cent of individual heterosis. However, two-way crossing does not provide any opportunity for the breeder to benefit from maternal or paternal heterosis, because the parents in a two-way cross are never themselves crossbred; they are always straightbred. In order to exploit maternal and/or paternal heterosis, other types of crossing must be used.

One of these is the **backcross**, which involves mating crossbred animals from a two-way cross back to one of the parental breeds:

$$(AB) \times A \qquad \text{or} \qquad (AB) \times B$$
$$\downarrow \qquad\qquad\qquad\qquad\qquad \downarrow$$
$$(AB)A \qquad\qquad\qquad\qquad (AB)B$$

With backcrossing, the crossbred parent is 100 per cent heterozygous, and hence shows 100 per cent parental heterosis. However, the backcross progeny are the result of the fusion of a gamete containing all, say, A genes (from the parental breed) and a gamete containing an average of one-half A genes and one-half B genes (from the crossbred parent). This means that at half of their loci, on average, backcross progeny have two A genes, i.e. are homozygous for genes from the A population, and at the other half of their loci, they have one A gene and one B gene, i.e. they are heterozygous. In other words, backcross progeny on average are 50 per cent less heterozygous than first-cross, AB, progeny. Consequently, they show on average only 50 per cent of individual heterosis.

A better way to exploit heterosis is to use a **three-way cross**, in which a first-cross animal, AB, is mated to an animal from a third population, C. Once again, because it is generally more profitable to improve female reproductive ability, a three-way cross is usually of the form

$$(AB)♀ \times C♂$$
$$\downarrow$$
$$(AB)C$$

This cross enables full utilization of maternal heterosis because the dam is 100 per cent heterozygous. It also enables full utilization of individual heterosis because the progeny are also 100 per cent heterozygous, being AC at one half of their loci, and BC at the other half, on average. It should be noted that even though first-cross and three-way-cross progeny both show full utilization of individual heterosis, in the sense that they are both 100 per cent heterozygous, they may not show the same amount of heterosis. The reason for this is that different crosses are involved in each case and, as noted earlier, the amount of heterosis is greater with some crosses than with others.

Because it is so successful at exploiting heterosis in the female parent and in the growing, commercial animal, and because it also enables exploitation of complementarity, the three-way cross is used widely throughout the world.

The final form of specific crossing is the four-way cross, in which the crossbred progeny from two separate two-way crosses are mated to produce commercial progeny:

$$
\begin{array}{ccc}
A \times B & & C \times D \\
\downarrow & & \downarrow \\
(AB) & \times & (CD) \\
& \downarrow & \\
& (AB)(CD) &
\end{array}
$$

Since both the male and female parent of the commercial progeny are crossbred, this cross enables full exploitation of both paternal and maternal heterosis, as well as individual heterosis. Once again, it should be noted that the actual amount of individual heterosis in the commercial progeny may not be the same as that observed in, for example, either of the two types of first-cross progeny.

## Rotational crossing

In all forms of specific crossing, both parents of the commercial progeny are either straightbred or are the crossbred progeny of straightbred parents. It follows that a commercial breeder who wishes to produce only the final commercial progeny has to obtain all breeding replacements, both male and female, from another source. Being obliged to introduce all breeding replacements from other populations is not always desirable, from a general management point of view and, especially in the case of pigs and poultry, from a disease point of view. It also deprives interested breeders of any possibility of breeding at least some of their own replacements.

**Rotational crossing** is an alternative form of regular crossing that overcomes some of these difficulties. It generally involves the use of males from two or three different populations, in regular sequence. If rotational crossing is continued in a commercial herd or flock for several years, and if all replacement females are bred in the herd or flock, all females will soon be crossbred, containing varying proportions of genes from the two or three populations from which males were obtained. Symbolically, we have the situation as illustrated in Table 18.1.

A major disadvantage of rotational crossing is that it does not allow any exploitation of complementarity, because the populations involved in the crossing cannot be restricted in use to a single purpose, as they are in specific crossing. Because of this, rotational crossing is a much more attractive

**Table 18.1** The two most common forms of rotational crossing, together with the proportions of genes from each parental breed, and average heterozygosity, in crossbred progeny in the early generations, and at equilibrium

**Two breed**

| | Proportion of genes from | | Average heterozygosity[1] |
|---|---|---|---|
| | A | B | |
| A × B | | | |
| [AB] × A | 1/2 | 1/2 | 1 |
| [(AB)A] × B | 3/4 | 1/4 | 1/2 |
| [((AB)A)B] × A | 3/8 | 5/8 | 3/4 |
| Equilibrium at generation: | | | |
| t | 1/3 | 2/3 | 2/3 |
| t + 1 | 2/3 | 1/3 | 2/3 |
| t + 2 | 1/3 | 2/3 | 2/3 |

**Three breed**

| | Proportion of genes from | | | Average heterozygosity[1] |
|---|---|---|---|---|
| | A | B | C | |
| A × B | | | | |
| [AB] × C | 1/2 | 1/2 | 0 | 1 |
| [(AB)C] × A | 1/4 | 1/4 | 1/2 | 1 |
| [((AB)C)A] × B | 5/8 | 1/8 | 1/4 | 3/4 |
| Equilibrium at generation: | | | | |
| t | 1/7 | 2/7 | 4/7 | 6/7 |
| t + 1 | 2/7 | 4/7 | 1/7 | 6/7 |
| t + 2 | 4/7 | 1/7 | 2/7 | 6/7 |

[1] Average heterozygosity of animals in square brackets, relative to a first-cross individual.

proposition where the populations available for crossing show little or no complementarity, but do show some economically useful heterosis.

## A comparison of different forms of regular crossing

Since the amount of heterosis is highly correlated with average heterozygosity, the easiest way to obtain an overall comparison of types of regular crossing is to compare them in terms of heterozygosity. This is done in Table 18.2.

In order to illustrate the practical implications of the information summarized in Table 18.2, we shall now consider some examples from particular species of domestic animals.

In beef cattle, a major determinant of profitability is the composite trait 'weight of calf weaned per cow joined'. Figure 18.1 shows the effects of heterosis on this trait, as observed in a large-scale crossing programme involving Herefords, Angus, and Shorthorns conducted in the USA. On average, there was 8.5 per cent individual heterosis and 14.8 per cent maternal heterosis, giving a total increase of 23.3 per cent in weight of calf weaned per cow joined. These are substantial benefits.

Given these results, and the levels of heterozygosity in Table 18.1, it is possible to calculate the benefits of other forms of regular crossing among the same three breeds. These are shown in Table 18.3. Once again, we can conclude that the practical and financial benefits of crossing are quite substantial.

**Table 18.2** Fraction of heterosis, as indicated by average heterozygosity, expected in the most common types of regular crossing

| Type of crossing | Fraction of heterosis | | |
|---|---|---|---|
| | Individual | Maternal | Paternal |
| Straightbred | 0 | 0 | 0 |
| Two-breed cross | | | |
| A♀ × B♂ | 1 | 0 | 0 |
| Backcross | | | |
| AB♀ × (A♂ or B♂) | 1/2 | 1 | 0 |
| (A♀ or B♀) × AB♂ | 1/2 | 0 | 1 |
| Three-breed cross | | | |
| AB♀ × C♂ | 1 | 1 | 0 |
| C♀ × AB♂ | 1 | 0 | 1 |
| Four-breed cross | | | |
| AB♀ × CD♂ | 1 | 1 | 1 |
| Rotational cross | | | |
| 2 sire breeds | 2/3 | 2/3 | 0 |
| 3 sire breeds | 6/7 | 6/7 | 0 |

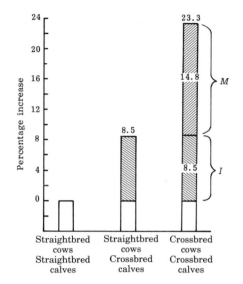

**Fig. 18.1** Heterosis in weight of calf weaned per cow joined, as a result of mating straightbred cows to bulls of a different breed (*centre*), or mating first-cross cows to bulls of a third breed (*right*). Results were obtained from all relevant crosses among Hereford, Angus, and Shorthorn cattle. *I* = individual heterosis; *M* = maternal heterosis.

**Table 18.3** Performance observed or expected from various types of regular crossing in cattle, sheep, and pigs

| Type of regular crossing | Heterosis utilized[1] | Weight of calf weaned per cow joined[2] | Weight of lamb weaned per ewe joined[2] | Pigs reared per sow per year[2] |
|---|---|---|---|---|
| Straightbred | nil | 100 | 100 | 100 |
| Two-breed cross | *I* | 108 | 107 | 106 |
| Backcross | $(1/2)\,I + M$ | 119 | — | — |
| Three-breed cross | | | | |
|   C♀ × AB♂ | *I* + *P* | — | 137 | — |
|   AB♀ × C♂ | *I* + *M* | 123 | 152 | 118 |
| Two-breed rotation | $(2/3)\,I + (2/3)\,M$ | 116 | — | 112 |
| Three-breed rotation | $(6/7)\,I + (6/7)\,M$ | 120 | — | — |
| Other | | | | |
|   AB♀ × AB♂ | $(1/2)\,I + M + P$ | — | 166 | — |

[1] *I* = individual heterosis; *M* = maternal heterosis; *P* = paternal heterosis.
[2] as a percentage of straightbred performance.

Similar conclusions can be drawn from crossing programmes in sheep and pigs, the results of which are shown in Table 18.3.

When interpreting these results, we must remember two things. First, performance of particular crosses between particular breeds are sometimes much better or much worse than the average figures given in Table 18.3, which should be taken only as a general guide. Second, the traits considered in Table 18.3 are closely associated with reproduction and/or viability and hence show substantial heterosis. Other traits less closely associated with reproduction and/or viability show less heterosis, and some traits (such as carcase traits) show essentially zero heterosis.

## Crossing to produce a synthetic

An alternative to regular crossing is to perform one or a few crosses between two or more populations in order to produce a single population of animals containing a mixture of genes from each population. A single population that is a mixture of various populations is called a **synthetic** or **composite**. Once a synthetic has been formed, the main aim is to improve it as rapidly as possible by selecting within it, following the procedures in Chapter 16. In many situations, the result of selection within a synthetic is a new breed. For example, the Santa Gertrudis, the Jamaican Hope, the Norwegian Red and White, the Luing, the Australian Milking Zebu, the Australian Friesian Sahiwal, and the Belmont Red are all cattle breeds formed comparatively recently by selection within a synthetic, and similar examples can be found in other species of domestic animals. Some synthetics are based almost entirely on just one traditional breed, and were founded with selected animals from a number of different strains within the breed. Others, such as many of the present-day broiler chicken populations maintained by breeding companies, are mixtures of several different breeds, each of which was thought to have at least some desirable traits in relation to the aim of the breeders concerned.

A particularly popular combination in the formation of synthetics in cattle has been that of *Bos taurus* with *Bos indicus*, in order to produce new breeds capable of improved production under tropical and semi-tropical conditions. The aim has usually been to combine the improved production ability of *Bos taurus* breeds with the heat tolerance and tick resistance of *Bos indicus* breeds.

Of course, if we go back far enough in time, it becomes evident that many of the long-established breeds that we know today started as synthetics of one form or another. In some cases, the crossing phase lasted a long time. But sooner or later, in most cases, the resultant synthetic was closed and a new breed began to emerge. Increasingly, it is being recognized that closing a synthetic for ever is not the best option. On the contrary, in most cases it is advantageous to introduce some new genetic variation from time to time, and this continues to be done in a number of cases.

The main guidelines to be followed in crossing to produce a synthetic are:

(1) Ensure that the animals used in the original crossings have the highest possible average breeding value for the relevant traits (it is no use starting a synthetic with inferior animals);
(2) Maximize variance in breeding values amongst the foundation animals in the synthetic, by using as many unrelated animals as possible from each of the contributing populations, bearing in mind the previous requirement that they should have the highest possible average breeding value.

With respect to heterosis, the simplest expectation is that if there are $n$ populations contributing equally to the synthetic, then $(1 - 1/n)$ of the heterosis present in the F1 (the first-cross progeny) is retained in the F2 (the progeny resulting from matings among F1s), and in subsequent generations. However, if the synthetic is not maintained at an adequate size, or if selection within the synthetic is very intense, inbreeding depression may whittle away the remaining heterosis. The main advantage of synthetics is that only one population has to be maintained, rather than the two or more parental populations required for a regular crossing programme.

## Grading-up

**Grading-up** involves a succession of backcrosses from one population into another population, with the aim of introducing a new gene or genes into one of the populations, or with the aim of substituting one population for the other.

### Introducing a new gene or genes

Suppose, for example, that some breeders wish to create a polled strain of a horned breed, and have one mutant animal that is heterozygous for the dominant polled gene, $P$, at their disposal. The polled animal does not necessarily have to belong to the same breed in which the polled strain is to be produced; its only requirement is to be able to produce fertile offspring when mated to members of that breed. The breeding programme to be followed in introducing the polled gene to a horned breed is called **introgression**, and is illustrated in Table 18.4. The procedure is very straightforward. All that is required is for all horned offspring to be culled each year so that only polled offspring remain to be mated back to the horned breed. A very critical requirement is that a large and representative sample of animals from the horned breed should be used in the backcrossing programme, to ensure that the polled strain has as much genetic variation as the horned breed from which it arose. In most situations, and especially if the above guideline has been followed, three or at the most four crosses, i.e. the original cross and

**Table 18.4** The use of grading-up to create a polled strain of a horned breed

| Generation | Mating programme | Average proportion of genes from horned breed in polled offspring |
|---|---|---|
| 0 | Polled × Horned | |
| 1 | Selected polled offspring } × Horned | $1/2 = (1/2)^1$ |
| 2 | Selected polled offspring } × orned | $3/4 = 1 - (1/2)^2$ |
| 3 | Selected polled offspring } × Horned | $7/8 = 1 - (1/2)^3$ |
| $t$ | | $1 - (1/2)^t$ |

two or three backcrosses, is sufficient to achieve the original aim. By this stage, the average proportion of genes from the horned breed in the new strain is either 7/8 (two backcrosses) or 15/16 (three backcrosses) and the polled offspring are indistinguishable from members of the horned breed, especially if there has been selection among polled offspring for traits associated with the horned breed, during grading-up.

The final phase of a grading-up programme for the introduction of a new gene depends on whether the gene is dominant or recessive. If it is recessive, the new strain can be formed immediately from all offspring exhibiting the trait; they will all breed true for the recessive gene. If, however, the gene is dominant, e.g. the polled gene, all offspring showing the trait are heterozygous and will not therefore breed true. The task is then to arrange matings among these animals, and in subsequent generations to distinguish carriers from non-carriers, with the aim of identifying and culling all carriers. The general requirements for this were outlined in Chapter 11.

DNA markers linked to the gene of interest can be of immense help during the final phase of introgression if the introgressed gene is dominant. If the gene is recessive, linked markers will be of substantial use during the back-crossing phase in enabling identification of carriers of the introgressed gene.

In practice, many introgression programmes involve the introduction of desirable quantitative traits rather than simply a single desirable gene. For example, there is currently much interest in introducing the high fecundity of Chinese pigs into European pigs. Exactly the same principles apply for introgressing a quantitative trait as for a single gene. And if sufficient DNA markers are available, they will be of substantial help in enabling the identification of the particular segments of chromosomes that are to be introgressed, i.e. the segments of chromosomes that carry fecundity genes from the Chinese pigs.

In fact, the use of DNA markers in introgression is likely to be one of the most immediate practical applications of DNA markers in animal breeding.

## Breed substitution

The late 1960s and early 1970s witnessed an awakening of world-wide interest in long-established continental European breeds of cattle such as Charolais and Simmental. A few animals and many doses of semen from a number of such breeds were exported to many countries in which these breeds were previously unknown, and in each country a race began to establish 'purebred' herds of these 'migrant' breeds as quickly as possible, by means of a grading-up procedure like that illustrated in Table 18.5.

In the early stages of establishing a breed using this type of grading-up, much controversy often arises as to the number of backcrosses that should be required before progeny are eligible for official registration as 'purebreds'. Such controversies illustrate a complete lack of understanding of the genetic basis of grading-up.

The most important point to realize about grading-up is that, except for half-breds, there is variation among the progeny of all other generations, with respect to the proportion of 'local' and 'migrant' genes.

For example, it is possible that a so-called three-quarter-bred could have more than 31/32 migrant genes. Equally likely, it could have just over 1/2 migrant genes. The reason for this is that segregation during the formation of gametes in half-breds and in all subsequent crosses gives rise to a spectrum of

**Table 18.5** Grading-up to a migrant breed, M, from any local animals, L

| Generation | Mating programme | Designation (grade) of animals in square brackets | Proportion of migrant genes in animals in square brackets | | |
|---|---|---|---|---|---|
| | | | Min.[1] | Av. | Max.[1] |
| 0 | L × M | | | | |
| 1 | [LM] × M | 1/2 bred | 1/2 | 1/2 | 1/2 |
| 2 | [(LM)M] × M | 3/4 bred | 1/2 | 3/4 | 1 |
| 3 | [((LM)M)M] × M | 7/8 bred | 1/2 | 7/8 | 1 |
| 4 | [(((LM)M)M)M] × M | 15/16 bred | 1/2 | 15/16 | 1 |
| 5 | etc. | 31/32 bred | 1/2 | 31/32 | 1 |

[1] Assuming no crossing-over.

different types of gametes, ranging theoretically from a gamete containing only local genes, to a gamete consisting solely of migrant genes (neglecting the effect of crossing-over). Thus, as shown in Table 18.5, the proportion of migrant genes in three-quarter-breds and all subsequent crosses can range from 1/2 to 1, if we neglect the effects of crossing-over. The most likely proportion of migrant genes in any cross is the average, which is the proportion that is used to describe that cross; and extreme deviations from these proportions are less likely than small deviations.

But the fact remains that by the time breeders have reached the second or third backcross, they may have offspring with proportions of migrant genes ranging from nearly 1/2 to nearly 1. Now, although breeders cannot tell exactly what proportion of migrant genes exists in any particular animal simply by looking at it, they can be certain that, on average, animals whose appearance corresponds more closely to the migrant breed are likely to have a larger than average proportion of migrant genes, within any particular grade.

And if breeders do any selection in favour of animals showing migrant-like appearance during their grading-up programme, by the time they have reached the second backcross, i.e. 7/8, their selected progeny will on average have a proportion of migrant genes far higher than 7/8, and probably higher than 31/32.

It is now obvious why the controversies about the required number of backcrosses are futile, even if the only aim of a grading-up programme was to obtain the highest possible proportion of migrant genes within a particular herd or flock.

But there is a more important reason why the debates are pointless. It is that breeders would improve economically important traits more rapidly if they stopped grading-up after the first or at most the second backcross, and concentrated solely on continual selection. In this way, the migrant genes are allowed to find their own optimum proportion for the particular production system.

Continual backcrossing simply removes all the local genes, and achieves nothing more than replicas of migrant animals that were alive 15 or 20 years ago. Such a programme implies that the local animals have absolutely nothing to offer by way of adaptation to local environments (both natural and managerial) that are often very different from those that exist in the country of origin of the migrant breed, In fact, of course, local animals are usually well-adapted to their local environment, and therefore they do have some genes that should make a useful contribution to the new breed being developed.

We can conclude that continual backcrossing in a grading-up programme is both unnecessary and undesirable.

## Preservation of rare or unwanted breeds

An important issue arises in situations where a breed that is native to a particular area appears to have no further use in that area or elsewhere, and consequently is in danger of being graded-up into extinction. The general question raised by this situation is whether such a breed should be preserved.

The arguments in favour of preservation are that we do not know what type of animals will be required in the future, and that we should therefore preserve all available genetic variation as an insurance against the unknown future. On the other hand, it is argued that breeders who aim to earn a living from animals cannot afford to look too far into the future; they appreciate the arguments in favour of preservation, but are not able to meet the relatively high cost of preserving populations that they are unlikely ever to utilize during their own lifetimes. Not surprisingly, therefore, the financial responsibility for preservation of unwanted breeds often falls on the public sector or on organizations set up specifically for that purpose. At both the international level, e.g. FAO, and at the local level, e.g. the Rare Breeds Trust in Great Britain, concerted efforts are being made to gather relevant data on breeds that seem threatened with extinction, and to act, where possible, to save them. In Ireland, for example, a conservation programme for the Kerry breed of cattle has been underway since 1982. It consists of a modest government subsidy for each calf registered, government support for the maintenance in a national park of the largest remaining herd, and access to software for the calculation of relationships between potential mates, with the aim of minimizing the rate of inbreeding.

Interestingly, the two areas that are probably of greatest concern are at either end of the spectrum of animal improvement. At one end we have a large variety of locally adapted native populations (often in developing countries) that are under threat from the influx of 'improved' breeds and strains from developed countries. And at the other end we have an increasing number of poultry selection lines that are discarded when yet another independent poultry breeder is taken over by a larger and often multinational breeding company.

There are no easy solutions to these problems. It is comforting, however, to see increasing activity in conservation around the world, led by the FAO's Global Animal Genetic Resources Programme, and to realize that more and more people are becoming concerned and are consequently giving more thought to possible solutions.

# Further reading

*Theory*

Cunningham, E. P. (1987). Crossbreeding—the Greek temple model. *Journal of Animal Breeding and Genetics*, **104**, 2–11.

Cunningham, E. P. and Connolly, J. (1989). Efficient design of crossbreeding experiments. *Theoretical and Applied Genetics*, **78**, 381–6.

Dempfle, L. (1990). Conservation, creation, and utilization of genetic variation. *Journal of Dairy Science*, **73**, 2593–600.

Hill, W. G. (1993). Variation in genetic composition in backcrossing programs. *Journal of Heredity*, **84**, 212–3.

Kinghorn, B. P., Shepherd, R. K., and Banks, R. G. (1989). A note on the formation of optimal composite populations. *Theoretical and Applied Genetics*, **78**, 318–20.

Solkner, J. (1993). Choice of optimality criteria for the design of crossbreeding experiments. *Journal of Animal Science*, **71**, 2867–73.

Solkner, J. and James, J. W. (1990). Optimum design of crossbreeding experiments. *Journal of Animal Breeding and Genetics*, **107**, 61–7, 411–420, 421–430.

Swan, A. A. and Kinghorn, B. P. (1992). Evaluation and exploitation of crossbreeding in dairy cattle. *Journal of Dairy Science*, **75**, 624–39.

## Crossing in practice

Cundiff, L. V., Nunezdominguez, R., Dickerson, G. E., Gregory, K. E., and Koch, R. M. (1992). Heterosis for lifetime production in Hereford, Angus, Shorthorn, and crossbred cows. *Journal of Animal Science*, **70**, 2397–410.

Derouen, S. M., Franke, D. E., Bidner, T. D., and Blouin, D. C. (1992). 2-breed, 3-breed, and 4-breed rotational crossbreeding of beef cattle—carcass traits. *Journal of Animal Science*, **70**, 3665–76.

Gregory, K. E., Cundiff, L. V., and Koch, R. M. (1992). Effects of breed and retained heterosis on milk yield and 200-day weight in advanced generations of composite populations of beef cattle. *Journal of Animal Science*, **70**, 2366–72.

Haley, C. S., Dagaro, E., and Ellis, M. (1992). Genetic components of growth and ultrasonic fat depth traits in Meishan and Large White pigs and their reciprocal crosses. *Animal Production*, **54**, 105–15.

Kuhlers, D. L., Jungst, S. B., and Little, J. A. (1994). An experimental comparison of equivalent terminal and rotational crossbreeding systems in swine—sow and litter performance. *Journal of Animal Science*, **72**, 584–90.

Morris, C. A., Cullen, N. G., Hickey, S. M., and Amyes, N. C. (1993). Evaluation of 3-breed composites alongside Angus controls for growth, reproduction, maternal, and carcass traits. *New Zealand Journal of Agricultural Research*, **36**, 341–8.

Pitchford, W. S. (1993). Growth and lambing performance of ewes from crosses between the Dorset Horn, Merino and Corriedale. *Livestock Production Science*, **33**, 127–39.

Thorpe, W., Kangethe, P., Rege, J. E. O., Mosi, R. O., Mwandotto, B. A. J., and Njuguna, P. (1993). Crossbreeding Ayrshire, Friesian, and Sahiwal cattle for milk yield and preweaning traits of progeny in the semiarid tropics of Kenya. *Journal of Dairy Science*, **76**, 2001–12.

Touchberry, R. W. (1992). Crossbreeding effects in dairy cattle—the Illinois experiment, 1949–1969. *Journal of Dairy Science*, **75**, 640–67.

Wohlfarth, G. W. (1993). Heterosis for growth rate in common carp. *Aquaculture*, **113**, 31–46.

Zarnecki, A., Norman, H. D., Gierdziewicz, M., and Jamrozik, J. (1993). Heterosis for growth and yield traits from crosses of Friesian strains. *Journal of Dairy Science*, **76**, 1661–70.

## Introgression

Hillel, J., Schaap, T., Haberfeld, A., Jeffreys, A. J., Plotzky, Y., Cahaner, A., and Lavi, U. (1990). DNA fingerprints applied to gene introgression in breeding programs. *Genetics*, **124**, 783–9.

Hillel, J., Gibbins, A. M. V., Etches, R. J., and Shaver, D. M. (1993). Strategies for the rapid introgression of a specific gene modification into a commercial poultry flock from a single carrier. *Poultry Science*, **72**, 1197–211.

Hospital, F., Chevalet, C., and Mulsant, P. (1992). Using markers in gene introgression breeding programs. *Genetics*, **132**, 1199–210.

## Conservation

Hall, S. J. G. and Ruane, J. (1993). Livestock breeds and their conservation—a global overview. *Conservation Biology*, **7**, 815–25.

Hare, D. (1992). Conservation of Canadian animal genetic resources. *Canadian Veterinary Journal*, **33**, 3–5.

Hodges, J. (1992). A global programme for animal genetic resources. *Livestock Production Science*, **32**, 94–7.

Loftus, R. and Scherf, B. (ed.) (1993). *World watch list for domestic animal diversity*. FAO, Rome.

Obata, T. and Takeda, H. (1993). Germplasm conservation of Japanese native livestock breeds (horses, cattle and goats). *Japan Agricultural Research Quarterly*, **27**, 8–12.

O'Huigin, C. and Cunningham, E. P. (1990). Analysis of breeding structure of the Kerry breed. *Journal of Animal Breeding and Genetics*, **107**, 452–7.

Reents, R., Meinikmann, H., and Glodek, P. (1992). Preservation of a genetic resource population of Old German Black and White cattle (DSR). *Archiv für Tierzucht*, **35**, 17–25.

Trail, J. C. M., Dieteren, G. D. M., and Teale, A. J. (1989). Trypanotolerance and the value of conserving livestock genetic resources. *Genome*, **31**, 805–12.

Travis, J. (1992). 3rd World—S(ave) O(ur) S(heep). *Science*, **255**, 678.

# 19 Selection and regular crossing

Traditionally, many stud breeders have regarded crossing as an insult to them and to their animals, and as a threat to their livelihoods. The aim of this chapter is to explain why these opinions are incorrect, and to illustrate that the most profitable future for both stud breeders and commercial breeders lies in breeding programmes that involve both selection and regular crossing.

## Selection

A selection programme within a population can lead to a steady improvement in average breeding value and hence in profitability. However, the average level of inbreeding also shows a steady increase, even if mating is entirely at random among the selected candidates. In addition, the greater the selection applied, the greater is the increase in average level of inbreeding. Thus, successful selection programmes in closed populations incur inbreeding depression which, as we saw in Chapter 13, has greatest effect on traits associated with viability and reproductive ability. If effective population size ($N_e$) is not too small, the increase in inbreeding depression may be unimportant from a practical point of view. However, if $N_e$ is relatively small, the steady increase in inbreeding depression may begin to adversely affect profitability.

Of course, this problem can be offset in practice by the occasional introduction of unrelated animals into the otherwise closed population. However, as soon as breeders start buying animals from other sources, the response in their own population is determined in part by the breeding values of the purchased animals; and if response to selection within their own population has been quite rapid, they may have difficulty finding other sources from which to purchase stock that match the average breeding value of their own stock. This is becoming an increasingly common dilemma.

## Selection and regular crossing

We saw in Chapter 18 that the traits that show the greatest inbreeding depression are those that also show the greatest heterosis when different populations are crossed. This observation immediately suggests a solution to the above dilemma: we can get the best of both worlds by continually selecting within each of several populations and by making regular crosses between them in order to produce the final commercial product.

In this way we are able to get the most out of all genetic variation; continual selection exploits variation in breeding values, $V_A$, and regular crossing exploits non-additive genetic variation, $V_D$ and $V_I$.

The major difficulty with breeding programmes involving both selection and regular crossing is the organizational and management problems associated with maintaining at least two different straightbred populations together with various crossbred populations. In some situations, this difficulty is overcome by co-operation amongst several breeders, with each breeder maintaining just one population. The financial benefits from combining continual selection with regular crossing are sufficient to make this extra effort well worthwhile in most circumstances.

An important practical point is that regular crossing can occur only if someone is maintaining and improving the straightbred lines. Thus, rather than presenting a threat to stud breeders, regular crossing actually provides them with a substantial incentive to maintain and improve their straightbred populations.

In discussing regular crossing in this section, we have concentrated solely on the benefits to be gained from heterosis. However, it was emphasized in Chapter 18 that there is more to crossing than just heterosis. In fact, it was pointed out that even in the absence of heterosis, certain crosses show complementarity. Thus, in certain circumstances, regular crossing may still be an economically viable proposition, even if there is negligible inbreeding depression in the relevant closed populations.

Furthermore, the benefits from complementarity can be enhanced by selection for different traits in the lines that are used in the crossing programme. If, for example, one line is always used as the sire of the final commercial generation in a three-way cross, it can be selected specifically for traits that are important in the commercial generation, e.g. growth rate and carcase quality. In contrast, a line that is used solely as the female parent of the F1 hybrid in a three-way cross, can be selected less for growth and carcase traits, and more for reproductive traits, probably utilizing information from relatives to help overcome the relatively low heritability of such traits. This leads to the development of specialized **sire lines** and **dam lines**.

Recalling some points made in Chapters 16 and 18, we can conclude that by carrying out selection within populations and regular crossing between populations, we are able to exploit additive gene effects within populations (through selection), additive gene effects between populations (through complementarity), and non-additive gene effects (through heterosis).

A final point should be made in relation to synthetics or composites. Sometimes, there are good reasons for crossing various populations on a once-only basis to produce a synthetic. Sooner or later, however, a synthetic has to be considered in the same category as any other population. Thus, even if inbreeding depression is not currently a problem in a particular synthetic, it may still be economically advantageous to use that synthetic in a regular crossing programme, if the synthetic exhibits useful complementarity with one or more other populations.

## Further reading

De Vries, A.G. and Van der Steen, H.A.M. (1990). Optimal use of nucleus and testing capacity in a pig breeding system with sire and dam lines. *Livestock Production Science*, **25**, 217–29.

Gama, L. T. and Smith, C. (1993). The role of inbreeding depression in livestock production systems. *Livestock Production Science*, **36**, 203–11.

Gempesaw, C. M., Wirth, F. F., and Bacon, J. R. (1992). A financial analysis of integration in aquaculture production—the case of hybrid striped bass. *Aquaculture*, **104**, 193–215.

Macbeth, G. M. and McPhee, C. P. (1986). An economic evaluation of breeding systems with selection and crossing of Large White and Landrace pigs in a closed herd. *Agricultural Systems*, **20**, 219–39.

# Biotechnology and the future

Much of this book has been concerned with the application of various forms of biotechnology to the breeding of animals. The aim of this chapter is to fill in the remaining gaps—to comment upon those aspects of biotechnology that have not been sufficiently covered in earlier chapters. In so doing, we shall be looking into the future, which is always a risky business. The predictions that follow, therefore, are made in the full knowledge that not all of them are likely to come to fruition.

## Artificial insemination (AI)

AI was the first form of reproductive technology to have large-scale practical implications for genetic improvement. Since it is basically a means of increasing the reproductive potential of males, AI enables fewer males to be selected as parents of the next generation. Its genetic effect, therefore, is to increase the intensity of selection of males. As soon as it became a practical reality in the dairy industry in the 1950s, breeding programmes were devised to enable its full genetical potential to be realized. Basically, these programmes involve progeny testing of dairy bulls, by distributing the semen from a team of young bulls across a number of participating herds, in each of which the daughters of the various young bulls are directly compared. Although this involves a long generation interval (because the bulls are not selected until their daughters have completed their first lactation), it results in a high accuracy of selection, and the potential genetic gain is substantially greater than that which is possible under natural mating. In dairy cattle, for example, AI can give rise to genetic improvement of around 1 per cent of the mean production per year. (While this may seem to be a very small figure, remember that the gain is cumulative, i.e. an additional gain of the same magnitude is achieved each year. Also, once each year's gain has been achieved, it remains for ever after, without the need for additional input to maintain it.)

Critics of AI have pointed to its potential for increasing the rate of inbreeding, with all the attendant disadvantages, especially in relation to autosomal recessive defects, as discussed in Chapter 13. AI certainly does have this potential, and, in closed populations, care must be taken to ensure that the effective population size is sufficiently large for the rate of inbreeding to be kept at an acceptably low level. In practice, most AI improvement programmes have a sufficiently large effective population size, and, in addition, intermittent immigration ensures that the level of inbreeding remains at satisfactorily low levels. What the critics of AI have generally failed to realize is that, at the level of commercial production, AI has the potential to *decrease* the rate of inbreeding, because it provides a far wider choice of unrelated males than is ever available under natural mating. This is very important, since it means that AI can be a very powerful tool for preventing the occurrence of inherited defects. Thus, rather than trying to condemn AI as a dangerous technology, as some well-meaning veterinary authorities try to do from time to time, all interested parties should be continually trying to encourage its correct use.

Given its many advantages, it seems likely that AI will continue to be used extensively in dairy improvement, and in any other form of animal production where the female reproductive cycle can be readily monitored or controlled.

## Multiple ovulation and embryo transfer (MOET)

Just as AI increases male reproductive potential, so does MOET increase female reproductive potential. Thus, the genetic consequence of MOET is an increase in female selection intensity. Alternatively, MOET can be used to decrease the female generation interval, by enabling replacements to be obtained from only the younger females in a population.

For industries in which the traditional form of improvement programme involves performance testing (e.g. beef and sheep), MOET offers considerable advantages, resulting in approximately 50 per cent additional response per year.

When superimposed on an AI improvement programme involving progeny-testing of males, MOET has relatively little effect, since the intensity of selection of females to breed the next team of males is already quite high. However, if MOET is used in circumstances where selection of males on the basis of progeny-testing is replaced by selection of males at a far younger age on the basis of their female sibs' performance, then, although the accuracy of selection is reduced, the generation interval is reduced to an even greater extent, with the result that the rate of genetic improvement per year is actually as great as, if not greater than, a progeny-testing programme.

Progeny-testing programmes are large-scale affairs, involving the recording of performance of thousands or tens of thousands of animals, and requiring the co-operation of many commercial farmers. In contrast, a MOET improvement programme can be conducted quite successfully in a nucleus population of just a few hundred animals, which can be run as a single herd or flock under the control of a just a few people. Since relatively few animals have to be recorded, it is feasible to measure traits additional to those traditionally measured. For example, in a dairy MOET nucleus, it is possible to measure individual food intake and various blood metabolites, and to genotype animals for relevant DNA markers. In contrast, in a state-wide or national progeny-testing programme, such additional activities are out of the question both economically and practically. In addition, because a MOET nucleus inevitably has substantial biotechnological expertise on hand, such herds or flocks are ideally placed to adopt new biotechnologies such as those discussed below. Finally, in developing countries, where large-scale recording schemes and widespread use of AI are almost out of the question, a MOET nucleus may be the only realistic way to conduct an improvement programme, because performance recording and the facilities and skills necessary for conducting MOET are required only in the nucleus. In all circumstances, the benefits of improvement in a MOET nucleus can be spread to the commercial level by the provision of natural-service bulls from the nucleus, or, if this source is insufficient to meet demand, from one or more multipliers. Alternatively, if the appropriate technology is available, AI of nucleus-bred males can be used.

Just as with AI, MOET has the potential to increase the rate of inbreeding. If it is used in a closed population, the effective population size must be sufficiently large to avoid an unacceptably high rate of inbreeding. In practice, again as with AI, occasional immigration is a very useful means of avoiding inbreeding problems. The challenge, of course, is to find unrelated animals of at least equal, and preferably, superior genetic merit. In practice, most MOET nucleus populations remain open for many years; each year, a proportion of the matings involve semen from outside bulls. If the resultant offspring have sufficiently high EBVs, they are retained, which means that the genes from the imported semen are incorporated into the nucleus. If the offspring are not good enough, they are culled.

In evaluating the potential of MOET, it helps to realize that this technology in effect changes a monotocous species into a polytocous species; in other words, MOET turns a cow into a sow. It follows that MOET is unlikely to have much effect on genetic improvement in naturally polytocous species. Consequently, cattle (both dairy and beef), sheep and goats are the species that have most to gain from the use of MOET nucleus populations.

## *In vitro* maturation (IVM) and *in vitro* fertilization (IVF) of ova

These two technologies have considerable potential. From the point of view of commercial animal production, they offer the potential for artificial insemination of semen to be replaced by artificial inembrionation of mass-produced specific-purpose embryos. Depending on the industry's needs, these embryos could be straightbreds, or F1 hybrids, or even 3-way or 4-way hybrids.

In relation to genetic improvement, IVM and IVF have the potential to reduce the variability in yield of embryos, and thereby increase the effectiveness of conventional MOET programmes. In addition, by enabling the collection of eggs from very young females, they hold the promise of reducing the generation interval and hence increasing the rate of improvement in a MOET nucleus.

IVM and IVF also raise new possibilities. For example, all selected males could be mated to all selected females, thereby creating a family of paternal half-sibs, a family of maternal half-sibs, and a family of full-sibs for each pair-wise combination of selected male and selected female. Improvement programmes using this mating design could achieve rates of response comparable with those achieved in MOET programmes.

## Embryo multiplication and transfer (EMT)

Large-scale EMT (previously called embryo cloning) has substantial potential for both improvement programmes and for commercial animal production. In the case of improvement programmes, EMT offers the possibility of obtaining extremely accurate EBVs for each of a number of different offspring (embryos) from the best nucleus matings, by clone-testing each embryo. Once the best clones have been identified, it is simply a matter of going to the freezer and extracting a few more embryos from those best clones, and growing them into adult animals, which are then mated to produce the next round of clones. Figure 20.1 illustrates how EMT could be incorporated into an improvement programme.

At the level of commercial production, EMT could have profound effects. For example, in the case of dairy production, sufficient cows could be in-embrionated with a female dairy hybrid (2-way, 3-way, or 4-way cross) to produce the next generation of commercial cows. This involves only a propor-tion of all dairy cows. The remainder could be given cloned embryos for use in the beef industry, e.g. F1 hybrid males for use as natural-service sires in beef herds, F1 hybrid females for use as dams in beef herds, or 3-way or 4-way cross slaughter-generation beef embryos.

An interesting consequence of the widespread practical application of EMT is that the average genetic merit of the clones that are used in commercial production is substantially higher than the average genetic merit of the nucleus herds from which they are chosen. This is the exact opposite of the lag which occurs in a traditional breeding pyramid, which was described in Chapter 17.

With the potential for large-scale benefits, it seems that EMT is certain to become a widespread reality in the future. However, there are some prob-lems that must be considered. Firstly, an immediate problem is that birth weights are substantially greater in cloned embryos than in normal embryos. Optimists argue that this is a technical hitch that can be overcome with further research and development. Others worry that it might be an insurmountable problem. More generally, there is concern that the widespread use of cloned animals will create problems associated with monoculture. If circumstances change, e.g. if a new and virulent form of a pathogen arises, whole popula-

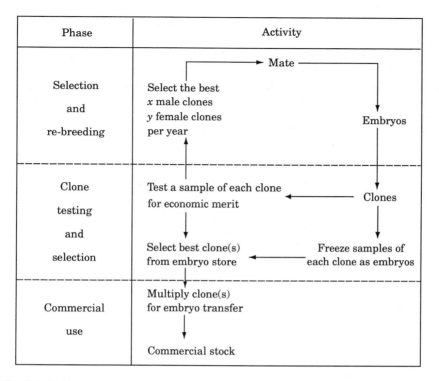

**Fig. 20.1** An improvement programme involving the use of EMT.

tions could be decimated. However, this argument overlooks the fact that a wide range of different clones will be available to commercial farmers. In addition, the clones will be used only at the commercial level; it will be absolutely necessary to maintain as much genetic variation as possible at the nucleus level, so that continual genetic improvement can be achieved, and to provide the range of genotypes that will be essential to provide for the changing circumstances certain to be encountered by commercial producers. A potentially serious problem with EMT is the concern felt by some people at the very thought of animal clones. The fact that many of our most widely-used agricultural plant species are clones, e.g. grapes, bananas, apples, may not provide any solace to people who believe that cloning animals is one step too far along the path of human intervention. These concerns should not be dismissed lightly.

## Control of sex ratio

In principle, the two main approaches to the control of sex ratio are sexing embryos (by the use of PCR with primers for sequences that occur only on the

Y chromosome) or using a variety of physical or physiological approaches to separate X-bearing sperm from Y-bearing sperm.

In relation to improvement programmes, the ability to manipulate sex ratio will not have a substantial impact. For example, if the sex ratio is altered in favour of males, the male selection intensity is obviously increased, but the female selection intensity is decreased.

If EMT becomes a reality, it would obviously be useful to know the sex of each clone before its large-scale propagation. However, since each clone will have undergone evaluation in the form of actual animals, the sex of each clone will be known as soon as the first animal is grown from that clone. Thus, there seems to be little need for sophisticated methods of determining sex of embryos.

In contrast, semen sexing, which is gradually edging towards at least partial success, may have some potential, e.g. in meat industries, where males are generally more profitable than females. However, semen sexing obviously requires the use of AI, which is not yet feasible in large-scale beef, lamb or pig production systems. In addition, the premium that meat farmers would be prepared to pay for sexed semen would be limited by the relatively small profit difference between the sexes. In dairy production, calculations have shown that producers could afford to pay approximately double the price for semen that would produce only female calves.

Probably the greatest potential for semen sexing is in IVM/IVF programmes, because it enables the production of single-sex embryo families.

An entirely different approach to altering the sex ratio involves use of the *SRY* gene or one of the other genes involved in mammalian sex determination. As described in Chapter 4, the importance of the *SRY* gene is that it appears to provide the initial trigger which causes the undifferentiated gonad in an embryo to develop into a testis rather than an ovary. If many copies of this gene could be inserted into autosomes by means of transgenesis, then, in addition to the 50 per cent of offspring that would be normal XY males, all XX animals which inherited one or more of these autosomes would be phenotypically male. However, they would also be sterile, which would confine their utility to the slaughter generation.

## Recombinant proteins

As described in Chapter 2, one of the benefits to arise from molecular technology has been the ability to entice one species (usually a microorganism, but also mammals—either cell cultures or transgenics) to mass-produce a protein from another species, including other microorganisms, mammals, and birds. Such proteins are called recombinant proteins.

One of the major uses of this technology has been the production of a new generation of vaccines directed against a wide range of pathogenic and parasitic diseases, following the cloning and appropriate expression of the gene(s) for the most antigenically protective protein portion of the pathogen or parasite. Some of these vaccines are already on the market, and are very successful; others have not been successful.

An interesting example of a recombinant protein is a vaccine against the cattle tick, *Boophilus microplus*. After the discovery that extracts from the gut of the tick provide protective immunity, extensive further studies eventually led to the partial sequencing of proteins in the protective extracts, which in turn enabled a DNA probe to be constructed (making use of the universal genetic code) corresponding to the tick gene for the protective protein. A tick genomic library was then screened with this probe, and eventually the appropriate tick gene was isolated, cloned, and expressed in *E. coli*.

Although vaccines are a very important example of the use of recombinant proteins, there are many other uses as well. In fact, the possibilities for recombinant proteins are endless. Unfortunately, so are the technical and financial challenges involved in translating an idea into a commercially viable product. There are also public concerns about the consumption of food from animals that have received recombinant proteins such as somatotropin (growth hormone). In addition, there is concern about the effect of such proteins on animals (will they be pushed too far?), and on the livelihood of farmers (will the dramatic increases in production per animal lead to a reduction in the number of viable farms?). In the case of bovine somatotropin (bST), there is also concern about the potential of the undisclosed use of bST in dairy herds to produce biased EBVs. The recent licensing of bovine and porcine somatotropin in several countries will provide test cases for the acceptance of this form of biotechnology.

## Transgenesis

The basic technology of transgenesis was described in Chapter 2. One of the initial major aims of transgenesis in farm animals was to obtain extra improvement in economically important traits, e.g. by inserting additional copies of the growth-hormone gene. However, the effects of the transgene need to be quite large before this use of transgenesis is more effective than conventional selection. The reason for this is that once the transgenic animal has been created, it takes several generations to introgress the transgene into a population, and to evaluate its effect. During this time, substantial additional gains will be made by conventional selection. Consequently, by the time the transgenic line is ready for commercial release, its non-transgenic competitors have made substantial additional progress by conventional selection.

In view of these substantial limitations, it seems likely that the greatest benefits of transgenesis in relation to animal production will come from introducing novel effects, such as utilizing novel foodstuffs, or overcoming problems associated with welfare (e.g. natural disease resistance) or pollution, or producing new forms of conventional animal products having a more desirable balance of amino acids. The potential for transgenesis in this area is limited only by our ability to devise novel approaches, and our knowledge of the existence and modes of function of genes.

In the shorter term, the most likely use of transgenesis will be in the production of human polypeptides required for pharmaceutical use. However, since just one or two transgenic animals will be sufficient to produce the world's requirements for various human proteins, this use of transgenesis is not likely to have an impact on practical animal production.

Important issues that must be faced in relation to transgenesis are the legal questions (who owns the transgene, and should transgenic animals be patented?) and the ethical and animal-welfare questions. As with EMT, many people feel that transgenesis is one step too far. Some scientists working with transgenesis are already devoting considerable time to informing other scientists and members of the public about what is happening, and in return are receiving useful feedback as to what is deemed to be acceptable. This is a laudable approach, and should be followed by scientists working in any area of biotechnology.

## Further reading

### General

Anon. (1993). International Symposium on Animal Biotechnology. *Molecular Reproduction and Development*, **36**, 220–90.

Anon. (1993). Issues arising from recent advances in biotechnology. *Veterinary Record*, **133**, 53–6.

Harlander, S. (1993). Genetic engineering of foods—a United-States perspective. *Trends in Food Science & Technology*, **4**, 301–5.

Hess, C. E. (1992). Biotechnology-derived foods from animals. *Critical Reviews in Food Science and Nutrition*, **32**, 147–50.

Robinson, J. J. and McEvoy, T.G. (1993). Biotechnology—the possibilities. *Animal Production*, **57**, 335–52.

Sellier, P. (1994). The future role of molecular genetics in the control of meat production and meat quality. *Meat Science*, **36**, 29–44.

Stelwagen, K., Gibbins, A. M. V., and McBride, B. W. (1992). Applications of recombinant DNA technology to improve milk production—a review. *Livestock Production Science*, **31**, 153–78.

Wilmut, I., Haley, C. S., and Woolliams, J. A. (1992). Impact of biotechnology on animal breeding. *Animal Reproduction Science*, **28**, 149–62.

Wilson, M. and Lindow, S. E. (1993). Release of recombinant microorganisms. *Annual Review of Microbiology*, **47**, 913–44.

### Multiple ovulation and embryo transfer

Bondoc, O. L. and Smith, C. (1993). Optimized testing schemes using nucleus progeny, adult MOET siblings, or juvenile MOET pedigrees in dairy cattle closed populations. *Journal of Animal Breeding and Genetics*, **110**, 30–40.

Christie, W. B., McGuirk, B. J., Strahie, R. J., and Mullan, J. S. (1992). Practical experience with the implementation of a MOET breeding scheme with dairy cattle. *Annales de Zootechnie*, **41**, 347–52.

Lohuis, M. M., Smith, C., and Dekkers, J. C. M. (1993). MOET results from a dispersed hybrid nucleus programme in dairy cattle. *Animal Production*, **57**, 369–78.

Mpofu, N., Smith, C., Van Vuuren, W., and Burnside, E. B. (1993). Breeding strategies for genetic improvement of dairy cattle in Zimbabwe. *Journal of Dairy Science*, **76**, 1163–1172, 1173–1181.

## Embryo multiplication and transfer

Colleau, J. J. (1992). Combining use of embryo sexing and cloning within mixed MOETs for selection on dairy cattle. *Génétique Sélection Evolution*, **24**, 345–61.

De Boer, I. J. M. and Van Arendonk, J. A. M. (1991). Genetic and clonal responses in closed dairy cattle nucleus schemes. *Animal Production*, **53**, 1–9.

## Control of sex ratio

Bishop, S. C. and Woolliams, J. A. (1991). Utilization of the sex-determining region Y gene in beef cattle breeding schemes. *Animal Production*, **53**, 157–64.

Halverson, J. L. and Dvorak, J. (1993). Genetic control of sex determination in birds and the potential for its manipulation. *Poultry Science*, **72**, 890–6.

Johnson, L. A., Cran, D. G., and Polge, C. (1994). Recent advances in sex preselection of cattle—flow cytometric sorting of X-chromosome and Y-chromosome bearing sperm based on DNA to produce progeny. *Theriogenology*, **41**, 51–6.

Kirkpatrick, B. W. and Monson, R. L. (1993). Sensitive sex determination assay applicable to bovine embryos derived from IVM and IVF. *Journal of Reproduction and Fertility*, **98**, 335–40.

## Recombinant proteins

Etherton, T. D., Krisetherton, P. M., and Mills, E. W. (1993). Recombinant bovine and porcine somatotropin—safety and benefits of these biotechnologies. *Journal of the American Dietetic Association*, **93**, 177–80.

Kimman, T. G. (1992). Risks connected with the use of conventional and genetically engineered vaccines. *Veterinary Quarterly*, **14**, 110-8.

## Transgenesis

Berkowitz, D. B. and Kryspinsorensen, I. (1994). Transgenic fish—safe to eat—a look at the safety considerations regarding food transgenics. *Bio/Technology*, **12**, 247–52.

Ebert, K. M. and Schindler, J. E. S. (1993). Transgenic farm animals—progress report. *Theriogenology*, **39**, 121–35.

Gama, L. T., Smith, C., and Gibson, J. P. (1992). Transgene effects, introgression strategies and testing schemes in pigs. *Animal Production*, **54**, 427–40.

Hafs, H. D. (ed.) (1993). Genetically modified livestock: progress, prospects and issues. *Journal of Animal Science*, **71**, (Suppl. 3), 1–56.

Martin, P. and Grosclaude, F. (1993). Improvement of milk protein quality by gene technology. *Livestock Production Science*, **35**, 95–115.
Perry, M. M. and Sang, H. M. (1993). Transgenesis in chickens. *Transgenic Research*, **2**, 125–33.

## Animal patents

Lesser, W. H. (ed.) (1990). *Animal patents*. Macmillan, London.

## Ethics and animal welfare

Anon. (1993). Symposium on biotechnology and animal welfare. *Livestock Production Science*, **36**, 1–119.
Loew, F. M. (1994). Beyond transgenics—ethics and values. *British Veterinary Journal*, **150**, 3–5.
Mepham, T. B. (1993). Approaches to the ethical evaluation of animal biotechnologies. *Animal Production*, **57**, 353–9.
Thompson, P. B. (1992). Designing animals—ethical issues for genetic engineers. *Journal of Dairy Science*, **75**, 2294–303.

# Books on particular species

## Cats

Robinson, R. (1991). *Genetics for cat breeders*, (3rd edn). Pergamon Press, Oxford.

## Dogs

Burns, M. and Fraser, M. N. (1966). *Genetics of the dog*, (2nd edn). Oliver and Boyd, Edinburgh.
Willis, M. B. (1976). *The German Shepherd dog: its history, development and genetics*. K & R Books, Leicester.
Hutt, F. B. (1979). *Genetics for dog breeders*. Freeman, San Francisco.
Clark, R. D. and Stainer, J. R. (ed.) (1983). *Medical and genetic aspects of purebred dogs*. Veterinary Medicine Publishing Company, Edwardsville, Kansas.
Willis, M. B. (1989). *Genetics of the dog*. H. F. & G. Witherby, London.
Robinson, R. (1990). *Genetics for dog breeders*. (2nd edn). Pergamon Press, Oxford.

## Fish

Ryman, N. and Utter, F. (ed.) (1987). *Population genetics and fishery management*. University of Washington Press, Seattle.
Gall, G. A. E. (ed.) (1993). *Genetics in aquaculture IV*. Elsevier, Amsterdam.
Purdom, C. E. (1992). *Genetics and fish breeding*. Chapman and Hall, London.

## Poultry

Hill, W. G., Manson, J. M., and Hewitt, D. (ed.) (1985). *Poultry genetics and breeding*. British Poultry Science Ltd, Longman Group, Harlow, England.
Cooke, F. and Buckley, P. A. (1987). *Avian genetics*. Academic Press, London.
Crawford, R. D. (ed.) (1990). *Poultry breeding and genetics*. Elsevier, Amsterdam.
Stevens, L. (1991). *Genetics and evolution of the domestic fowl*. Cambridge University Press, Cambridge.

## Sheep

Turner, H. N. and Young, S. S. Y. (1969). *Quantitative genetics in sheep breeding*. Macmillan, Melbourne.
South Australian Coloured Sheep Owners Society (1979). *Breeding coloured sheep and using coloured wool*. Peacock Publications, Hyde Park, South Australia.

Day, G. and Jessup, J. (ed.) (1984). *The history of the Australian Merino*. Heinemann, Melbourne.
Land, R. B. and Robinson, D. W. (ed.) (1985). *The genetics of reproduction in sheep*. Butterworth, London.
Garrna, J. and White, L. (1985). *Merinos, myths, and Macarthurs*. Australian National University Press, Canberra.
McGuirk, B. J. (ed.) (1987). *Merino improvement programs in Australia*. Australian Wool Corporation, Melbourne.
Massy, C. (1990). *The Australian Merino*. Viking O'Neill, Sydney.

## Cattle

Hinks, C. J. M. (1983). *Breeding dairy cattle*. Farming Press, Ipswich, England.
Schmidt, G. M., Van Vleck, L. D., and Hutjens, M. F. (1988). *Principles of dairy science*, (2nd edn). Prentice-Hall International, Englewood Cliffs, New Jersey.

## Horses

Lasley, J. F. (1970). *Genetic principles in horse breeding*. University of Missouri Press, Columbia.
Jones, W. E. (1982). *Genetics and horse breeding*. Lea and Febiger, Philadelphia.
Evans, J. W., Borton, A., Hintz, H. F., and Van Vleck, L. D. (1986). *The horse*, (2nd edn). Freeman, San Francisco.

# Index

Italic numbers denote illustrations